CARDIOVASCULAR ACTIONS OF SULFINPYRAZONE:
Basic and
Clinical Research

CARDIOVASCULAR ACTIONS OF SULFINPYRAZONE: Basic and Clinical Research

Edited by

Maurice McGregor, M.D.
J. Fraser Mustard, M.D., Ph.D.
Michael F. Oliver, M.D.
Sol Sherry, M.D.

Proceedings of
an International Symposium,
Hamilton, Bermuda,
May 21-23, 1979

Published by

Symposia Specialists
Inc.

MEDICAL BOOKS

Symposia Specialists, Inc.
1470 N.E. 129th Street
Miami, FL 33161

CIBA-GEIGY Corporation
556 Morris Ave.
Summit, NJ 07901

Library of Congress Catalog Card Number 79-93243
International Standard Book Number 0-88372-133-3

Printed in the United States of America

Contents

Contributors

Chairmen

MAURICE McGREGOR, M.D., Professor of Medicine, McGill University; Senior Physician, Royal Victoria Hospital, Montreal, Quebec, Canada.

J. FRASER MUSTARD, M.D., PH.D., Professor of Pathology; Dean, Faculty of Health Sciences, McMaster University, Hamilton, Ontario, Canada.

MICHAEL F. OLIVER, M.D., Duke of Edinburgh Professor of Cardiology, University of Edinburgh and the Royal Infirmary of Edinburgh, Edinburgh, Scotland.

SOL SHERRY, M.D., Professor and Chairman, Department of Medicine, Temple University School of Medicine, Philadelphia, Pennsylvania.

Speakers

PETER CLOPATH, D.Sc., Research Department, Pharmaceuticals Division, CIBA-GEIGY Limited, Basle, Switzerland.

JOEL D. COOPER, M.D., Associate Professor of Surgery, Department of Surgery, University of Toronto Faculty of Medicine, Toronto, Ontario, Canada.

JOHN D. FOLTS, PH.D., Associate Professor of Medicine, Cardiovascular Section, Clinical Research Center, University of Wisconsin, Madison, Wisconsin.

LAURENCE A. HARKER, M.D., Professor of Medicine, Department of Medicine, University of Washington School of Medicine, Seattle, Washington.

STUART W. JAMIESON, M.B., Fellow, Department of Cardiovascular Surgery, Stanford University School of Medicine, Stanford, California.

GERALD J. KELLIHER, PH.D., Associate Professor, Pharmacology and Medicine, The Medical College of Pennsylvania, Philadelphia, Pennsylvania.

ERWIN H. MARGULIES, PH.D., Medical Department, Pharmaceuticals Division, CIBA-GEIGY Corporation, Summit, New Jersey.

JOHN W. D. McDONALD, M.D., PH.D., Department of Medicine, The University of Western Ontario, London, Ontario, Canada.

CHRISTOS B. MOSCHOS, M.D., Professor of Medicine, College of Medicine and Dentistry—New Jersey Medical School, Newark, New Jersey.

KLAUS MÜLLER, PH.D., Research Department, Pharmaceuticals Division, CIBA-GEIGY Limited, Basle, Switzerland.

HENRY J. POVALSKI, M.S., Research Department, Pharmaceuticals Division, CIBA-GEIGY Corporation, Summit, New Jersey.

DAVID L. SACKETT, M.D., Professor of Medicine, Departments of Clinical Epidemiology and Biostatistics, McMaster University, Hamilton, Ontario, Canada.

PETER P. STEELE, M.D., Associate Professor, University of Colorado Medical Center; Chief, Cardiology, Veterans Administration Hospital, Denver, Colorado.

ROBERT B. WALLIS, PH.D., Horsham Research Centre, CIBA-GEIGY Pharmaceuticals Division, Horsham, England.

PETER N. WALSH, M.D., PH.D., Associate Professor of Medicine, Specialized Center for Thrombosis Research, Temple University School of Medicine, Philadelphia, Pennsylvania.

ALAN M. WHITE, PH.D., Horsham Research Centre, CIBA-GEIGY Pharmaceuticals Division, Horsham, England.

MARY P. WIEDEMAN, PH.D., Professor of Physiology, Temple University School of Medicine, Philadelphia, Pennsylvania.

Discussants

K. D. BUTLER, PH.D., Horsham Research Centre, CIBA-GEIGY Pharmaceuticals Division, Horsham, England.

D. INNES CARGILL, PH.D., Research Department, Pharmaceuticals Division, CIBA-GEIGY Corporation, Ardsley, New York.

WILLIAM D. CASH, PH.D., Research Department, Pharmaceuticals Division, CIBA-GEIGY Corporation, Ardsley, New York.

J. G. DOMENET, M.D., CIBA-GEIGY Pharmaceuticals Division, Macclesfield, England.

ROY A. ELLIS, M.D., Vice President—Medical Director, Pharmaceuticals Division, CIBA-GEIGY Corporation, Summit, New Jersey.

F. FONTANILLES, M.D., Medical Department, Pharmaceuticals Division, CIBA-GEIGY Limited, Basle, Switzerland.

JOHN GORDON, PH.D., Institute of Animal Physiology, Agricultural Research Council, Babraham, Cambridge, England.

G. P. McNICOL, M.D., PH.D., Professor and Head, Department of Medicine, The University of Leeds, Leeds, England.

C. RICHARD MINICK, M.D., New York Hospital, Cornell Medical Center, New York, New York.

RONALD D. ROBSON, PH.D., Research Department, Pharmaceuticals Division, CIBA-GEIGY Corporation, Summit, New Jersey.

Foreword

In this volume are presented the results of newly completed research into the cardiovascular actions of sulfinpyrazone (Anturane). Sulfinpyrazone was introduced by the Geigy Corporation in the late 1950's as a uricosuric agent for the treatment of gout — a purpose for which it is still widely used. A whole new area of research into the actions of the drug opened up in 1965 with publication of a paper by Smythe, Ogryzlo, and Mustard, entitled "The Effect of Sulfinpyrazone (Anturan) on Platelet Economy and Blood Coagulation in Man," in which the authors reported their chance finding that sulfinpyrazone corrected shortened platelet survival in gout patients. As a result of this fortuitous discovery, over the next 5 years extensive experimental research, led by Fraser Mustard and Marian Packham in Canada, was conducted into the effects of sulfinpyrazone and other similar agents on platelets and vessel walls.

Clinical studies were started in this same 5-year period by John Blakely, Ed Genton, Peter Steele, Jack Hirsh, and Geoff Evans, with the assistance of Michael Gent in methodology and statistics. During this period Fraser Mustard was unable to stimulate the interest of the Geigy Corporation in this new research, in spite of repeated efforts to do so. However, in 1971 Geigy, now part of CIBA-GEIGY, awoke to the new possibilities for their drug and decided to support and coordinate the diverse research efforts.

Another milestone was the symposium held in 1972 at McMaster University on "Platelets, Drugs and Thrombosis." The proceedings of this symposium contained the first published results of the clinical work conducted since 1965. The year 1972 also marked the initiation of the extensive Canadian Cooperative Trial in which the effects of aspirin and sulfinpyrazone were compared in the preventive treatment of patients with transient ischemic attacks and threatened stroke.

A second symposium, "Platelets, Thrombosis, and Inhib-itors," which reviewed the entire field at that time, was held in 1973 in Honolulu, and the same year a major review article by Mustard, Kinlough-Rathbone, and Packham, "Pathogenesis and Clinical Trials," appeared.

With the impetus of Canadian clinical involvement a New Drug Submission was made in 1974 to the Health Protection Branch in Canada. In October this submission on sulfinpyrazone was approved, permitting its use in thromboembolic conditions. Early in 1975 the drug entered into general use by Canadian physicians for its new indication.

In April 1975 the CIBA-GEIGY Corporation, after some hesitation because of the size, scope, and cost of the project, decided to sponsor an extensive study to be conducted jointly by its companies in the United States and Canada, but guided and controlled by an independent academic policy committee. In this study, called the Anturane Reinfarction Trial, the effects of sulfinpyrazone were compared with those of placebo on the subsequent survival of patients who had recently suffered an acute myocardial infarction. During the same year a series of three review articles by Genton, Gent, Hirsh, and Harker on "Platelet-Inhibiting Drugs in the Prevention of Clinical Thrombotic Disease" appeared in the *New England Journal of Medicine* and another major review article by Mustard and Packham, "Platelets, Thrombosis, and Drugs," appeared.

The initial results of the Anturane Reinfarction Trial, published in February 1978 in the *New England Journal of Medicine*, suggested a major benefit from treatment with sulfinpyrazone for patients who had suffered a recent acute myocardial infarction. This effect was particularly striking in preventing sudden cardiac death in these patients during the early months after the acute myocardial infarction. During the same year and in the same journal the published results of the Canadian Cooperative Trial suggested that aspirin, but not sulfinpyrazone, reduced the frequency of transient cerebral ischemic attacks and of progression to stroke.

The mechanisms of action of sulfinpyrazone that account for its clinical effects are still not defined but the search to define them has spawned a wealth of research into sulfinpyrazone's effects in various experimental situations. In this volume the reports on this research have been grouped in four sections: Effect on Platelet Function; Platelet-Vessel Wall Interaction; Experimental Animal Studies; and Clinical Studies. Summaries of these sections have been provided by the four editors of this volume: Drs. J. Fraser Mustard, Maurice McGregor, Michael F. Oliver, and Sol Sherry, and a summary of all the research reported has been provided by Dr. Sherry.

This volume constitutes the proceedings of a symposium sponsored by the CIBA-GEIGY Corporation and held in Hamilton, Bermuda, May 21-23, 1979. We are deeply indebted to the four editors of this volume, not only for their efforts toward the publication, but also for acting as chairmen of the symposium and moderating the discussions that appear at the end of each chapter. Thanks are also due to the members of the CIBA-GEIGY Organizing Committee: Drs. Ronald D. Robson, Erwin H. Margulies, and Alan M. White, and Dr. Daniel B. Leach, who brought together the distinguished speakers and other participants. We are grateful to Mr. Alvin Skuro of CIBA-GEIGY who made local arrangements for the symposium, Mr. Robert F. Orsetti who made arrangements for the publication, and Ms. Lucinda M. Pitcairn who edited the manuscripts and discussions.

Roy A. Ellis, M.D.
Vice President — Medical Director
Pharmaceuticals Division
CIBA-GEIGY Corporation
Summit, New Jersey

Effect on Platelet Function

Inhibition of Platelet Involvement in the Sublethal Forssman Reaction by Sulfinpyrazone

K. D. Butler, Ph.D. and A. M. White, Ph.D.

Introduction

The guinea pig is a Forssman antigen-positive animal. The Forssman antigen is mainly localized in the lungs where it is found in all cell types of the alveoli, the endothelium of blood vessels, connective tissues and on the surface of muscle cells [1]. Intravenous injection of Forssman antibody is known to result in a rapid antigen-antibody reaction in the lungs manifested as bronchospasm [2] and as vascular lesions showing platelets adhering to the subendothelium [3, 4]. Death as a result of Forssman shock has been shown to be complement- and platelet-dependent [5, 6]. Tsai et al. [6] demonstrated that drugs that inhibit platelet secretion, such as aspirin [7] and sulfinpyrazone [8], afford protection against the lethal reaction. We undertook to determine if thrombocytopenia induced by sublethal doses of Forssman antibody would likewise be inhibited by sulfinpyrazone, aspirin, and another inhibitor of platelet secretion, indomethacin.

Materials and Methods

Animals

Guinea pigs (Dunkin-Hartley, 350 to 500 g) were obtained from Hacking and Churchill, Huntingdon, England. Guinea pigs

K. D. Butler, Ph.D. and A. M. White, Ph.D., Horsham Research Centre, CIBA-GEIGY Pharmaceuticals Division, Horsham, West Sussex, England.

3

genetically C4-deficient were obtained from a breeding colony maintained in our own laboratories.

Preparation and Administration of Forssman Antiserum

Sheep erythrocyte stroma suspended in Freund's Complete Adjuvant were used to immunize New Zealand White rabbits. The animals were given subcutaneous injections with stroma from 10^9 sheep erythrocytes and two weeks later a boosting dose of stroma from 10^9 cells. Four weeks after the booster injection, the animals were skin-tested with stroma from 10^8 cells. Those animals displaying a positive response, indicated by an Arthus reaction with a hemorrhagic central area, were bled one week after the skin test. Blood was allowed to clot and serum was removed after centrifugation. The antiserum was administered intravenously into the marginal ear vein of ether-anesthetized guinea pigs.

Dose response curves were constructed for all batches of antisera used for inducing Forssman reactions. Doses were chosen which would induce 50% to 80% thrombocytopenia against which to test drugs.

Platelet Counts

Blood (4.5 ml) was taken from ether-anesthetized animals by cardiac puncture into a 5-ml plastic syringe containing 3.8% trisodium citrate (0.5 ml). The anticoagulated blood was inverted three times in the syringe and then centrifuged in graduated plastic or siliconized glass centrifuge tubes at 200 g for 15 min at 4°C. The platelet-rich plasma (PRP) was removed with a siliconized Pasteur pipette and the platelet concentration was determined using a Coulter counter Industrial Model D. The platelet count per cubic millimeter of whole blood was calculated as

$$\frac{\text{No. platelets/ml PRP} \times \text{vol PRP (ml)}}{\text{Vol blood} - \text{vol anticoagulant (ml)}}$$

The SE of the platelet-counting procedure was ± 1.3%.

Administration of Drugs

For intravenous injection 1 g each of aspirin, sulfinpyrazone and the metabolites of sulfinpyrazone (Fig. 1), i.e., sulfin-

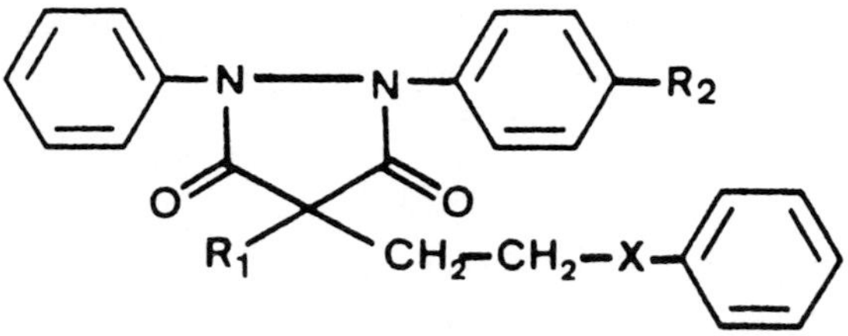

Compound	R_1	R_2	X
G 28 315 (Sulphinpyrazone)	H	H	SO
G 25 671	H	H	S
G 31 442	H	H	SO_2
G 32 642	H	OH	SO

FIGURE 1.

pyrazone sulfone (G 31442), p-hydroxy sulfinpyrazone (G 32642), and the thioether (G 25671), were each dissolved in an equivalent of 1N NaOH, adjusted to pH 7.4 with acid or alkali, and made up to 10 ml with physiological saline to give a final concentration of 100 mg/ml. In the case of indomethacin, 70 mg was dissolved in 1N NaOH (2.1 ml), adjusted to pH 7.4 with acid or alkali as required, and made up to 7 ml with saline to give a final concentration of 10 mg/ml.

For oral administration drugs were suspended in 20% wt/vol polyethylene glycol "6000" and approximately 0.5 ml of suspension was given to each animal.

Platelet Isolation and Labeling

Guinea pigs were bled by cardiac puncture into 3.8% trisodium citrate (1 part citrate:9 parts blood) and the platelets were isolated and labeled with ^{51}Cr and infused as previously described [9].

Measurement of Radioactivity in Whole Blood and in Different Organs

Blood (2 ml) was removed by cardiac puncture while the animal was under ether anesthesia. The animal was then killed by opening the chest. Organs were removed, washed free of surface blood, and blotted dry. The blood and organs were then placed in preweighed plastic vials for measurement of radioactivity in a Beckman Biogamma Counter.

Complement Depletion

Circulating complement levels in guinea pigs were depleted by intraperitoneal injections of anticomplementary factor from cobra venom (Cordis Laboratories) in a daily dose of 200 U/kg for three days. The animals were used experimentally 24 h after the final dose of cobra venom factor.

Statistical Analysis

The inhibition of thrombocytopenia was analyzed for statistical significance using Student's t test for unpaired data.

Results

Time Course of Thrombocytopenia

The results from groups of guinea pigs given injections of 0.2 ml, 0.3 ml, or 0.5 ml Forssman antiserum, bled by cardiac puncture, and killed at various time intervals after the challenge are shown in Figure 2. After injection of 0.2 ml of antiserum, the platelet count fell rapidly to produce a pronounced thrombocytopenia, which was maximal 3 min after the challenge. After this time the platelet count slowly returned to normal and animals given this low dose of antiserum did not die from Forssman shock. With a higher sublethal dose of antibody (0.3 ml), the thrombocytopenia, although reversible, was more severe. With the highest dose (0.5 ml), there was no significant return of the platelet count towards normal levels before the animals died.

The effect of cobra venom factor on the thrombocytopenia in the sublethal Forssman reaction is shown in Table 1. As can be seen, depletion of the circulating complement levels prevented the development of the thrombocytopenia and a similar result was obtained in genetically C4-deficient animals. As can be seen in these animals there was no thrombocytopenia due to 0.2 ml antiserum. With 0.5 ml Forssman antiserum the effect in these animals was equivalent to a sublethal challenge in genetically intact animals.

Percent control

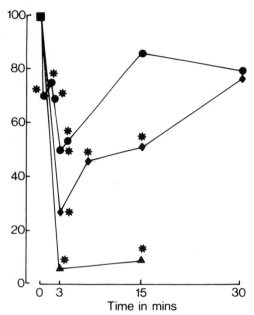

FIG. 2. Platelet count at different times after 0.5 ml (—▲——▲—), 0.3 ml (—◆——◆—), and 0.2 ml (—●——●—) Forssman antiserum IV. *Significant difference (p≤0.05) from values at time zero.

Table 1. Effects of Forssman Antiserum on Circulating Platelet Count in C4-Deficient Guinea Pigs, Guinea Pigs Treated with Cobra Venom Factor (CVF), and Untreated Controls

| Type of Guinea Pig | Platelet Count (1,000/cu mm) After Forssman Antiserum at Doses of | | |
	0 ml	0.2 ml	0.5 ml
C4-Deficient	284 ± 23	271 ± 27*	119 ± 19*
Normal	240 ± 10	109 ± 13	10 ± 1
CVF-Treated	323 ± 35	385 ± 39*	NI
Normal	294 ± 18	179 ± 13	NI

CVF was given intraperitoneally in doses of 200 U/kg daily for 3 days. Blood samples were taken 3 min after intravenous injection of antiserum. Results are mean ± SE for five animals in each group. NI = Not investigated. *p ≤ 0.05.

Platelet Sequestration

The distribution of radioactivity among various organs after the intravenous injection of antibody is shown in Table 2. There was a rapid increase in the amount of radioactivity present in the lungs after both doses (0.2 ml and 0.3 ml) of antibody (maximal after 3 min) followed by a slower decrease. In addition to the increase in ^{51}Cr in the lungs, there was a slower increase in the radioactivity in the liver. This reached a maximum 15 min after challenge and subsequently declined. However, the radioactivity still remained significantly elevated above control levels 30 min after challenge. There was no increase in the amount of radioactivity found in the heart or kidney after either dose of antiserum (Table 2).

Effect of Platelet Inhibitory Drugs
on the Acute Thrombocytopenia

The results obtained with sulfinpyrazone, aspirin, and indomethacin are shown in Table 3. Sulfinpyrazone (100 mg/kg) administered intravenously 30 or 60 min prior to the animals receiving a sublethal injection of Forssman antiserum inhibited the development of thrombocytopenia by 59% and 100%, respectively. Aspirin and indomethacin at doses of 100 mg/kg and 10 mg/kg, respectively, had no effect.

Table 2. ^{51}Cr Distribution in Normal Guinea Pigs after Intravenous Administration of Forssman Antiserum

Organ	^{51}Cr (counts/min per g tissue) at Intervals (min)			
	0	3	15	30
	After 0.2 ml Antiserum			
Blood	2,566 ± 261	1,265 ± 221*	1,308 ± 214*	1,622 ± 145*
Heart	642 ± 61	621 ± 85	562 ± 97	531 ± 117
Lung	1,087 ± 126	5,647 ± 1,324*	1,731 ± 356	1,227 ± 83
Liver	1,797 ± 139	2,031 ± 199	3,562 ± 661*	2,598 ± 299*
Kidney	860 ± 89	704 ± 38	627 ± 67	626 ± 66
	After 0.3 ml Antiserum			
Blood	2,504 ± 121	844 ± 142*	857 ± 188*	1,116 ± 257*
Heart	548 ± 78	487 ± 202	340 ± 90	272 ± 97
Lung	1,389 ± 157	9,717 ± 1,008*	4,107 ± 990	1,488 ± 462
Liver	1,505 ± 130	1,932 ± 253	3,205 ± 530*	2,529 ± 309*
Kidney	1,397 ± 71	1,141 ± 25*	1,235 ± 172	1,005 ± 54*

Results are expressed as counts/min per gram wet weight of tissue or per gram of blood and are mean ± SE for five animals. *p ≤ 0.05.

Table 3. Effect of Sulfinpyrazone, Aspirin, and Indomethacin on
Acute Thrombocytopenia Induced by Forssman Reaction

Drug and Time Administered (IV) Before Challenge	Dose (mg/kg)	Platelet Count (1,000/cu mm)			Inhibition (%)
		Before Challenge (Control)	After Challenge		
			Untreated	Treated	
Sulfinpyrazone					
60 min	100	189 ± 28	85 ± 15	194 ± 28	100**
	50	266 ± 6	150 ± 10	152 ± 19	1
30 min	100	218 ± 14	121 ± 16	179 ± 10	59.4*
	50	219 ± 24	89 ± 16	61 ± 10	0
Aspirin					
60 min	100	323 ± 25	147 ± 35	137 ± 20	0
30 min	100	337 ± 25	67 ± 22	36 ± 15	0
Indomethacin					
60 min	10	285 ± 19	167 ± 17	150 ± 28	0
30 min	10	337 ± 25	67 ± 22	68 ± 22	0.5

Guinea pigs were challenged with Forssman antiserum 3 min before measurement of platelet count. Results are mean ± SE for five animals. Controls did not receive medication. *$p \leq 0.05$. **$p \leq 0.01$.

From Table 4 it can be seen that the sulfone (G 31442) of sulfinpyrazone inhibited the thrombocytopenia by 62% when administered 60 min prior to challenge in a dose of 100 mg/kg. The p-hydroxy derivative (G 32642) was less active, being found to inhibit the thrombocytopenia by only 53% 30 min after intravenous administration of a dose of 200 mg/kg. It was not possible to test the thioether (G 25671) at a dose of 200 mg/kg, but at an intravenous dose of 100 mg/kg it did not have any effect, showing that it is the least active of the three compounds in this test system (Table 4).

The effect of sulfinpyrazone could be overcome if the antiserum dose was increased to one which would normally result in the death of the animal (Table 5). Animals were given sulfinpyrazone 100 mg/kg (IV) 60 min prior to injection of increasing doses of antiserum. Sulfinpyrazone inhibited development of thrombocytopenia induced by either 0.2 or 0.3 ml antiserum but not that induced by the higher dose of 0.4 ml. If the animals were not sacrificed so that blood samples for platelet counts could be obtained, control animals given this dose of antiserum died 10 to 15 min after administration of the antiserum, whereas in those pretreated with sulfinpyrazone, death was prevented although thrombocytopenia still occurred.

Table 4. Effect of Three Analogs of Sulfinpyrazone on
Acute Thrombocytopenia Induced by Forssman Reaction

Drug and Time Administered (IV) Before Challenge	Dose (mg/kg)	Platelet Count (1,000/cu mm)			Inhibition (%)
		Before Challenge (Control)	After Challenge Untreated	Treated	
G 31442 (sulfone)					
60 min	100	284 ± 27	74 ± 19	204 ± 26	61.7**
	50	337 ± 25	67 ± 22	45 ± 19	0
30 min	200	242 ± 17	135 ± 9	46 ± 18	
	100	219 ± 24	48 ± 12	102 ± 39	31.9
G 32642 (p-hydroxy)					
60 min	200	242 ± 17	135 ± 9	119 ± 26	0
	100	284 ± 24	74 ± 19	162 ± 31	41.4
30 min	200	242 ± 17	135 ± 9	192 ± 20	52.8*
	100	219 ± 24	48 ± 12	104 ± 22	32.8
G 25671 (thioether)					
60 min	100	267 ± 19	132 ± 20	156 ± 37	17.7
30 min	100	219 ± 24	48 ± 12	43 ± 12	0

Guinea pigs were challenged with Forssman antiserum 3 min before measurement of platelet count. Results are mean ± SE for five animals. Controls did not receive medication. *$p \le 0.05$. **$p \le 0.01$.

A number of other control substances were studied. It was found that intravenous doses of phenylbutazone up to 100 mg/kg, mepyramine up to 2 mg/kg, methysergide up to 2 mg/kg, and heparin up to 1000 U/kg did not inhibit the thrombocytopenia.

When sulfinpyrazone was administered at various times before the animals were challenged with antibody, the inhibitory effect was no longer apparent after 6 h in this test system (Table 6).

Table 5. Effect of Sulfinpyrazone (100 mg/kg IV) Administered One Hour
Before Challenge with Various Doses of Forssman Antiserum

Antiserum (ml)	Platelet Count (1,000/cu mm)	
	Control	Sulfinpyrazone-Treated
0	189 ± 28	191 ± 12
0.2	85 ± 15	194 ± 28**
0.3	19 ± 4	177 ± 28***
0.4	13 ± 2	24 ± 9

Results are mean ± SE for five animals. **$p \le 0.01$. ***$p \le 0.001$.

Table 6. Effect of Sulfinpyrazone (100 mg/kg IV) Administered at Various Times Before Challenge with Forssman Antiserum (0.3 ml)

Time Between Drug and Challenge	Platelet Count (1,000/cu mm) After Challenge	Inhibition (%)
20 min	155 ± 33	28
1 h	200 ± 17	50**
2 h	242 ± 36	71*
4 h	193 ± 11	47**
6 h	160 ± 31	30
18 h	162 ± 53	31
Control Values		
Before Challenge	299 ± 13	
After Challenge	99 ± 23	

Results are mean ± SE for five animals. *$p \leq 0.02$. **$p \leq 0.01$.

Effect of Platelet Inhibitory Drugs on Platelet Sequestration in the Lungs

The effect of sulfinpyrazone (100 mg/kg) on the distribution of ^{51}Cr into various organs of guinea pigs following intravenous administration of 0.2 ml Forssman antiserum is shown in Table 7. The drug partially inhibited the increase in ^{51}Cr in the lungs of challenge animals. Aspirin had no effect (Table 8).

Discussion

Not all of the factors involved in the pathogenesis of the Forssman reaction are known. It is clear from the work of

Table 7. ^{51}Cr Distribution after Sulfinpyrazone (100 mg/kg IV) Administration One Hour Before Challenge with Forssman Antiserum

Organ	^{51}Cr (counts/min per g tissue) Before Challenge Control	After Challenge Untreated	Sulfinpyrazone-Treated
Blood	1700 ± 113	972 ± 88*	1375 ± 241
Lung	902 ± 72	2976 ± 311*	1588 ± 247†
Heart	466 ± 131	344 ± 49	324 ± 74

Results are expressed as counts/min per gram wet weight of tissue and are mean ± SE for five animals. Controls did not receive sulfinpyrazone. *Statistically significant difference ($p \leq 0.05$) from controls. †Statistically significant difference ($p \leq 0.05$) from controls and from untreated animals after challenge.

Table 8. ^{51}Cr Distribution after Aspirin (100 mg/kg IV) Administration
One Hour Before Challenge with Forssman Antigen

| Organ | ^{51}Cr (counts/min per g tissue) | | |
| | Before Challenge Control | After Challenge | |
		Untreated	Aspirin-treated
Blood	5706 ± 298	1952 ± 116*	1594 ± 97*
Lung	2478 ± 197	42046 ± 2359*	39994 ± 2833*
Heart	783 ± 131	798 ± 65	920 ± 212

Results are expressed as counts/min per gram wet weight of tissue or per gram of blood and are mean ± SE for five animals. Controls did not receive aspirin. *Statistically significant difference (p < 0.05) from controls.

Taichman and Tsai [4] that platelets are an essential component in the genesis of the secondary vascular lesions that occur during this reaction. However, these workers did not consider that platelets were involved in the production of primary lesions on the vascular endothelium. From the studies described here it is apparent that there is also platelet involvement even when Forssman antibody is administered in sublethal doses. The extent of involvement is related to the dose of antiserum administered. The thrombocytopenia and associated platelet accumulation in the lungs proved to be reversible, with most of the platelets apparently returning, in due course, to the circulation.

The finding that in C4-deficient guinea pigs the endothelial damage (J.R.J. Baker et al., unpublished data) and thrombocytopenia after a lethal dose of Forssman antiserum were equivalent only to those in a sublethal reaction in normal animals indicated that the alternate pathway of complement could support a limited degree of endothelial cell injury. It also confirmed the findings of May and Frank [10] that sequential complement activation is required for full demonstration of the cellular damage in this reaction.

The fall in platelet count and platelet sequestration in various vascular beds during the nonlethal Forssman reaction does not appear to be dependent on platelet prostaglandin synthesis. If this was the case, then indomethacin, aspirin, and sulfinpyrazone would all be expected to inhibit these processes, with indomethacin being more potent than aspirin, which in turn would be more potent than sulfinpyrazone, as seen for inhibition of platelet prostaglandin synthesis and the thrombocytopenia in the Arthus reaction [9].

The distinction between the effects of aspirin and sulfinpyrazone is perhaps our most interesting finding, since it represents an addition to a list of other important pharmacological differences between these substances. Within the platelet they have rather similar actions since they are both inhibitors of platelet prostaglandin synthesis [11, 12] and hence, under appropriate circumstances, inhibitors of platelet secretion.

When the platelet interacts with its environment *in vivo*, however, the situation is apparently very different. Aspirin, while extending platelet survival in rabbits, has been reported not to influence shortened platelet survival in man at a dose which certainly inhibited platelet function [13]. Sulfinpyrazone has been shown to reverse shortened platelet survival when administered in a number of clinical situations, including gout [14], coronary artery disease [15], transient cerebral ischemic attacks [16], and rheumatic heart disease [17]. Aspirin (up to 10^{-4} M) does not protect ^{51}Cr-labeled human umbilical vein endothelial cells in culture against ^{51}Cr leakage induced by homocysteine, whereas sulfinpyrazone has this property at concentrations of 10^{-6} M or more [18]. Aspirin is considerably more potent than sulfinpyrazone as an inhibitor of PGI_2 production by pig aortic endothelial cells in culture [19].

With regard to pharmacological properties related to side effects, aspirin is a more potent inhibitor of stomach prostaglandin and thromboxane synthesis than is sulfinpyrazone [20], possibly explaining the low ulcerogenic potential of sulfinpyrazone.

Recently, in an animal model relating to the development of senile arthrosis, an interesting effect of sulfinpyrazone has been observed (G. Wilhelmi, personal communication). Groups of C57Bl mice, which develop spontaneous arthroses, were treated orally for 4 months with sulfinpyrazone at doses of 15 mg/kg per day and 50 mg/kg per day. Their knee joints were then examined histologically after serial sectioning [21, 22]. A marked trend towards reduction in incidence of arthrosis and severity of arthrotic lesions was seen when a comparison with histology from joints of untreated animals was made. It has already been shown that aspirin, also given orally at doses of 50 mg/kg and 150 mg/kg, increased the incidence of arthrosis and severity of lesions using the same animal model [23].

References

1. Tanaka, N. and Leduc, E.C.: A study of the cellular distribution of Forssman antigen in various species. J. Immunol. 77: 182-212, 1956.
2. Pelczarska, A.B. and Roszkowski, A.P.: Inhibitors of Forssman guinea-pig "anaphylaxis." J. Pharmacol. Exp. Ther. 185: 116-126, 1973.
3. Böhm, G.M., Vugman, I., Valeri, V. et al: Ultrastructural alterations to pulmonary blood vessels in acute immunological lung lesions in rats, mice and guinea pigs. J. Pathol. 11: 95-100, 1973.
4. Taichman, N.S. and Tsai, C.-C.: Platelets, drugs and intravascular immune reactions. In Hirsh, J., Cade, J.F., Gallus, A.S. and Schonbaum, E. (eds.): Platelets, Drugs and Thrombosis. Basle:S. Karger, 1975, pp. 169-181.
5. Spear, G.S. and Kihara, I.: Complement and heterophile shock. John Hopkins Med. J. 126: 210-216, 1970.
6. Tsai, C.C., Taichman, N.S., Pulver, W.H. et al.: Heterophile antibodies and tissue injury. III. Am. J. Pathol. 72: 179-196, 1973.
7. O'Brien, J.R.: Effects of salicylates on human platelets. Lancet 1: 779, 1968.
8. Packham, M.A., Warrior, E.S., Glynn, M.F. et al.: Alteration of the response of platelets to surface stimuli by pyrazole compounds. J. Exp. Med. 126: 171-188, 1967.
9. Butler, K.D., Pay, G.F., Roberts, J. M. et al.: The effect of sulphinpyrazone and other drugs on the platelet response during the acute phase of the active Arthus reaction in guinea pigs. Thrombosis Res. 15: 319-340, 1979.
10. May, J.E. and Frank, M.M.: Complement-mediated tissue damage: Contribution of the classical and alternate complement pathways in the Forssman reaction. J. Immunol. 108: 1517-1525, 1972.
11. Smith, J.B. and Willis, A.L.: Aspirin selectively inhibits prostaglandin production in human platelets. Nature New Biol. 231: 235, 1971.
12. Ali, M. and McDonald, J.W.D.: Effect of sulfinpyrazone on platelet prostaglandin synthesis and platelet release of serotonin. J. Lab. Clin. Med. 89 :868-875, 1977.
13. Harker, L.A. and Slichter, S.J.: Studies of platelet and fibrinogen kinetics in patients with prosthetic heart valves. N. Engl. J. Med. 283: 1302-1305, 1970.
14. Smythe, H.A., Ogryzlo, M.A., Murphy, E.A. et al.: The effect of sulfinpyrazone (Anturan®) on platelet economy and blood coagulation in man. Canad. Med. Assoc. J. 92: 818-821, 1965.
15. Steele, P., Battock, D. and Genton, E.: Effects of clofibrate and sulfinpyrazone on platelet survival time in coronary artery disease. Circulation 52: 473-476, 1975.

16. Steele, P., Carroll, J., Overfield, D. et al.: Effect of sulfinpyrazone on platelet survival time in patients with transient cerebral ischemic attacks. Stroke 8: 396-398, 1977.

17. Steele, P., Weily, H.S., Davies, H. et al.: Platelet survival in patients with rheumatic heart disease. New Engl. J. Med. 290: 537-539, 1974.

18. Harker, L.A., Wall, R.I., Harlan, J.M. et al.: Sulfinpyrazone prevention of homocysteine-induced endothelial cell injury and arteriosclerosis. Clin. Res. 26: 554A, 1978.

19. Gordon, J.L. and Pearson, J.D.: Effects of sulphinpyrazone and aspirin on prostaglandin I_2 (prostacyclin) synthesis by endothelial cells. Br. J. Pharmacol. 64: 481-483, 1978

20. Ali, M., Zamecnik, J., Cerskus, A.L. et al.: Synthesis of thromboxane B_2 and prostaglandins by bovine gastric mucosal microsomes. Prostaglandins 14: 819-827, 1977.

21. Wilhelmi, G. and Faust, R.: Suitability of the C57 black mouse as an experimental animal for the study of skeletal changes due to ageing, with special reference to osteo-arthrosis and its response to Tribenoside. Pharmacology 14: 289-296, 1976.

22. Wilhelmi, G.: Effect of C 21524-Su (Pirprofen) on spontaneous osteo-arthrosis in the mouse. Pharmacology 16: 268-272, 1978.

23. Wilhelmi, G.: Fördernde und hemmende Einflüsse von Tribenosid und Acetylsalicylsäure auf die spontane Arthrose der Maus. Arzneim. Forsch. 28: 1724-1726, 1978.

Discussion

Dr. Minick: Do the Forssman and the Arthus reactions cause similar changes in endothelial cells?

Dr. White: There are minor endothelial changes in the sublethal Forssman reaction, but in the Arthus reaction only intralumenal deposits of platelets are seen.

Dr. Minick: Have you, or has anyone, tested the effect of these drugs in larger blood vessels, rather than the microcirculation, in association with immunologically induced injuries such as immune complex disease?

Dr. White: Not extensively, to my knowledge.

Dr. Minick: The types of reactions in the microvasculature and the large arteries may differ somewhat.

Dr. White: They are rather different; I think this is true.

Dr. McDonald: Have you tested phenylbutazone in the spontaneous arthrosis model? Is it active?

Dr. White: I am not aware of any results with phenylbutazone; no.

Dr. Wiedeman: How critical, do you think, is the dose that we give these animals?

Dr. White: I think that the dose is critical and that it is important to know what the plasma levels are. With the doses that we've given both intravenously and orally one would have expected the plasma levels to be much higher than the 20 μg/ml reached as a maximum during therapeutic dosage of 800 mg/day, but we know from subsequent pharmacokinetic work that this is not so.

Dr. Clopath: You found no effect with the thioether analog of sulfinpyrazone in the Forssman reaction, but the biotransformation, as well as the pharmacokinetics, of those two drugs might be very different. I don't know how sensible it is to pretreat the animals 30 min before the challenge without testing other periods of pretreatment.

Dr. White: In an ideal world one would do that. My colleague, Dr. Wallis, will address at greater length the question of sequential treatment before immunological challenge. He will also say something about the effect of the thioether over a sustained period of time.

Dr. Domenet: You said that 100 mg/kg or more of aspirin did not inhibit the Forssman reaction; have you tried a lower dose?

Dr. White: Yes, we have tested the response to the full dose range.

Mr. Povalski: The differences between the two compounds, aspirin and sulfinpyrazone, in the Forssman and Arthus reactions are very striking. Could you speculate on the possible reasons?

Dr. White: I think that in the Arthus reaction you have platelet aggregation either as a response to interaction with antigen-antibody complexes around the walls of the vessels, or, particularly in the guinea pig, as a response to C3a anaphylatoxin. It has been shown recently by Becker in Germany that there are platelet binding sites for C3a in this species, of both low and high affinity. In the light of subsequent evidence we were particularly fortunate, perhaps, in choosing the guinea pig for investigation of the platelet response to the Arthus reaction.

In the case of the Forssman reaction, we don't see platelets as intralumenal aggregates; we see them along the walls of the vasculature. We can hypothesize that the reaction starts with an antigen/antibody reaction on the vasculature, somehow damaging the endothelium. After edema is established, then perhaps platelets accumulate in some way adjacent to the damage. That is speculation, however, and we haven't been able to prove it.

Dr. Mustard: In your experiments what happens to the leukocyte count in the Forssman reaction?

Dr. White: There is no change.

Sustained Effects
of Sulfinpyrazone

K. D. Butler, Ph.D., W. Dieterle, Ph.D.,
E. D. Maguire, B.Sc., G. F. Pay, M.I.Biol.,
R. B. Wallis, Ph.D. and A. M. White, Ph.D.

Introduction

Sulfinpyrazone was first thought to affect platelet function in 1965, when Smythe et al. [1] showed that shortened platelet survival in patients with gout was prolonged as a result of treatment with this drug. Since that time the effect of this substance has been examined in many animal and human models of pathological conditions involving platelet thromboembolism, and these studies have been recently reviewed [2]. However, some of the possible reasons for the observed effects of sulfinpyrazone on platelet-mediated phenomena have only recently come to light. One of the major areas of interest is its effect on platelet prostaglandin biosynthesis.

In 1977 Ali and McDonald [3] showed that sulfinpyrazone competitively inhibited human platelet prostaglandin synthetase and almost certainly the cyclooxygenase [4] in a broken cell preparation with a K_i of 35 μg/ml. Our own data (unpublished) confirm that similar inhibitory potency is found in an intact cell system using platelet-rich plasma (PRP). Here the inhibition of sodium arachidonate-induced aggregation is competitively inhibited with an A_2 of 50 μg/ml. Both of these parameters (K_i and A_2) represent the concentrations of sulfinpyrazone which require a doubling of the sodium arachidonate concentration in

K. D. Butler, Ph.D., Research Centre, CIBA-GEIGY Pharmaceuticals, Horsham, England; W. Dieterle, Ph.D., Research Department, Pharmaceutical Division, CIBA-GEIGY, Ltd., Basle, Switzerland; E. D. Maguire, B.Sc., G. F. Pay, M.I.Biol., R. B. Wallis, Ph.D. and A. M. White, Ph.D., Research Centre, CIBA-GEIGY Pharmaceuticals, Horsham, England.

19

order to retain the normal response. It is therefore reasonable to assume that the sulfinpyrazone largely equilibrates with the cellular compartment in which prostaglandin synthesis takes place. After ingestion of a single 200-mg dose of sulfinpyrazone in man (i.e., the same as that used three or four times per day in the major clinical trials), the maximum plasma concentration of the drug is only 14 to 23 μg/ml [5]. This concentration of sulfinpyrazone would be expected to inhibit prostaglandin synthesis only slightly. The small amount of evidence to hand [6, 7], substantiated by us in this paper, suggests that there is no build-up in the plasma concentration of unchanged drug during prolonged dosage. Therefore it seemed logical, if inhibition of platelet cyclooxygenase contributes to the clinical effectiveness of the drug, to look in the plasma for other substances derived from sulfinpyrazone, which are more potent inhibitors of platelet prostaglandin synthesis than the unchanged drug. We have done this using inhibition of sodium arachidonate-induced platelet aggregation and inhibition of malondialdehyde (MDA) production *ex vivo* as more sensitive methods than inhibition of collagen-induced platelet secretion [3] or collagen-induced platelet aggregation [8]. We were encouraged in our attempts because we were able to confirm through the use of these more sensitive techniques the demonstration that sulfinpyrazone has a sustained effect in rabbits [9].

Studies relating to the inhibition by sulfinpyrazone of platelet function in experimental animal models have involved us in the use of the Arthus [8, 10] and Forssman reactions [11] in guinea pigs. The findings reported here relate the time course of *in vivo* events subsequent to the administration of sulfinpyrazone with *ex vivo* events in this species and in man, again using sodium arachidonate-induced platelet aggregation. A preliminary communication relating to the human study has been published [12]. Evidence is also presented here which is consistent with the thioether (G 25671) being an active metabolite of the parent compound responsible for the prolonged effect of sulfinpyrazone in the guinea pig.

Materials and Methods

Guinea pigs used in biological studies (Dunkin Hartley, 350 to 500 g) were obtained from Hacking and Churchill, Huntingdon, U.K. Metabolic studies were carried out in male Dunkin Hartley Pirbright (200 to 300 g) guinea pigs. Human volunteers who had taken no nonsteroidal anti-inflammatory drugs, including aspirin, for at least 2 weeks prior to the studies gave signed informed consent.

Sulfinpyrazone was obtained from Geigy Pharmaceuticals, Macclesfield, U.K. For oral administration to guinea pigs it was suspended in polyethylene glycol "6000" solution (20% wt/vol) at such a concentration that approximately 0.5 ml was administered to each animal. For intravenous administration it was suspended in 0.9% NaCl and solubilized by adjusting the pH to 7.5 with 0.1 M NaOH. Oral administration to man was by sugar-coated tablets. Sulfinpyrazone metabolites and ^{14}C-sulfinpyrazone were obtained from CIBA-GEIGY Ltd., Basle, Switzerland.

Arachidonic acid, obtained from Sigma U.K., was dissolved in 0.1 M Na_2CO_3 and stored under oxygen-free N_2 in an injection vial at $4°C$ prior to use. ADP was obtained from Sigma U.K. Collagen solution was obtained from Hormon Chemie, München, B.R.D.

Blood samples were obtained from guinea pigs by cardiac puncture under ether anesthesia. Blood (9 ml) was drawn into 3.8% wt/vol trisodium citrate (1 ml). Blood samples from human subjects were taken from the antecubital vein and immediately diluted with 1/10 volume 0.1 M citric acid adjusted to pH 6.5 with NaOH and containing 0.078 M D-glucose.

Platelet aggregation was measured by the standard methods previously described [8]. Aggregation rates were measured by drawing tangents to the initial part of the aggregation traces and calculating the percentage change per minute. In view of the more complex nature of the traces when human PRP is stimulated with sodium arachidonate, the results were substantiated either by measuring the minimum concentration of sodium arachidonate which caused aggregation or by measuring the concentration which caused the trace to cross 5% of the chart width in exactly 1 min. Dose-response curves of at least six different agonist concentrations were plotted in all cases. ED_{50} was defined as the concentration of agonist which causes 50% of the maximal response achievable by increasing the agonist concentration. Platelet counts of each sample were measured and found not to be statistically significantly different between treated and control groups.

Platelet counts subsequent to the induction of the Arthus reaction in guinea pigs were measured as previously described [10]. The Forssman reaction was elicited in guinea pigs and platelet counts were measured as described in the previous paper [11].

Sulfinpyrazone concentration was measured by the spectrophotometric method of Burns et al. [13] unless otherwise stated.

MDA biosynthesis was measured in samples of washed human platelets. Platelets were washed by first forming platelet aggregates through the addition of ADP (20 μl, 1 mg/ml) to PRP (4 ml) and agitation of the mixture with a siliconized Pasteur pipette [14]. When large aggregates had been obtained, 4 ml of 0.94 mM NaH_2PO_4 containing 72 mM NaCl and 53 mM EDTA adjusted to pH 6.5 was added, and the suspension was centrifuged at 170 g for 5 min at 20°C. The supernatant fluid was discarded and the platelet pellet was resuspended in 0.94 mM NaH_2PO_4 containing 137 mM NaCl, 2.68 mM KCl, 2.34 mM $MgCl_2 \cdot 6H_2O$ and 5.56 mM glucose adjusted to pH 6.5. MDA production was induced by addition of 10 μM sodium arachidonate and incubation of the platelets with shaking at 37°C for 15 min in a water bath. MDA was estimated by the thiobarbituric acid method [15], by comparison with standards as described by Smith et al. [16]. Data were analyzed by Student's t test or paired t test, as appropriate.

The metabolism of ^{14}C-sulfinpyrazone in the guinea pig was studied after a single dose of 100 mg/kg IV. Blood was withdrawn from four animals each at various times up to 24 h, and plasma was prepared from the individual samples.

Total radioactivity was measured in all samples of plasma. Unchanged sulfinpyrazone and the metabolites G 31442, G 32642, GP 52097, and CGP 17385 (Fig. 1) were specifically determined by multiple inverse isotope dilution analysis [5]. So that unknown metabolites might be isolated, the plasma pool was extracted with 1,2-dichloroethane at pH 1 under N_2. The radioactive compounds in the extract were separated and purified by high-resolution liquid chromatography [7].

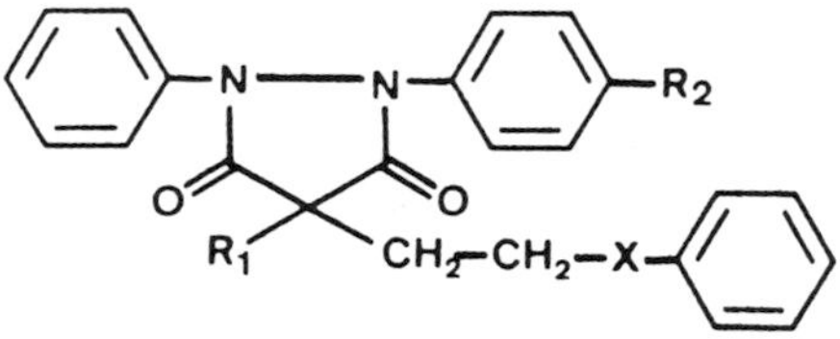

Compound	R_1	R_2	X
G 28 315 (Sulphinpyrazone)	H	H	SO
G 25 671	H	H	S
G 31 442	H	H	SO_2
G 32 642	H	OH	SO
GP 52 097	OH	H	SO
CGP 17 385	H	OH	SO_2

FIG. 1. Structures of sulfinpyrazone and its known metabolites.

Results

*Effects of Sulfinpyrazone
in Guinea Pigs Ex Vivo*

The ability of sulfinpyrazone to inhibit sodium arachidonate-induced platelet aggregation *ex vivo* was employed to study the time course of the effects of the drug in guinea pigs.

Both oral and intravenous doses of sulfinpyrazone to guinea pigs caused inhibition of sodium arachidonate-induced platelet aggregation *ex vivo*. Inhibition lasted for at least 24 h even with moderate doses of the drug and maximal inhibition occurred approximately 6 h after dosing (Fig. 2). The effect of different doses of the drug was then investigated near the time of maximal inhibition (i.e., 7 h). Inhibition of sodium arachidonate-induced aggregation *ex vivo* appeared to be competitive and was statistically significant with oral doses as low as 3 mg/kg at this time point (Fig. 3).

ADP-induced platelet aggregation was not inhibited even after the highest dose of sulfinpyrazone.

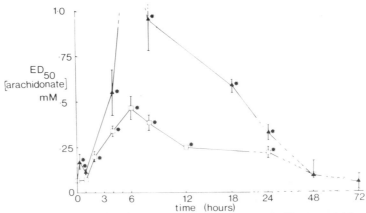

FIG. 2. Time course of effects of sulfinpyrazone on sodium arachidonate-induced aggregation *ex vivo* in the guinea pig. Sulfinpyrazone 30 mg/kg PO (□) or 100 mg/kg IV (▲) was administered at time 0 to groups of five guinea pigs. Blood was withdrawn at the times indicated and the aggregation rate of the PRP measured using sodium arachidonate as the agonist. The concentration of sodium arachidonate required to cause 50% maximal aggregation rate (ED_{50}) was determined for each sample and plotted ± standard error. Asterisks denote statistically significant inhibition ($p < 0.05$). Reprinted, with permission, from Butler et al. [8].

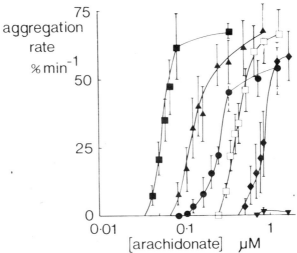

FIG. 3. Effect of sulfinpyrazone on platelet aggregation *ex vivo* 7 h after administration to guinea pigs. PRP was prepared from groups of five control animals (■) or animals treated with sulfinpyrazone 3 mg/kg PO (▲), 10 mg/kg PO (●), 30 mg/kg PO (□), 100 mg/kg PO (◆) or 300 mg/kg PO (▼). Platelet aggregation was measured and plotted ± standard errors. Reprinted, with permission, from Butler et al. [8].

Effect of Sulfinpyrazone on the Arthus
Reaction in Guinea Pigs In Vivo

The thrombocytopenia caused by inducing an Arthus reaction in guinea pigs reaches a maximum approximately 20 min after the antigenic challenge [10].

Sulfinpyrazone caused sustained inhibition of the thrombocytopenia; this inhibition was maximal when the drug was administered 4 to 6 h before the antigenic challenge (Fig. 4).

Only relatively high doses of the drug, i.e., 200 mg/kg PO, are inhibitory after 1 h [10]. However, oral doses as low as 30 mg/kg inhibited at 4 to 18 h and 10 mg/kg inhibited at 4 h (Fig. 4).

Effect of Sulfinpyrazone
in Man Ex Vivo

A single dose of 400 mg caused inhibition of sodium arachidonate-induced primary platelet aggregation 2 h later when the aggregation rate was measured by drawing a tangent

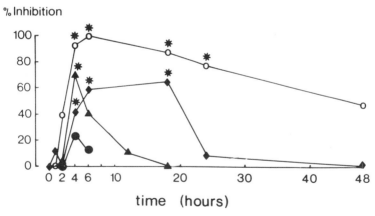

FIG. 4. Effect of sulfinpyrazone on the thrombocytopenia induced by the Arthus reaction in guinea pigs. Sulfinpyrazone was administered orally to groups of five animals in doses of 100 mg/kg (○), 30 mg/kg (♦), 10 mg/kg (▲), or 3 mg/kg (●) at time 0. The Arthus reaction was induced at the time indicated. The platelet counts of challenged animals (i.e., 0% inhibition) varied from 0.84 to 1.1×10^8 platelets/ml and of unchallenged animals (i.e., 100% inhibition) from 2.64 to 3.51×10^8 platelets/ml. Asterisks denote statistically significant inhibition of thrombocytopenia (p < 0.05). Reprinted, with permission, from Butler et al. [8].

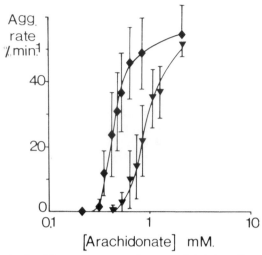

FIG. 5. Effect of sulfinpyrazone on human platelet sodium arachidonate-induced aggregation 2 h after drug administration. Blood samples were withdrawn from five volunteers either immediately before (♦) or 2 h after (▼) oral administration of 400 mg sulfinpyrazone. Platelet-rich plasma was prepared and the aggregation rate induced by sodium arachidonate measured at different agonist concentrations. Results are ± standard error.

to the initial part of the aggregation trace (i.e., between 5% and 10% of the chart width)(Fig. 5). Log sodium arachidonate concentration versus response curves were shifted to higher sodium arachidonate concentrations and the curves were parallel to control curves. Similar results were obtained if the lowest concentration of sodium arachidonate to cause platelet aggregation was measured. After 2 h the median effective dose (ED_{50}) for sodium arachidonate was shifted from $480 \pm 46\ \mu M$ to $936 \pm 119\ \mu M$ (p<0.01) (Fig. 5).

Figure 6 shows that both sodium arachidonate-induced platelet aggregation and MDA biosynthesis were inhibited for 72 h and 24 h, respectively, after the single dose. The dose-response curves of platelet primary aggregation induced by ADP were not affected at any time points measured. The plasma concentration of sulfinpyrazone was maximal at 2 h and rapidly declined to an undetectable level by 24 h. Again the inhibition of sodium arachidonate-induced aggregation was

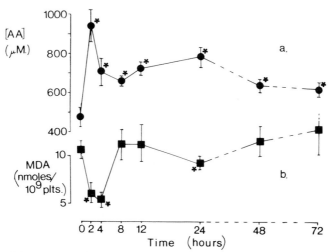

FIG. 6. Effect of sulfinpyrazone on platelet function *ex vivo* in man. Curve *a* (●) is the ED_{50} for sodium arachidonate-induced aggregation compared to control at time 0. Curve *b* (■) is the MDA production induced by sodium arachidonate (10 μM). Results are shown ± standard error. Asterisks denote statistically significant ($p < 0.05$) difference from control.

manifested as a shift in the concentration versus response curve, giving rise to an increase in the ED_{50} for the sodium arachidonate agonist.

A single (200 mg) dose of sulfinpyrazone had no significant effect on aggregation of human platelets induced by sodium arachidonate *ex vivo* at 1 h or at 24 h.

Although the inhibitory effect of sulfinpyrazone in man (5 mg/kg, PO) is not as large as that found in the guinea pig with a smaller dose of 3 mg/kg, the effect in man was longer lasting and consequently might be expected to build up during therapy with multiple doses of the drug. Figure 7 shows that this is the case when a dosage schedule of 200 mg given four times daily is used, but slow build-up is less noticeable when a dosage of 400 mg twice daily is used. In the study seven volunteers took 200 mg of sulfinpyrazone and blood samples were taken before dosage on the first day and 3 to 4 h after the first tablet on days 2, 3, 4, and 5. On the seventh day of the study, sulfinpyrazone

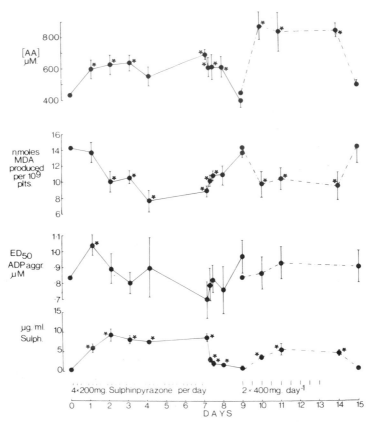

FIG. 7. Effect of therapeutic dosage schedules of sulfinpyrazone on human platelet function *ex vivo*. Sulfinpyrazone (200 mg four times daily) was administered to a group of seven male volunteers for 7 days (———) or 400 mg twice daily to a group of five male volunteers for 5 days (—·—·). Doses were taken at the times indicated by vertical lines at the bottom of the figure. Blood samples were taken at the times indicated (•) and concentration of sodium arachidonate needed to induce platelet aggregation with a time lag of 1 min, biosynthesis of MDA, and the ED_{50} for ADP-induced platelet aggregation were measured. Sulfinpyrazone concentration was measured in samples of plasma. Results are mean ± standard error. Asterisks denote results statistically significantly different ($p < 0.05$) from those at day 0 (———) or day 9 (-----).

dosage was terminated and blood samples were taken 4, 8, and 12 h afterwards and on days 8 and 9. The aggregation response measured as the concentration of sodium arachidonate causing aggregation with a time lag of 1 min returned to the control value by day 9. The MDA biosynthesis induced by sodium arachidonate had returned to the control value by day 9. Three of these volunteers and two who had not taken sulfinpyrazone previously started a regimen of 400 mg of sulfinpyrazone twice daily on day 9. Blood samples were taken before starting the drug on day 9 and 12 h after a sulfinpyrazone dose (i.e., when the plasma drug level was low) on days 10 and 11. On day 13 dosing was terminated, and blood samples were taken 12 h and 36 h afterwards, at which time the response of the platelets had again returned to the control level.

Spectrophotometric measurement of the plasma concentrations of sulfinpyrazone showed that there were always less than 9 μg/ml and 5.5 μg/ml in the 200 mg four times daily and 400 mg twice daily studies, respectively. These concentrations are too low to cause any significant direct inhibition of platelet function when measured *in vitro* where at least 20 μg/ml are required [8].

The responsiveness of PRP to ADP was changed very little during the study but one statistically significant result occurred 1 day after commencing treatment with 200 mg of sulfinpyrazone given four times daily (Fig. 7).

Metabolism of Sulfinpyrazone
in Guinea Pigs

The plasma concentrations of total ^{14}C and of the individually determined compounds in guinea pigs after an intravenous 100 mg/kg dose are given in Figure 8. Plasma concentration as measured by radioactivity decreased initially from 415 μg/ml (10 min) to 54 μg/ml (1 h) but rose again after 1 h and reached a maximum level of 269 μg/ml at 6 h. The concentration of intact sulfinpyrazone rapidly declined from 361 μg/ml (10 min) to 9.4 μg/ml (3 h). Again, an increase was observed thereafter with a maximum of 18.7 μg/ml at 5 h, which can be explained by enterohepatic recycling of sulfinpyrazone. The sulfone metabolite G 31442 (Fig. 1) showed a concentration minimum of 2.8 μg/ml after 1 h and a maximum

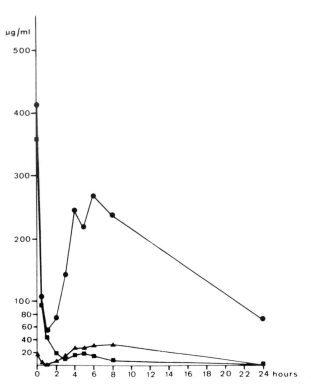

FIG. 8. Concentration of radioactive products in plasma after intravenous dosing of ^{14}C-sulfinpyrazone to four guinea pigs. Total radioactivity (●) and concentration of unchanged sulfinpyrazone (■) and of the sulfone metabolite G 31442 (▲) are plotted against time. The metabolites G 32642, GP 52097, and CGP 17385 were present at low levels not exceeding 1 µg/ml at times beyond 30 min and are therefore not included.

plateau of 27.9 to 33.1 µg/ml between 4 and 8 h. The metabolites G 32642, GP 52057, and CGP 17385 (Fig. 1) were present at low levels not exceeding 1 µg/ml at times beyond 30 min. Judged from the area under the concentration-time curve (0 to 24 h), these three compounds accounted for only 0.3%, 0.2%, and 0.1%, respectively, of total ^{14}C. The values for sulfinpyrazone and the sulfone metabolite correspond to 8.2% and 11.3%, leaving about 80% of the plasma radioactivity unidentified (Fig. 8).

Since the percentage of unidentified material in plasma was highest between 3 and 24 h, all samples from this time interval were pooled. About 80% of the ^{14}C-content of the plasma pool was extractable. Liquid chromatography yielded one major compound which was identified by mass spectrometric analysis as the thioether G 25671. The mass spectrum showed the molecular ion (m/e 388) and the same fragmentation pattern as the authentic compound. Thus, the major circulating metabolite in the guinea pig has been identified as the thioether of sulfinpyrazone, G 25671 (Fig. 1).

Discussion

The plasma concentration of sulfinpyrazone in guinea pigs could be as high as 1.5 mg/ml immediately after the intravenous injection of a dose of 100 mg/kg to a 400-g animal. The drug is metabolized at a considerable rate; at 1 h the plasma level drops to 54 μg/ml and at 6 to 7 h to a level well below the K_i for inhibition of platelet cyclooxygenase. Presumably for this reason only high doses of the drug (200 mg/kg PO) were inhibitory 1 h after dosing [8]. The plasma concentration 1 h after an oral dose of 200 mg/kg was 2.6 μg/ml (J. Godbillon, unpublished data, using the method of Lecaillon and Souppart [7]). In vivo inhibition of platelet function at this time was seen only after this oral dose and higher ones [10]. However, considerably lower doses (minimum 10 mg/kg) were capable of having an inhibitory effect 6 to 7 h after dosing, but not at earlier times.

These data are all consistent with the formation of a metabolite in this species which is more potent towards inhibition of cyclooxygenase-mediated platelet function than the parent compound. Such a metabolite does not appear to inhibit the platelet involvement in the Forssman reaction, which is not cyclooxygenase-dependent [11], since the time course of inhibition relates more closely to the pharmacokinetics of the parent molecule than to those of metabolites.

After injection of ^{14}C-sulfinpyrazone to guinea pigs, a large proportion of circulating radioactivity is in the form of the thioether (G 25671). Subtraction of the concentration of sulfinpyrazone and its previously identified metabolites G 31442, G 32642, GP 52097, and CGP 17385 from the total plasma radioactivity at each time point (Fig. 8) leaves approximately 80% of the ^{14}C label unaccounted for. The difference is maximal at approximately 6 h and the major component is G 25671.

G 25671 is a potent inhibitor of sodium arachidonate-induced platelet aggregation *in vitro* (approximately 12 times more potent than sulfinpyrazone). It also inhibits collagen-induced platelet aggregation but has no effect on the primary phase of ADP-induced aggregation (unpublished data). G 25671 also inhibits the thrombocytopenia caused by the Arthus reaction but not that caused by the Forssman reaction [11]. It is therefore likely that the sustained effect of sulfinpyrazone in the guinea pig is due to metabolism of the parent molecule to its thioether G 25671.

In the human studies platelet effects are similar. Twenty-four hours after a single oral dose of 200 mg [5] or even 800 mg (P. Imhof et al., unpublished data), the plasma concentration declines to a level below the limits of detection of the methods used in this paper. However, we see disturbances of platelet function at this time which strongly suggest that platelet prostaglandin synthesis is still inhibited.

Multiple dosing with sulfinpyrazone (200 mg four times daily or 400 mg twice daily) in man causes a small increase in the inhibitory effect over that seen after a single dose. Thus, prostaglandin-dependent platelet function remains competitively inhibited after one dose, up to the time that a subsequent dose is taken [12]. The sustained effect of sulfinpyrazone in man is less pronounced than that found in the guinea pig with similar doses. Whether this is due to a small amount of metabolism of sulfinpyrazone to G 25671 is still under investigation.

These results, which, in the human studies, include measurement of MDA production as an indirect indicator of the integrity of the prostaglandin pathway, are consistent with the results of Ali and McDonald [4], in that they support the view that sulfinpyrazone exerts its platelet inhibitory effects through competitive inhibition of prostaglandin synthesis. Such suppression is likely to constitute an important aspect of the mode of action of the drug, although other properties such as ability to protect the endothelium [17] may also have great significance.

Acknowledgments

We thank Mr. R.J. Jones, Mr. A.A. Turnbull, and Miss D. Zelaschi for skilled technical assistance and Drs. J. Turney, M. Weston, L. Williams, and F. Woods for the use of their laboratory facilities during the multiple-dose human study.

References

1. Smythe, H.A., Ogryzlo, M.A., Murphy, E.A. et al.: The effect of sulphinpyrazone (Anturan®) in platelet economy and blood coagulation in man. Canad. Med. Assoc. J. 92: 818-821, 1965.
2. Margulies, E.H. and White, A.M.: Sulfinpyrazone. *In* Goldberg, M.E. (ed.): Pharmacological and Biochemical Properties of Drug Substances, Vol. 2. Washington, D.C.: American Pharmaceutical Association, 1979, pp. 255-278.
3. Ali, M. and McDonald, J.W.D.: Effects of sulfinpyrazone on platelet prostaglandin synthesis and platelet release of serotonin. J. Lab. Clin. Med. 89: 868-875, 1977.
4. Ali, M., Cerskus, A.L., Zanecnik, J. et al.: Synthesis of prostaglandin D_2 and thromboxane B_2 by human platelets. Thromb. Res. 11: 485-496, 1977.
5. Dieterle, W., Faigle, J.W., Mory, H. et al.: Biotransformation and pharmacokinetics of sulphinpyrazone (Anturan) in man. Eur. J. Clin. Pharmacol. 9: 135-145, 1975.
6. Rosenfeld, J., Buchanan, M., Powers, P. et al.: Determination of sulphinpyrazone in patient plasma by gas chromatography. Thromb. Res. 12: 247-255, 1978.
7. Lecaillon, J.-B and Souppart, C.: Quantitative assay of sulphinpyrazone in plasma and urine by high performance liquid chromatography. J. Chromatog. 121: 227-234, 1976.
8. Butler, K.D., Wallis, R.B. and White, A.M.: A study of the relationship between *ex vivo* and *in vivo* effects of sulphinpyrazone in the guinea pig. Haemostasis 8: 353-360, 1979.
9. Buchanan, M.R., Rosenfeld, J. and Hirsh, J.: The prolonged effect of sulphinpyrazone on collagen-induced platelet aggregation *in vivo*. Thromb. Res. 13: 883-892, 1978.
10. Butler, K.D., Pay, G.F., Roberts, J.M. et al.: The effect of sulphinpyrazone and other drugs on the platelet response during the acute phase of the active Arthus reaction in guinea pigs. Thromb. Res. 15: 319-340, 1979.
11. Butler, K.D. and White, A.M.: Inhibition of the platelet involvement in the sublethal Forssman reaction by sulphinpyrazone and not by aspirin. This volume.
12. Maguire, E.D., Pay, G.F., Turney, J. et al.: Inhibition of human platelet function induced by sulphinpyrazone. VIIth International Congress on Thrombosis and Haemostasis (Abst. No. 0232), 1979.

13. Burns, J.J., Yü, T.F., Ritterband, A., et al.: A potent new uricosuric agent, the sulfoxide metabolite of the phenylbutazone analogue, G 25671. J. Pharmacol. Exp. Ther. 119: 418-426, 1957.
14. Mohammed, S.F., Reddick, R.L. and Mason, R.G.: Characterization of human platelets separated from blood by ADP-induced aggregation. Am. J. Pathol. 79: 81-94, 1975.
15. Stuart, M.J., Murphy, S. and Oski, F.A.: A simple nonradioisotope technique for the determination of platelet life-span. New Engl. J. Med. 292: 1310-1313, 1975.
16. Smith, J.B., Ingerman, C.M. and Silver, M.J.: Malondialdehyde formation as an indicator of prostaglandin production by human platelets. J. Lab. Clin. Med. 88: 167-172, 1976.
17. Harker, L.A., Wall, R.J., Harlan, J.M. et al.: Sulphinpyrazone prevention of homocysteine-induced endothelial cell injury and arteriosclerosis. Clin. Res. 26: 554, 1978.

Discussion

Dr. Sherry: It would appear that the assumption is being made that the effect of sulfinpyrazone or its metabolites relates almost entirely to their extracellular concentration. Is it at all possible that we are dealing with an effect due to the intracellular concentration? If so, what data do you have along that line?

Dr. Wallis: Yes, we incubated whole blood *in vitro* with ^{14}C-sulfinpyrazone and found that the concentration of sulfinpyrazone in the platelets was very little more than you would find in the plasma. That was an *in vitro* experiment, however; we haven't yet performed it *ex vivo*. Adding sulfinpyrazone to platelet-rich plasma is surely an indication of how much the platelets are inhibited, because we're measuring a cellular event, caused by arachidonic acid, that is dependent on the plasma concentration, that is, the concentration of sulfinpyrazone outside the platelet. When you add sulfinpyrazone to platelet-rich plasma the effect is no greater after 0.5 h than after 1 min.

Dr. McDonald: Does the thioether account for approximately 80% of the metabolites in the guinea pig?

Dr. Wallis: Yes.

Dr. McDonald: Does the sulfone account for the major part of the metabolites in man, as far as you know, with the thioether being about 10%?

Dr. Wallis: Yes, in man the metabolism is very slight. In the plasma we find mainly sulfinpyrazone; the metabolites make up only a small percentage, 4% or 5%, of the total. The maximum that the thioether could account for would be about 10% of that. We are re-examining data from human subjects after therapeutic dosage to find out what this percentage is.

Dr. McDonald: Is the potency of the thioether roughly tenfold that of sulfinpyrazone?

Dr. Wallis: Yes.

Dr. Folts: You mentioned that ADP-induced aggregation was not affected in the guinea pig or in man by sulfinpyrazone or its derivatives. Do you know of any species in which it is?

Dr. Wallis: By sulfinpyrazone, no.

Dr. Folts: I have found that it appears to be effective in the dog, but dog platelets may be different.

Dr. Wallis: The dog is an unusual animal; it appears not to have a thromboxane A_2 receptor on the platelet, for instance.

Dr. Gordon: You stated that the effect against the Arthus reaction was maximal after about 6 h, as opposed to 2 h against the Forssman reaction (although that was after an IV injection of sulfinpyrazone). Do you, therefore, conclude that the effect against the Arthus reaction is due primarily to the thioether metabolite, whereas the effect against the Forssman reaction is not?

Dr. Wallis: Yes, the effect against the Forssman reaction after 2 h was due to sulfinpyrazone itself.

Dr. Gordon: Would you also conclude that the reason the effect is maximal 2 h after IV injection against the Forssman reaction, rather than after a few minutes, is due to the enterohepatic recirculation?

Dr. Wallis: Quite likely, yes, because the sulfinpyrazone concentration after IV dosage decreases very rapidly, within a few minutes, and then comes back into the circulation by the enterohepatic recirculation.

Dr. Mustard: When platelets that are exposed to sulfinpyrazone are washed, the effect is lost. Does the metabolite, which presumably inhibits the cyclooxygenase, bind to platelets more firmly than does sulfinpyrazone?

Dr. Wallis: In fact, we have evidence to the contrary; it's very easy to wash the effects of G 25671 out of the platelets. We did an experiment in rabbits in which just a centrifugation, wash, and resuspension of the platelets in control plasma removed about 90% of the activity.

Effects of Sulfinpyrazone
on Synthesis of Prostaglandins
and Thromboxanes by Platelets
In Vitro and *In Vivo*

John W. D. McDonald, M.D., Ph.D., Muslim Ali, Ph.D.
and Andrew L. Cerskus, M.S.

Sulfinpyrazone has been shown to normalize shortened platelet survival in certain animal models of thrombosis and in a limited number of clinical studies. It may also influence platelet—endothelial cell interaction *in vitro*. These effects of sulfinpyrazone are regarded as perhaps unique to the drug. However, in some controlled clinical trials, platelet survival has not been found to be shortened in patients with cerebrovascular and cardiovascular disease, and sulfinpyrazone was without effect on platelet survival. The relationship of platelet survival to the syndrome of sudden death in patients with ischemic heart disease remains uncertain. It is possible that inhibition of platelet cyclooxygenase activity and thromboxane formation, an effect which is not unique to sulfinpyrazone but shared with nonsteroidal anti-inflammatory drugs, may account for at least part of the efficacy of sulfinpyrazone.

Figure 1 summarizes the role of prostaglandins and thromboxanes in platelet function. Aggregating agents, such as collagen, generate free arachidonic acid from platelet membrane phospholipid by the activation of phospholipase A_2. Arachi-

John W. D. McDonald, M.D., Ph.D., Muslim Ali, Ph.D. and Andrew L. Cerskus, M.S., Department of Medicine, The University of Western Ontario, London, Canada.

This research was supported by the Medical Research Council of Canada and the Ontario Heart Foundation.

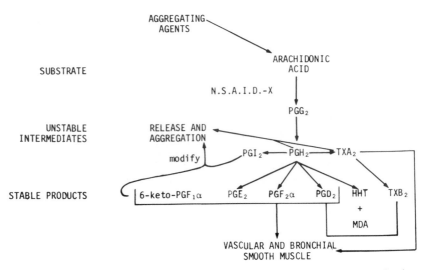

FIG. 1. Relationships between platlet function and prostaglandin synthesis.

donic acid is substrate for fatty acid cyclooxygenase, which
catalyzes formation of the unstable prostaglandins G_2 and H_2
(PGG_2 and PGH_2). Thromboxane synthetase catalyzes the
further metabolism of PGH_2 to thromboxane A_2 (TXA_2),
another highly unstable compound. PGG_2, PGH_2 and TXA_2
cause platelets to release their granule contents and to aggregate, TXA_2 being the most potent of the three compounds in
this respect.

TXA$_2$ is also a potent constrictor of coronary and cerebral
arteries [1]. The recent demonstration by Lewy et al. [2] of
elevated thromboxane levels in plasma of patients with Prinzmetal's angina suggests that the material may be of importance
in human disease. PGH_2 is further metabolized to stable
prostaglandins, of which PGD_2 may be the most important with
respect to platelets. PGD_2 inhibits aggregation and could play a
role in limiting the process. It also constricts bronchial and
vascular smooth muscle. Conversion of PGH_2 to heptadecatri-
enoic acid (HHT) and malondialdehyde (MDA) has no known
physiological significance, but the measurement of MDA has
been a useful technique in some laboratories for measuring
activity of the pathway.

Moncada et al. [3] demonstrated the conversion by blood
vessels of PGH_2 to another unstable material, prostacyclin,

which has now been desginated PGI_2. PGI_2 is important in platelet physiology because it stimulates platelet adenylate cyclase and elevates platelet cyclic AMP, thereby inhibiting aggregation [4, 5]. It shares this property with D and E prostaglandins, but it is more potent. It is also a powerful vasodilator. Therefore, it antagonizes both platelet aggregation and vasoconstriction caused by TXA_2. PGI_2 is converted to 6-keto-$PGF_{1\alpha}$ and TXA_2 is converted to stable thromboxane B_2 (TXB_2). It is possible to measure the activity of the pathways for prostacyclin synthesis and thromboxane synthesis by radioimmunoassay of the stable end products, 6-keto-$PGF_{1\alpha}$ and TXB_2.

The source of PGH_2 for vascular PGI_2 synthesis is not certain. Moncada et al. [3] originally suggested that vessels mainly use platelet-generated PGH_2, but Powell and Solomon [6] and others provided evidence that the vessels themselves also contribute PGH_2 for PGI_2 synthesis. Synthesis of PGI_2 may partly account for the resistance of normal endothelium to platelet adherence and aggregation. Aspirin and other non-steroidal anti-inflammatory drugs inhibit the platelet release reaction and aggregation by inhibiting cyclooxygenase activity and therefore blocking the generation of PGH_2 and TXA_2. It has been pointed out by Moncada [3] and others that any drug active at this step may be a two-edged sword, since it also causes inhibition of synthesis of potentially protective PGI_2. One challenge to those interested in this field might be the development of nonsteroidal anti-inflammatory drugs which would have a potent action on platelet cyclooxygenase activity but be relatively weak in their effects on vascular cyclo-oxygenase activity, so that they do not interfere with PGI_2 synthesis. There are a limited number of examples of tissue specificity of inhibitors in the prostaglandin field [7].

Kinlough-Rathbone et al. [8] have shown that there are other pathways for aggregation of platelets which do not involve the metabolism of arachidonic acid and the formation of thromboxanes. This is particularly true for thrombin-induced aggregation and also for part of the aggregating effect of collagen.

Zucker found that with low concentrations of collagen, sulfinpyrazone inhibits the release of serotonin from platelets [9]. Packham and associates [10] originally showed that sulfinpyrazone inhibits collagen-induced release from platelets and that the extent of inhibition is dependent on the concentrations of collagen used. In later experiments [11] it was shown that sulfinpyrazone is a very weak inhibitor of thrombin-induced release from platelets and that an effect could only be shown with low concentrations of thrombin.

In *in vitro* studies [12] we demonstrated that sulfinpyrazone is a reasonably potent inhibitor of collagen-induced serotonin release, if the collagen concentration is at a level that induces release of only about 20% of the labeled serotonin. We also studied a small group of patients who were entered in the Canadian Stroke Study [13]. Over a range of collagen concentrations which induced about 20% serotonin release in platelets from patients taking placebo, release was inhibited by about 50% in those patients taking sulfinpyrazone, 200 mg four times daily. As reported by others, there was no effect at higher collagen concentrations.

We repeated the experiment in normal volunteer subjects [12]. Serotonin release was inhibited significantly by the ingestion of sulfinpyrazone, 200 mg four times daily for 24 h, the test being done about 2 h after the last dose of the drug. The inhibition increased when the sulfinpyrazone dose was increased to 400 mg four times daily for 24 h. These results demonstrate an *ex vivo* dose-dependent effect of the drug.

For an investigation of the nature of the inhibitory effect, washed platelets were incubated with ^{14}C-labeled arachidonic acid and the formation of labeled TXA_2 and PGD_2 was determined as an estimate of cyclooxygenase activity. Sulfinpyrazone was shown to be a competitive inhibitor, strongly inhibiting cyclooxygenase activity at lower arachidonic acid concentrations, with the inhibition diminishing as the arachidonic acid concentration increased. With low arachidonic acid concentrations (2 and 10 μM), significant inhibitory effects of sulfinpyrazone are demonstrable at very low concentrations of the drug (2.5 and 5 μM). These results showed that sulfinpyrazone inhibition of cyclooxygenase activity probably accounts for the inhibition by sulfinpyrazone of collagen-induced serotonin and ADP release. It could also account for other effects of the drug on platelets. Gerrard and White [14] showed that the cyclic endoperoxides, G_2 and H_2, mediate changes in platelet function which are independent of the release reaction. Effects on other tissues may occur because TXA_2 is a potent vasoconstrictor.

In the presence of a strong collagen stimulus the arachidonic acid concentration generated may be sufficiently high to overcome the inhibitory effect of sulfinpyrazone and, perhaps more importantly, to activate the mechanism of aggregation which is independent of prostaglandin and thromboxane synthesis. With dilute collagen, the arachidonic acid concentration generated is low enough that the inhibitory effect of sulfinpyrazone is manifest and the nonprostaglandin pathway is less important. There is no basis upon which to conclude that high collagen and arachidonic acid concentration, or the reverse, is more representative of *in vivo* platelet activation. Indeed, this could vary among pathological conditions.

Inhibition by sulfinpyrazone of thromboxane formation could theoretically be the result of inhibition of cyclooxygenase activity or of thromboxane synthetase activity. The evidence that the drug is a cyclooxygenase inhibitor is that synthesis of PGD_2 is also inhibited by sulfinpyrazone. Furthermore, we have shown that sulfinpyrazone antagonizes the irreversible inhibition of platelet cyclooxygenase activity caused by aspirin (Table 1). Under conditions in which 50 μM of aspirin inhibited platelet cyclooxygenase activity by 93%, inhibition by 50 μM of sulfinpyrazone was 64%. When the two agents were combined,

Table 1. Effects of Aspirin and Sulfinpyrazone
on Platelet Cyclooxygenase Activity

Drug	Concentration (μM)	Inhibition (%)
Aspirin	50	93
Sulfinpyrazone	50	64
Aspirin +	50	
Sulfinpyrazone	50	64
Aspirin	500	93
Sulfinpyrazone	500	82
Aspirin +	500	
Sulfinpyrazone	500	82

Suspensions of washed intact platelets were preincubated with aspirin and sulfinpyrazone for 10 min prior to the addition of ^{14}C-arachidonic acid (10 μM).

the inhibitory effect approximated that seen with sulfinpyra-zone. The effect was also observed with higher concentrations of the two drugs. The interpretation of these experiments is that sulfinpyrazone occupies the site on the cyclooxygenase enzyme that is acetylated by aspirin. Therefore, the effect of sulfinpyrazone is at the level of inhibition of cyclooxygenase activity and it shares this property with the nonsteroidal anti-inflammatory drugs.

Figure 2 shows the relative potency of a number of these drugs on platelet cyclooxygenase activity. Sulfinpyrazone is of similar potency, or within the same general range, as aspirin and phenylbutazone, while indomethacin, fenoprofen, and naprox-en are more potent. It would be interesting to have similar dose-response data for vascular cyclooxygenase activity.

One pharmacokinetic consideration to be considered in the design of future clinical trials is the effect of the metabolites of sulfinpyrazone. Buchanan et al. [15] provided evidence that the maximum inhibitory effect of sulfinpyrazone on *in vivo* collagen-induced platelet aggregation occurs 18 h after admin-istration of the drug, when sulfinpyrazone is not detectable in

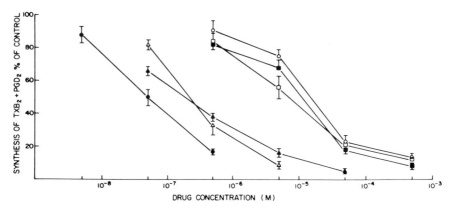

FIG. 2. Effects of nonsteroidal anti-inflammatory drugs on synthesis of TXB_2 and PGD_2 by washed platelets. Synthesis of TXB_2 and PGD_2 from arachidonate-^{14}C (10 μM) during 1-min incubations was determined after preincubation for 10 min with indomethacin ($\bullet$——$\bullet$) or acetylsalicylic acid ($\circ$——$\circ$), and for 2 min with naproxen ($\blacktriangle$——$\blacktriangle$), fenoprofen ($\triangle$——$\triangle$), phenylbutazone ($\square$——$\square$), or sulfinpyrazone ($\blacksquare$——$\blacksquare$). Results represent the mean ($\pm$ SEM) of three to eight independent experiments.

the plasma. One suggestion is that the accumulation of active sulfinpyrazone metabolites could account for this effect. We have studied the effect of two metabolites of sulfinpyrazone supplied by the CIBA-GEIGY Corporation, the structures of which are shown in Figure 3. We tested these for their potency as inhibitors of collagen-induced serotonin release and of cyclooxygenase activity *in vitro*. The sulfone is approximately ten times as potent an inhibitor of collagen-induced serotonin release as the parent compounds, while the structural change in the other metabolite results in almost complete loss of potency. Over a narrower concentration range, the same holds true for inhibition of cyclooxygenase activity (Figs. 4 and 5).

Intravenous infusion of arachidonic acid to rabbits produces respiratory distress, profound hypotension, intravenous platelet aggregation, and death. Nonsteroidal anti-inflammatory drugs, including aspirin, indomethacin, and sulfinpyrazone, protect

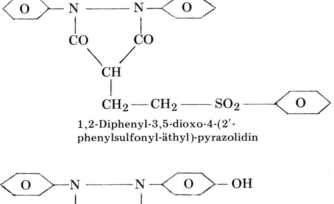

1,2-Diphenyl-3,5-dioxo-4-(2'-
phenylsulfonyl-äthyl)-pyrazolidin

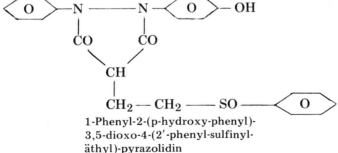

1-Phenyl-2-(p-hydroxy-phenyl)-
3,5-dioxo-4-(2'-phenyl-sulfinyl-
äthyl)-pyrazolidin

FIG. 3. Two metabolites of sulfinpyrazone.

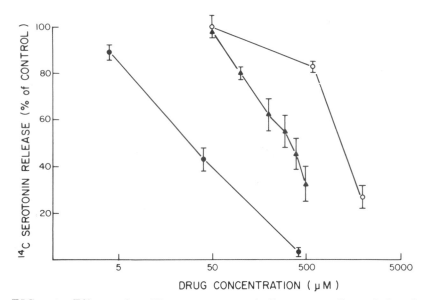

FIG. 4. Effect of sulfinpyrazone metabolites on collagen-induced serotonin-^{14}C release. Release was induced by the addition of acid-soluble collagen (0.2 µg) to platelet-rich plasma after 5 min of preincubation with 1,2-Diphenyl-3,5-dioxo-4-(2-phenylsulfonyl-athyl)-pyrazolidin (●——●), sulfinpyrazone (▲——▲), or 1-phenyl-2-(p-hydroxy-phenyl)-3,5-dioxo-4-(2-phenyl-sulfinyl-athyl)-pyrazolidin (○——○). Saline was added to control samples. Release was determined 4 min after the addition of collagen. Results represent the mean (± SEM) of five determinations.

against these effects. To determine whether this process is accompanied by measurable thromboxane and prostaglandin synthesis, we pretreated female rabbits with saline, aspirin, or sulfinpyrazone. We then injected arachidonic acid in a dose of 1.4 mg/kg into the marginal ear vein over a period of 1 min, as described by Silver et al. [16]. Control animals received a saline infusion.

At 2 min after the start of the injection, carotid arterial blood was aspirated into indomethacin solution, and platelet-rich plasma was prepared in EDTA. The content of TXB_2 was determined by radioimmunoassay.

The infusion caused intense intravascular platelet aggregation, most easily monitored by a decrease in peripheral blood platelet count (Table 2). The majority of the animals died. Protection against death and *in vivo* platelet aggregation was

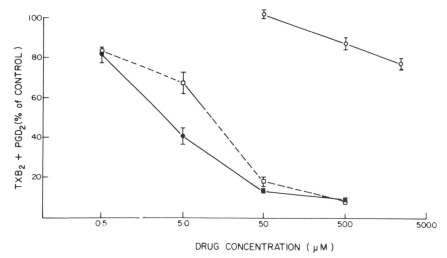

FIG. 5. Effect of sulfinpyrazone metabolites on the synthesis of TXB_2 and PGD_2 by washed platelets. Synthesis of TXB_2 and PGD_2 from arachidonate-^{14}C (10 μM) during 1-min incubations was determined after preincubation for 2 min with 1,2-Diphenyl-3,5-dioxo-4-(2-phenylsulfonyl-athyl)-pyrazolidin (●——●), sulfinpyrazone (□——□) or 1-phenyl-2-(p-hydroxy-phenyl)-3,5-dioxo-4-(2-phenyl-sulfinyl-athyl)-pyrazolidin (○——○). Results represent the mean (± SEM) of three to seven independent experiments.

afforded by large doses of aspirin. This protection may be somewhat less complete with the smaller dose of aspirin. Sulfinpyrazone in a lower dose is approximately equally as effective as a high dose of aspirin.

TXB_2 was not detectable by radioimmunoassay in the plasma of the animals prior to the arachidonate infusion. The infusion resulted in very high levels of circulating TXB_2. This increase was completely blocked by large doses of aspirin and by sulfinpyrazone. The block appeared to be less complete with the lower dose of aspirin but the difference is not statistically significant. TXB_2 was detectable in about half of the animals treated with low-dose aspirin.

We have no proof that thromboxane synthesis is the cause of death in these animals. The effectiveness of the nonsteroidal anti-inflammatory drugs suggests that involvement of one or more prostaglandins or TXB_2 is involved in some way. There does appear to be a relationship between the degree of

Table 2. Arachidonate Infusion in Rabbits

Treatment Group	n	Reduction in Blood Pressure (%)	Reduction in Platelet Counts (%)	Mortality	Increase in Plasma TXB_2 (ng/ml)	Increase in Plasma 6-keto-$PGF_{1\alpha}$ (ng/ml)
Control	10	99.5 ± 0.5	80.6 ± 5.2	9/10	142.0 ± 41.0	3.3 ± 0.7
Aspirin, 250 mg/kg	8	28.1 ± 13.4	20.1 ± 5.5	1/8	21.0 ± 21.0 0 (7 rabbits) 168 (1 rabbit)	1.4 ± 0.3
Aspirin, 25 mg/kg	11	48.1 ± 15.0	43.1 ± 11.4	5/10	2.5 ± 1.4	4.9 ± 1.9
Sulfinpyrazone, 30 mg/kg	10	52.5 ± 8.4	21.6 ± 8.2	0/10	0	1.6 ± 0.3

Rabbits were treated with aspirin or sulfinpyrazone by intraperitoneal injection 45 min prior to infusion of arachidonate, 1.4 mg/kg. The control group received the same sodium carbonate/saline solution used as vehicle for the drugs. Results are mean ± SEM.

thromboxane synthesis, platelet aggregation, and mortality. Figure 6 shows that death of the animals was usually associated with a drop in platelet count of greater than 60% and with thromboxane levels of greater than 10 ng/ml.

Profound hypotension is the rule in these animals unless they are pretreated with nonsteroidal anti-inflammatory drugs or sulfinpyrazone. This may result from formation of a prostaglandin rather than thromboxane. TXB_2 may be only a marker of the series of reactions of arachidonate metabolism.

We also measured the levels of the prostacyclin metabolite, 6-keto-$PGF_{1\alpha}$ in these animals. Unlike thromboxane, 6-keto-$PGF_{1\alpha}$ was detectable by radioimmunoassay in the plasma of a fairly high proportion of animals before the arachidonate infusion. Levels of 6-keto-$PGF_{1\alpha}$ increased after the arachidonic acid infusion in all treatment groups. This increase appeared to be inhibited by both aspirin and sulfinpyrazone.

We have also infused collagen into rabbits to produce intravascular platelet aggregation and thromboxane formation. The degree of platelet aggregation, as measured by a drop in

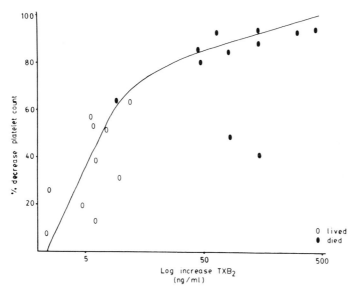

FIG. 6. Arachidonate infusion in rabbits. Relationship between the degree of thromboxane synthesis, platelet aggregation, and mortality.

platelet count, is shown in Table 3. Again, aspirin and sulfinpyrazone appeared to be effective in preventing death. The drugs appeared to be less effective in preventing the drop in platelet count than they were in the arachidonic acid experiments. This result is not unexpected, since it is known from the work of Kinlough-Rathbone et al. [17] that collagen produces platelet aggregation by a mechanism independent of the arachidonate pathway. It is of some interest that the drugs appear to be about as effective in preventing death as they were with the arachidonate infusions. This suggests that the prostaglandin and thromboxane formation during collagen-induced platelet aggregation, rather than the degree of platelet aggregation per se, is of importance in causing death in these animals.

Thromboxane levels produced by collagen infusion were much lower than those observed in the arachidonate experiments. We did not demonstrate a statistically significant reduction of thromboxane synthesis with sulfinpyrazone when mean values were compared. The results presented in this way may be quite misleading. In three of the six sulfinpyrazone-treated animals, no elevation of thromboxane occurred, whereas it occurred in all of the control animals. In one of the three in which an elevation occurred, the level was up to 10 ng/ml. There probably is a significant effect of sulfinpyrazone. The fact that sulfinpyrazone blocked any increase in 6-keto-$PGF_{1\alpha}$ levels indicates that it was exerting an effect on cyclooxygenase activity *in vivo* in this experiment.

In the control animals 6-keto-$PGF_{1\alpha}$ was elevated significantly by the collagen infusion, and aspirin appeared to have an inhibitory effect on that increase. In this particular group of six animals, none had a measurable level of 6-keto-$PGF_{1\alpha}$ prior to collagen infusion.

In conclusion, sulfinpyrazone inhibits thromboxane synthesis by human platelets *in vitro*. When platelet aggregation is induced *in vivo* in rabbits by thromboxane formation from arachidonic acid, sulfinpyrazone protects the animals against aggregation and death and blocks thromboxane synthesis. One may speculate that in man intravascular platelet aggregation occurs in the coronary circulation. This process results in ischemia and perhaps in arrhythmia, because of obstruction by platelet microemboli or thromboxane-induced vasoconstriction,

Table 3. Collagen Infusion in Rabbits

Treatment Group	n	Reduction in Blood Pressure (%)	Reduction in Platelet Counts (%)	Mortality	Increase in Plasma TXB$_2$ (ng/ml)	Increase in Plasma 6-keto-PGF$_{1\alpha}$ (ng/ml)
Control	8	90.3 ± 7.0	86.9 ± 1.2	6/8	2.5 ± 0.5	1.4 ± 0.3
Aspirin, 250 mg/kg	6	37.7 ± 6.6	59.8 ± 8.1	0/6	0	0.4 ± 0.2
Aspirin, 25 mg/kg	6	66.3 ± 17.6	80.0 ± 4.3	3/6	1.3 ± 0.6	0.5 ± 0.2
Sulfinpyrazone, 30 mg/kg	6	44.0 ± 4.6	74.3 ± 3.2	0/6	2.4 ± 1.6	0.1 ± 0.1

Rabbits were pretreated with aspirin or sulfinpyrazone by intraperitoneal injection 45 min prior to infusion of collagen 60 µg/kg. The control group received the same sodium carbonate/saline solution used as vehicle for the drugs. Results are mean ± SEM.

or both. The ability of sulfinpyrazone to protect postmyocardial infarct patients from sudden death could relate to the inhibition of this process.

References

1. Needleman, P., Minkes, M. and Raz, A.: Thromboxanes: Selective biosynthesis and distinct biological properties. Science 193: 163-165, 1976.
2. Lewy, R.I., Smith, J.B., Silver, M.J., Saia, J., Walinsky, P. and Wiener, L.: Detection of thromboxane B_2 in peripheral blood of patients with Prinzmetal's angina. Prostaglandins and Medicine 5: 243-248, 1979.
3. Moncada, S., Higgs, E.A. and Vane, J.R.: Human arterial and venous tissues generate prostacyclin (Prostaglandin X), a potent inhibitor of platelet aggregation. Lancet 1: 18-21, 1977.
4. Gorman, R.R., Bunting, S. and Miller, O.V.: Modulation of human platelet adenylate cyclase by prostacyclin (PGX). Prostaglandins 13: 377-388, 1977.
5. Tateson, J.E., Moncada, S. and Vane, J.R.: Effects of prostacyclin (PGX) on cyclic AMP concentrations in human platelets. Prostaglandins 13: 389-397, 1977.
6. Powell, W.S. and Solomon, S.: Formation of 6-oxoprostaglandin $F_{1\alpha}$ by arteries of the fetal calf. Biochem. Biophys. Res. Commun. 73: 815-822, 1977.
7. Flower, R.J.: Drugs which inhibit prostaglandin biosynthesis. Pharmacol. Rev. 26: 33-66, 1974.
8. Kinlough-Rathbone, R.L., Reimers, H.K., Mustard, J.F. and Packham, M.A.: Sodium arachidonate can induce platelet shape change and aggregation which are independent of the release reaction. Science 192: 1011-1012, 1976.
9. Zucker, M.B. and Peterson, J.: Effect of acetylsalicylic acid, other nonsteroidal anti-inflammatory agents and dipyridamole on human blood platelets. J. Lab. Clin. Med. 76: 66-75, 1970.
10. Packham, M.A., Warrior, E.S., Glynn, M.E., Senyi, A.S. and Mustard, J.F.: Alteration of the response of platelets to surface stimuli by pyrazole compounds. J. Exp. Med. 126: 171-188, 1967.
11. Packham, M.A. and Mustard, J.F.: The effect of pyrazole compounds on thrombin-induced platelet aggregation. Proc. Soc. Exp. Biol. Med. 130: 72-75, 1969.
12. Ali, M. and McDonald, J.W.D.: Effects of sulfinpyrazone on platelet prostaglandin synthesis.and platelet release of serotonin. J. Lab. Clin. Med. 89: 868-875, 1977.
13. McDonald, J.W.D., Stuart, R.K. and Barnett, H.J.M.: Effects of aspirin and sulfinpyrazone on platelet prostaglandin synthesis. In Manning, G.W. and Haust, M.D. (eds.): Atherosclerosis. New York: Plenum Press, 1977, pp. 222-224.
14. Gerrard, J.M. and White, J.G.: The influence of prostaglandin endoperoxides on platelet ultrastructure. Am. J. Pathol. 80: 189-196, 1975.

15. Buchanan, M.R., Rosenfeld, J. and Hirsh, J.: The biphasic effect of sulfinpyrazone on platelet function (Abst.). Thromb. Haemostas. 38: 66, 1977.

16. Silver, M.J., Hoch, W., Kocsis, J.J., Ingerman, C.M. and Smith, J.B.: Arachidonic acid causes sudden death in rabbits. Science 183: 1085-1087, 1974.

17. Kinlough-Rathbone, R.L., Packham, M.A., Reimers, H.-J., Cazenave, J.-P. and Mustard, J.F.: Mechanisms of platelet shape change, aggregation and release induced by collagen, thrombin or A23,187. J. Lab. Clin. Med. 90: 707-719, 1977.

Discussion

Dr. White: You rightly pointed out that in different pathological situations it is uncertain whether platelets are aggregating in response to what might be called a high or low collagen concentration. Even in the high-collagen, or thrombin, situation, sulfinpyrazone and, indeed, aspirin still do inhibit the concomitant production of prostaglandins, even though they themselves would not inhibit the overall aggregation process. We have shown this, as have others. This is sometimes overlooked.

Dr. McDonald: The data on the collagen infusion would support that, too. Intense platelet aggregation may not be the entire cause of the altered physiology in the animals. Thromboxane formation may be at least as important; you can inhibit that and apparently spare the lives of a significant number of rabbits.

Dr. Gordon: We published a short paper recently on the comparative effects of sulfinpyrazone and aspirin on the production of prostacyclin by cultured vascular endothelial cells (Br. J. Pharmacol. 64: 481, 1978). These data were obtained using a bioassay of platelet aggregation, that is, adding endothelial cells to platelet-rich plasma. We then repeated the same kind of experiment, using a radioimmunoassay for 6-keto-PGF$_{1\alpha}$, the stable product of prostacyclin. Sulfinpyrazone prevented the formation of 6-keto-PGF$_{1\alpha}$ in these endothelial cell cultures, but only at concentrations around 50 to 100 μM, whereas aspirin was extraordinarily effective, having an ED$_{50}$ around 1 μM. We decided to repeat the experiment using rings of aorta from the animals from which we had derived the endothelial cells instead of cultured endothelial cells. Sulfinpyrazone showed the same order of activity against the production of prostaglandin in the rings as it did in the cultured endothelial cells, whereas aspirin was much less effective.

Dr. McDonald: Perhaps aspirin doesn't have the same ability to acetylate in the rings as it would have in the thinner endothelial cell preparation, and there is difficulty in getting adequate exposure to the drug.

Dr. Gordon: We've looked at the kinetics, and aspirin's effectiveness was not greatly altered by prolonged incubation. It took 20 min or so to reach its maximal effectiveness in the cultured cells and possibly 30 min in the rings. We had exactly the same thought as you, but the experiments we performed did not substantiate the idea.

Dr. Wallis: When you did those experiments, were the cells in the presence of any plasma proteins or were they in a washed system?

Dr. Gordon: We used conventional culture medium, which contains 10% by volume of fetal calf serum.

Dr. Wallis: Since sulfinpyrazone is about 95% bound to the albumin, your 100 μM figure in the presence of only 10% serum (or plasma) is a little bit misleading from the blood levels that you'd expect to get from sulfinpyrazone. Those blood levels of 100 μM are about 40 μg/ml, which is about double the normal plasma concentration anyway, and since there is less plasma binding, this would seem to indicate that sulfinpyrazone *in vivo* has very little effect on prostacyclin production.

Dr. Gordon: I agree.

Dr. Harker: The other possibility is that much of the effect may be mediated through smooth muscle cell. Have you done control experiments with smooth muscle cells in culture?

Dr. Gordon: Yes, but not in as much detail as with the endothelial cells. The effectiveness of both drugs against smooth muscle cells in culture was comparable to their effects against endothelium in culture.

Dr. Sherry: Is there a direct effect of sulfinpyrazone on thromboxane A_2 synthetase?

Dr. McDonald: I can't exclude that there could be an effect on thromboxane synthetase, but the effect that we have observed would seem clearly to be on the cyclooxygenase. There are two lines of evidence for this. One is that synthesis of prostaglandin D_2 is also inhibited; that occurs below the branch point and shouldn't involve the thromboxane synthetase enzyme. Secondly, sulfinpyrazone competes, apparently, for binding sites with aspirin.

Dr. Sherry: At the present moment, then, it is still unclear whether sulfinpyrazone has a direct effect on the thromboxane A_2 synthetase?

Dr. McDonald: It clearly inhibits the cyclooxygenase, and if it has any effect on the thromboxane synthetase, it must be very small by comparison.

Dr. Sherry: I was intrigued by observations that sulfinpyrazone negates the effect of aspirin on the cyclooxygenase. Has that been demonstrated *in vivo* as well as *in vitro*? This is of particular relevance to the Canadian Neurological Study.

Dr. McDonald: In *ex vivo* studies with platelets from some of the transient ischemic attack (TIA) patients in the control study, it did appear that patients taking a combination of sulfinpyrazone and aspirin had slightly lower levels of inhibition of cyclooxygenase activity than those taking aspirin alone. You can't demonstrate any sulfinpyrazone effect in this system, because these are washed platelets and when you remove the plasma you remove the sulfinpyrazone effect. A study in platelet-rich plasma would provide an answer to that question.

Dr. Sherry: Wouldn't it be important, then, to test it in platelet-rich plasma?

Dr. McDonald: Yes, I think it would. Dr. Mustard has pointed out that an interference by sulfinpyrazone with aspirin effect could be important in the vascular tissue, as well. In other words, sulfinpyrazone might protect the vascular tissue from the "harmful" effect of aspirin on inhibition of PGI_2 synthesis.

Dr. Cargill: We have looked at PGI_2 synthesis in the aortic rings from rabbits that have been dosed with either aspirin or sulfinpyrazone. We don't know what the plasma levels of the drugs were, but aspirin completely inhibited PGI_2 synthesis, whereas sulfinpyrazone had very little effect at 2 h after the last dose. In aspirin-treated animals 24 h after the last dose there was a marked reduction in the inhibition of PGI_2 synthesis.

Dr. Cash: The question was raised by Dr. Sherry about a possible inhibitory effect of sulfinpyrazone directly upon thromboxane synthetase. My colleague, Dr. Ku, at the Ciba-Geigy Corporation in Ardsley, has looked at this in a lysed platelet preparation under conditions where imidazole, substituted imidazoles, and other known inhibitors produce a striking effect upon thromboxane synthetase. Sulfinpyrazone is extremely weak; the inhibitory concentration, 50% (IC_{50}) is considerably higher than the IC_{50} that one measures for it against cyclooxygenase. Therefore we agree with Dr. McDonald that sulfinpyrazone acts primarily at the level of cyclooxygenase.

Dr. Clopath: Did you measure circulating prostacyclin in those rabbits into which you injected arachidonic acid, and if so, what was the result?

Dr. McDonald: No, we measured only the 6-keto-$PGF_{1\alpha}$. The PGI_2 would be included in the 6-keto-$PGF_{1\alpha}$; it is quantitatively converted there. There was an increase with arachidonic acid that was blunted by the inhibitors.

Dr. Mustard: I'm surprised that you were measuring 6-keto-$F_{1\alpha}$ in your animals given aspirin, because if you give animals a high dose of aspirin, take out the aortas, and expose the aortas to arachidonic acid, they cannot produce any inhibitor of platelet function. What do you think is being measured — the specific product or some other contaminants?

Dr. McDonald: There is some cross-reactivity in the radioimmunoassay. I suppose that if there were very high levels of, say, $PGF_{2\alpha}$ (but there are thought not to be) we could pick this up as low levels of 6-keto-$PGF_{1\alpha}$; but PGI_2 is probably a circulating hormone. We studied the plasma about 45 min after the aspirin injection, and there could still have been some 6-keto there from prior synthesis. We haven't done time studies.

Effect of Sulfinpyrazone on Complement-Mediated Pulmonary Dysfunction in Sheep

J. D. Cooper, M.D., S. W. Fountain, M.D., E. Menkes, M.D. and B. A. Martin

In the course of prolonged extracorporeal perfusion through a silicone rubber membrane oxygenator in sheep, the onset of oxygenator perfusion is associated with a transient but marked rise in pulmonary vascular resistance, a transient leukopenia, and a significant loss in circulating platelets.

We have designed studies to elucidate the cause of the increase in pulmonary vascular resistance and its relationship, if any, to the concomitant leukopenia and thrombocytopenia.

Background

We have developed a standard animal model which isolates the effects of the blood-oxygenator interaction from other factors which may cause hematologic changes.

We have previously described this animal model [1]. In summary, Suffolk sheep, weighing 30 kg, are cannulated for veno-venous perfusion, with the jugular vein used for access. Blood is drawn off from the inferior vena cava via a cannula inserted down the right jugular vein. Oxygenated blood is returned to the superior vena cava via a left jugular vein catheter. Carotid artery and Swan-Ganz pulmonary artery cannulae also are inserted for monitoring of blood pressure, determination of arterial blood gases, pulmonary artery and

J. D. Cooper, M.D., S. W. Fountain, M.B., E. Menkes, M.D. and B. A. Martin, Department of Surgery, University of Toronto Faculty of Medicine, Toronto, Canada.

pulmonary wedge pressures, and cardiac output by the thermodilution method (Cardiac Output Model 9510, Edwards Laboratories, Santa Ana, CA). The animals are sedated with ketamine
for the cannulation and then allowed to recover completely
before they are attached to the extracorporeal circuit.

For the initial 2 h, perfusion is conducted with the
oxygenator excluded from the circuit by means of a shunt
around it. This period of control perfusion permits the animal
to adjust to the hemodilution from the priming solution and
permits adjustment of the heparin administration (approximately 0.5 to 1.0 mg/kg per hour) to produce an activated
clotting time of approximately 400 sec, equivalent to a
Lee-White clotting time of just under 2 h. At the end of the
control perfusion the membrane oxygenator is abruptly introduced into the circuit by unclamping the oxygenator and
clamping the shunt around it. Platelet and leukocyte counts are
then measured at frequent intervals, along with constant
monitoring of the arterial pulmonary artery and pulmonary
wedge pressures.

Our standard perfusion model is associated with a platelet
loss of approximately 60% to 70% of circulating platelets within
the first 30 min, followed by a gradual rise. We have attempted
to modify the early platelet loss by various means. We found
that administration of 1500 mg of sulfinpyrazone intravenously
during the control perfusion prior to oxygenator insertion
produced a marked platelet-sparing effect [1].

The results of these experiments are depicted in Figure 1.
Four animals were pretreated with sulfinpyrazone prior to
oxygenator insertion while three animals received no such
pretreatment prior to oxygenator insertion. In both groups of
animals, platelet aggregation in response to ADP markedly
diminished during the first 2 h of oxygenator perfusion.
Thereafter, however, the animals pretreated with sulfinpyrazone
showed consistently superior platelet aggregation than did the
control animals.

The pulmonary artery pressures for the two groups of
animals are displayed in Figure 2. The control animals show a
marked rise in pulmonary artery pressure. This was associated
with a fall of approximately 20% in the cardiac output,
indicating that the rise in pulmonary artery pressure was due

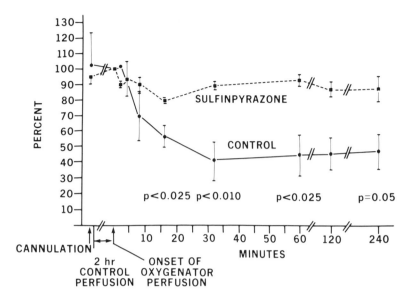

FIG. 1. Platelet count (mean ± SEM), as a percentage of preinfusion value, in three sheep undergoing standard oxygenator perfusion and in four sheep receiving sulfinpyrazone prior to oxygenator insertion. All values are corrected for changes in hematocrit.

exclusively to a rise in pulmonary vascular resistance. In the animals pretreated with sulfinpyrazone, no significant pulmonary vascular response follows oxygenator insertion.

In both groups of animals, the leukocyte count fell to 20% of baseline values within the first 15 min. It returned to normal within 1 h in the sulfinpyrazone-treated group, but only after several hours in the control group.

At the time of these experiments, we did not know the cause of the pulmonary vascular response to oxygenator perfusion. We assumed that since sulfinpyrazone had a platelet-sparing effect, it might also be blocking a platelet release phenomenon responsible for the pulmonary vascular response.

It was subsequently demonstrated by Craddock and his associates [2] that exposure of blood to dialyzer membranes activates the complement system with resulting peripheral leukopenia and pulmonary leukostasis. They also demonstrated [3] that the infusion of complement-activated plasma in sheep produced a rise in pulmonary artery pressure and a fall in

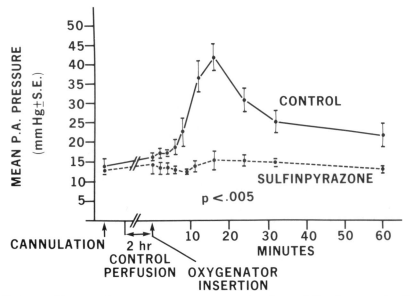

FIG. 2. Mean pulmonary artery pressure in sheep following onset of membrane oxygenator perfusion. The control group (n = 3) received no sulfinpyrazone. Sulfinpyrazone group (n = 4) received 1500 mg of sulfinpyrazone intravenously prior to oxygenator insertion.

arterial oxygen tension (PaO_2), concomitant with a transient leukopenia.

Activation of the complement system has been demonstrated following incubation of sheep blood with the silicone membrane used for fabrication of membrane oxygenators [4]. It therefore seems likely that the pulmonary vascular response and transient leukopenia occurring during oxygenator perfusion in sheep is due to activation of the complement system. It was postulated by Craddock and co-workers [5] that the rise in pulmonary artery pressure following infusion of complement-activated plasma in sheep was due to the observed entrapment of leukocytes in the pulmonary circulation (pulmonary leukostasis). Our observations that sulfinpyrazone eliminated the pulmonary response without altering the initial leukopenic response suggested that leukostasis alone did not explain the pulmonary response following complement-activation. Further studies were designed to investigate the relationship between complement-mediated leukopenia and alterations in pulmonary vascular resistance and pulmonary gas exchange.

Materials and Methods

Based upon initial reports by Craddock et al. [3], initial experiments were conducted in rabbits. New Zealand white rabbits, weighing approximately 3 kg, were temporarily anesthetized for insertion of carotid artery and central venous cannulae. In several it was also possible to insert a #4 French Swan-Ganz catheter into the pulmonary artery through an internal jugular vein. (This technique was described to us by Dr. J. B. Forrest of McMaster University, Hamilton, Ontario.)

Heparinized plasma (1 U/ml) was then prepared and the complement system was activated by incubating plasma with zymosan (I.C.N. Pharmaceuticals, Cleveland, Ohio) at a ratio of 5 mg of zymosan per milliliter of plasma, a combination which produces maximal activation of the complement system. This incubation was carried out for 30 min at $37°C$, following which the plasma was centrifuged to remove the zymosan. The plasma was reinfused into the central venous cannula of the rabbits at a rate of 1 ml/min for 15 min. Arterial blood samples were drawn for measurement of PaO_2, carbon dioxide tension (PCO_2), and pH prior to infusion and thereafter at frequent intervals. Figure 3 demonstrates the leukopenia produced by the plasma infusion in seven rabbits. No significant change in the PaO_2 occurred during or after the infusion of complement-activated plasma (Fig. 4). In the three rabbits having Swan-Ganz cannulae, no change in pulmonary artery pressure occurred with the plasma infusion.

Analysis of the complement-activated plasma [6] showed complete loss of hemolytic complement (CH_{50}) and immunoelectrophoretic analysis of C3 showed increased anodal mobility indicative of C3 activation.

We next repeated the experiment in sheep. Suffolk sheep weighing approximately 30 to 40 kg were cannulated with a carotid artery cannula, a central venous cannula, and a modified Swan-Ganz thermodilution catheter.

When the animals had recovered fully from the sedation used for the cannulation, heparinized plasma (1 U/ml) was collected and 20 ml of complement-activated plasma was prepared as for the rabbit experiments. The activated plasma was then reinfused through the central venous cannula for 4 min at a rate of 5 ml/min. This was done in seven sheep (Group I). In seven additional sheep (Group II), 2 g of sulfinpyrazone

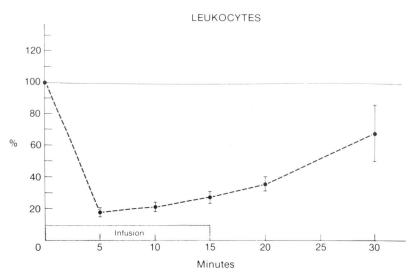

FIG. 3. Leukocyte counts (mean ± SEM) in seven rabbits during and after infusion of complement-activated plasma. Counts are expressed as a percentage of preinfusion value.

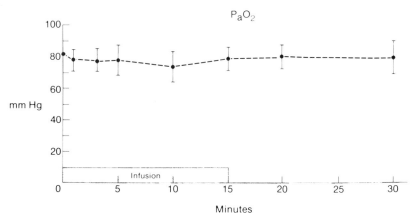

FIG. 4. Arterial oxygen tension (PaO_2) in seven rabbits during and after infusion of complement-activated plasma. No significant change in PaO_2 occurred in this group of animals.

(CIBA-GEIGY, Dorval, PQ) was administered intravenously to the sheep after blood had been drawn for plasma preparation, but at least 30 min prior to reinfusion of the activated plasma.

For the sheep experiments, hemodynamic monitoring and frequent determinations of arterial blood gases and leukocyte count were performed as for the rabbits. In addition, the platelet count was determined at frequent intervals, and in some experiments, platelet aggregation in response to ADP (1 mg/ml) and to a suspension of bovine collagen was determined.

Results

The leukopenia produced by activated plasma infusion was similar for the two groups of sheep (Fig. 5). However, the pulmonary vascular response was markedly different in the two groups of animals. Control animals had a marked rise in pulmonary artery pressure and pulmonary vascular resistance, whereas animals pretreated with sulfinpyrazone showed no such rise in response to infusion of activated plasma (Fig. 6). Cardiac output decreased slightly from the preinfusion value in the

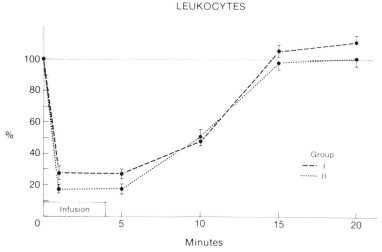

FIG. 5. Leukocyte counts (mean ± SEM), as a percentage of preinfusion value, in sheep during and after infusion of complement-activated plasma. Group I animals (n = 7) received no sulfinpyrazone. Group II (n = 7) received sulfinpyrazone prior to plasma infusion.

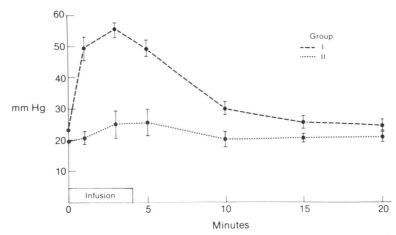

FIG. 6. Mean pulmonary artery pressure (mean ± SEM) in sheep during and after infusion of complement-activated plasma. Group I (n = 7) received no sulfinpyrazone. Group II (n = 7) received pretreatment with sulfinpyrazone. The difference between the two groups is statistically significant for all postinfusion values with the exception of the 20-min point. At 1 min and at 3 min, p< 0.001.

control animals, from 6.6 L/min prior to infusion to 5.3 L/min at the height of the pulmonary response. The pretreated animals showed no significant change in cardiac output.

PaO$_2$ results are shown in Figure 7. Pretreated animals showed no significant change, whereas control animals showed a significant arterial hypoxemia, maximal at 5 min following the onset of plasma infusion. There was no significant change in PaCO$_2$ for either group.

No significant change in platelet count occurred in either group of animals. Similarly, there was no change in platelet aggregation in response to ADP produced by plasma infusion. In sulfinpyrazone-treated animals, platelet aggregation in response to ADP was slightly diminished following sulfinpyrazone administration, but no further change was produced by subsequent plasma infusion. Platelet responsiveness to collagen, however, did diminish markedly following administration of sulfinpyrazone.

Discussion

We assume that the pulmonary vascular and leukopenic responses to membrane oxygenator perfusion in sheep are

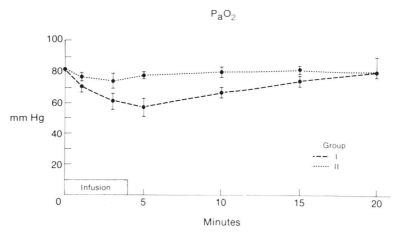

FIG. 7. Arterial oxygen tension (PaO_2) (mean ± SEM) in sheep during and after infusion of complement-activated plasma. Group I (n = 7) received no sulfinpyrazone. Group II (n = 7) received pretreatment with sulfinpyrazone. All animals were spontaneously breathing room air. The differences between Group I and Group II were statistically significant at the 5- and 10-min points (p<0.01).

related to activation of the complement system by exposure of blood to the membrane surface. The thrombocytopenia is presumably related to platelet trauma, common to all forms of extracorporeal perfusion, with resultant platelet adhesion and aggregation. The platelet-sparing effect of sulfinpyrazone in the oxygenator experiments presumably relates to diminished platelet sensitivity. The elimination of pulmonary vascular response in these sheep pretreated with sulfinpyrazone is likely to be related to a different mechanism of action of sulfinpyrazone.

The infusion of complement-activated plasma in animals has previously been demonstrated to produce pulmonary capillary engorgement with polymorphonuclear leukocytes [2]. Similar pathologic observations have been observed in humans following cardiopulmonary bypass [7]. Pulmonary dysfunction and pulmonary leukostasis have been associated in a variety of pathologic conditions [8, 9], but the exact relationship between the leukostasis and the pulmonary dysfunction remains unclear.

In the rabbit experiments no pulmonary dysfunction resulted from the pulmonary leukostasis caused by complement activation, whereas in sheep a marked rise in pulmonary artery pressure and a significant decline in PaO_2 resulted. The reason for this species difference is not known, but the rabbit experiments demonstrate that pulmonary leukostasis alone cannot explain the pulmonary dysfunction produced by infusion of complement-activated plasma. The plasma infusion experiments in sheep confirmed our previous observations, namely that pulmonary vascular response can be blocked with sulfinpyrazone, while the leukopenic response is unaltered. This does not imply, however, that pulmonary leukostasis is not related to pulmonary dysfunction. It has been demonstrated, for example that the C5a fraction of complement is responsible for leukocyte aggregation [10], and that anaphylatoxins produced by C3 and C5 components cause release of histamine from mast cells, contraction of smooth muscle, and increased capillary permeability [11]. Furthermore, complement activation is known to cause release of histamine [12] and lysozomal enzymes [13] from human leukocytes. The finding of Craddock and co-workers that complement-activated plasma produces no pulmonary response in sheep rendered acutely neutropenic with colchicine [3] further supports a role for leukocytes in the pathogenesis of the pulmonary response to complement-activation.

The mechanism of action of sulfinpyrazone in blocking the pulmonary response has not been identified. However, the observation that sulfinpyrazone does block collagen-induced platelet aggregation suggests that inhibition of prostaglandin synthesis is likely occurring. Ali and McDonald [14] have demonstrated that platelet prostaglandin synthesis is strongly inhibited by sulfinpyrazone. Presumably such inhibition may occur in leukocytes and in vessel walls as well.

To further explore the possibility that inhibition of prostaglandin synthesis will block complement-mediated pulmonary dysfunction, we are conducting experiments utilizing the cyclooxygenase inhibitor, indomethacin, prior to challenging sheep with complement-activated plasma. Based on preliminary results, it appears that a daily oral dose of 10 mg/kg will accomplish the same protection as was afforded by sulfinpyrazone pretreatment.

It is apparent that pulmonary leukostasis per se cannot be invoked as the cause of pulmonary dysfunction following infusion of complement-activated plasma. The role of leukocytes in the production of pulmonary dysfunction requires further elucidation.

Acknowledgments

The authors are grateful to Mr. S. R. Gregory and Miss J. Masterson for technical assistance, and to Dr. J. O. Minta of the Department of Experimental Pathology, University of Toronto, for performance of immunologic studies.

References

1. Birek, A., Duffin, J., Gynn, M.F.X. and Cooper, J.D.: The effect of sulfinpyrazone on platelet and pulmonary responses to onset of membrane oxygenator perfusion. Trans. Am. Soc. Artif. Intern. Organs 22: 94-100, 1976.
2. Craddock, P.R., Fehr, J., Dalmasso, A.P., Brigham, K.L. and Jacob, H.S.: Hemodialysis leukopenia; pulmonary vascular leukostasis resulting from complement activation by dialyzer cellophane membranes. J. Clin. Invest. 59: 879-888, 1977.
3. Craddock, P.R., Fehr, J., Brigham, K.L., Kronenberg, R.S. and Jacob, H.S.: Complement and leukocyte-mediated pulmonary dysfunction in haemodialysis. New Engl. J. Med. 296:14, 769-774, 1977.
4. Lindsay, R.M., Friesen, M., Cooper, J.D., Birek, A., Scott, K. and Linton, A.L.: Platelet-foreign surface interactions with oxygenator membranes. *In* Kenedi, R.M., Courtney, J.M., Gaylor, J.D.S. and Gilchrist, T. (eds.): Proceedings of a Seminar on the Clinical Applications of Membrane Oxygenators and Sorbent-Based Systems. University of Strathclyde, Scotland, August, 1976, pp. 248-261.
5. Craddock, P.R., Jacob, H.S. and Brigham, K.L.: Pulmonary dysfunction in hemodialysis, letter. N. Engl. J. Med. 298: 283, 1978.
6. Kabat, E.A. and Mayers, M.M. (eds.): Experimental Immunochemistry. Springfield, IL: Charles C Thomas, 1971, pp. 135-139.
7. Wilson, J.W.: The pulmonary cellular and subcellular alterations of extracorporeal circulation. Surg. Clin. North Am. 54: 1203-1221, 1974.
8. Hechtman, H.B., Lonergan, E.A. and Shepro, D.: Platelet and leukocyte lung interactions in patients with respiratory failure. Surgery 83: 155-163, 1978.
9. Turino, G.M., Rodriquez, J.R. and Greenbaum, L.M.: Mechanisms of pulmonary injury. Am. J. Med. 57: 493, 1974.
10. Craddock, P.R., Hammerschmidt, D., White, J.G., Dalmasso, A.P. and Jacob, H.S.: Complement (C5a)-induced granulocyte aggregation in-vitro: a possible mechanism of complement-mediated leukostasis and leukopenia. J. Clin. Invest. 60: 260-264, 1977.
11. Vallota, E.H. and Muller-Eberhard, H.J.: Formation of C3a and C5a anaphylatoxins in whole human serum after inhibition of the anaphylatoxin inactivator. J. Exp. Med. 137: 1109-1123, 1973.

12. Grant, J.A., Dupree, E., Goldman, A.S., Schultz, D. and Jackson, A.L.: Complement-mediated release of histamine from human leukocytes. J. Immunol. 114: 1101-1106, 1975.
13. Goldstein, I.M., Brai, M., Osler, A.G. and Weissman, G.: Lysozomal enzyme release from human leukocytes: mediation by the alternate pathway of complement-activation. J. Immunol. 1111: 33-37, 1973.
14. Ali, M. and McDonald, J.W.D.: Effects of sulfinpyrazone on platelet prostaglandin synthesis and platelet release of serotonin. J. Lab. Clin. Med. 89: 868-875, 1977.

Discussion

Dr. McDonald: Could you summarize again briefly the comparison of the dose responses of sulfinpyrazone and indomethacin?

Dr. Cooper: Indomethacin, 10 mg/kg per day for 48 h, with the last dose given in the morning, will block the response; a dose of 2.5 mg/kg per day will not. With sulfinpyrazone, the standard model uses a single injection of 1500 mg, which is equivalent to 50 mg/kg for these 30-kg sheep. In the one experiment with sulfinpyrazone PO, a dose of 20 mg/kg per day was used, and it did not block the response. In two experiments where we gave IV titrations, when we reached 1 g, that is, 30 mg/kg, we seemed to be getting the effect.

Dr. McDonald: Indomethacin, then, would seem to be about five to ten times more potent?

Dr. Cooper: I haven't yet determined blood levels for the two drugs; when we get those determined, perhaps we can make better comparisons.

Dr. McDonald: I would just note briefly that in your early experiments with indomethacin, which failed to produce a result, it was the time after the last dose that the experiment was carried out, rather than the dose itself, that was responsible.

Dr. Cooper: I think that is correct. At first I was under a misconception in regard to indomethacin and did not give a dose on the morning of the experiment, but had given it for three days in advance. When we started giving a dose of it on the morning of the experiment, we did get the effect.

Dr. Sherry: Dr. Cooper's interesting observations raise a question that many of us would like an answer to, that is, what is the effect of sulfinpyrazone on prostaglandin synthesis by tissues other than the platelet? Here we see an observation which may be related to the leukocytes, and we are much concerned about what effect sulfinpyrazone may have on cardiac muscle prostaglandin synthesis.

Dr. Cooper: I think I can point to Dr. McDonald as probably giving you a better response than I can.

Dr. McDonald: We haven't done many studies with leukocytes. Certainly with the gastric mucosa, sulfinpyrazone inhibits prostaglandin synthesis, and it is probably considerably weaker than aspirin and indomethacin in that respect. I am sure you will find some inhibition by sulfinpyrazone of prostaglandin synthesis in every tissue. When these drugs have been studied in more than 25 tissues of the rat, they all inhibit in all tissues. The differences in their efficacy are pretty slight, as a rule; only occasionally can you find a drug which has practically no effect in one tissue and is very potent in another.

Dr. Mustard: In Craddock's work in Harry Jacob's laboratory, the thesis is that the activation of complement, C5, is a factor in the adherence of leukocytes to the vessel wall and that superoxide formation by those leukocytes alters the endothelium. Your data would not be compatible with sulfinpyrazone interfering with the C5 activation of the leukocytes adhering to the endothelium, but they might be compatible with some effect on superoxide production and subsequent effects on the endothelium. Has anybody studied the effect of sulfinpyrazone on superoxide production?

Dr. Cooper: I don't know. This whole model could be causing a platelet release phenomenon without causing aggregation or loss of platelets, but the fact that it's reproducible time after time in the same animal without measurable change in platelets makes me think that, in fact, it's not specifically blocking a platelet-mediated effect in these animals. Secondly, when the sheep's blood was put into an isolated circuit and pumped around the small oxygenator, the one effect of sulfinpyrazone was to protect against leukocyte loss on the surfaces, as opposed to the control model. Thus I have very indirect evidence, and this isn't in my particular field of expertise.

Dr. Mustard: I would agree that your data strongly favor the leukocyte as the mediator rather than the platelets. Dr. White, do you want to try to answer the superoxide question?

Dr. White: Some years ago Jim Gerrard in Jim White's laboratory showed that nitrotetrazolium blue was a potent inhibitor of the prostaglandin pathway in platelets, and recently, he has shown that vitamin E plus nitrotetrazolium blue absorbs free radicals very strongly; they have a synergistic effect. We have referred the problem of whether sulfinpyrazone and it's metabolites do absorb free radicals to an authority, namely, Professor Slater in Brunel University, and we're waiting for his results. It is something of which we've been aware and about which we are trying to get answers.

Effect on Platelet Function:
General Discussion

J. Fraser Mustard, M.D., Ph.D., Moderator

Dr. Robson: Dr. McDonald implied that there is not always a good correlation between platelet aggregation and death in his rabbit experiments, and he suggested that thromboxane synthesis may be causative. I wonder if the same could apply to Dr. Cooper's experiments in sheep? Could this pulmonary vasoconstriction really be caused by thromboxane? Again, Dr. McDonald mentioned that Prinzmetal's angina has an elevated thromboxane level. Has anybody tested aspirin or sulfinpyrazone in this angina, since if it's due to thromboxane, it might well be amenable to treatment with these drugs?

Dr. Cooper: Dr. McDonald has kindly offered to do some assays for a thromboxane B_2 response to the infusion of complement-activated plasma in the indomethacin-treated, the sulfinpyrazone-treated, and the untreated animals. It is hoped that these assays will tell us whether there is at least a correlation with the pulmonary vascular response.

Dr. McDonald: I can just add that Dr. Cooper gave us several hundred samples from his experiments, so that we could analyze them in a blinded fashion. We selected two bundles and assayed them, hoping that we might get some interesting information for this meeting. Unfortunately, all the samples came from animals treated with indomethacin, and the thromboxane levels, although measurable in most samples, were very low. If only we had had a few which hadn't been treated with indomethacin, in which thromboxane levels would have been somewhat higher, it would have been interesting. I think the fact that indomethacin and sulfinpyrazone are both effective, and indomethacin is roughly five times as potent as sulfinpyrazone, suggests very strongly that a prostaglandin or thromboxane is involved in that part of the response blocked by these drugs, that is, the pulmonary artery hypertension.

Dr. Mustard: I would like clarification from Dr. Cooper on one point. Does aspirin have an effect in the sheep system?

Dr. Cooper: Only a platelet-sparing effect. The pulmonary vascular response had not been previously described in the sheep. In fact, aspirin has been tried by others in an attempt to preserve platelets but proved of no value. As far as pulmonary responses to complement activation, I have not tried experiments with aspirin nor know of anyone who has.

Dr. McDonald: In regard to the question about use of aspirin in patients with Prinzmetal's angina, in the report by Smith and his colleagues in *Prostaglandins in Medicine* in which elevated thromboxane levels were reported, aspirin treatment did reduce the plasma thromboxane levels. I don't think it's clear whether it had any clinical effect on the patients. Dr. McGregor might be able to tell us whether anyone has tested it in a systematic way.

Dr. McGregor: I haven't heard of it.

Dr. Clopath: In regard to the question raised by Dr. Sherry about the effects of sulfinpyrazone on prostaglandins, I have done various experiments in swine treated with 30 mg/kg of aspirin or sulfinpyrazone. When prostacyclin-generating capacity was measured according to the Moncada bioassay in the pulmonary artery, the thoracic aorta, and the abdominal aorta, and for the vessel walls, both drugs had an identical effect in reducing prostacyclin generation by half from 8 pg/mg of wet weight tissue per minute. I have no results yet for the kidneys.

Dr. Oliver: While coronary artery spasm may be produced by some prostaglandin change (TXA_2, perhaps), the reverse might also be true. Using a model of experimental myocardial ischemia, with occlusions of branches of the coronary arteries, we became interested some time ago in looking at PGE_1 release, identifiable in the coronary sinus. One can induce the release of this particular prostaglandin by waves of regional ischemia.

Dr. Wiedeman: Dr. Cooper, in the oxygenator system, did sulfinpyrazone prevent leukocyte adherence to the glass that you were circulating it through?

Dr. Cooper: The source of the leukocyte loss during perfusion — and this is true for any type of extracorporeal perfusion, be it renal dialysis, cardiopulmonary bypass, or whatever — is associated with an initial total loss of poly-morphonuclear leukocytes. I presume that this perfusion is analogous to the human situation, that is, that there is presumably a temporary loss of polys into capillaries in the lung. We did measure the leukocyte loss across the membrane, between blood going in and out, and that is not the source of the loss. The standard model of perfusion produces a temporary transient leukopenia, with a selective loss of polys, a rise in pulmonary vascular resistance, a fall in PO_2, and a 70% loss of platelets, with gradual recovery to the baseline situation. Animals pretreated with sulfinpyrazone show the same initial loss of leukocytes but a much more rapid rebound, so that at 30 or 60 min, there is a return to baseline levels. In untreated animals, it takes 3 or 4 h for a return to baseline levels. The pulmonary artery response and the PO_2 fall are eliminated as well in those animals pretreated with sulfinpyrazone.

Dr. Sherry: On one hand, in this session we have been told about the action of sulfinpyrazone on prostaglandin pathways, and it's apparent that it has an effect much like aspirin or indomethacin. On the other hand, differences between sulfin-pyrazone and aspirin have been reported in a number of models. Would the panel be willing to speculate as to why they believe that sulfinpyrazone acts differently from other prostaglandin inhibitors?

Dr. White: It is quite clear from the papers in this symposium that there are areas in which these two drugs are very similar, and other areas in which they're different. At this point, we can only give pharmacological evidence of the differences; we cannot relate them to chemical findings.

Dr. Wallis: You all know that aspirin acetylates platelets. With no acetylsalicylic acid present in the surrounding blood to affect them, acetyl platelets, that is, platelets which have the acetyl group on them, would be expected to be different from platelets in sulfinpyrazone-containing plasma because the effect of sulfinpyrazone is competitive. The effect of the acetyl group attached to the platelet wouldn't be expected to be competi-tive; you wouldn't expect to be able to retain a normal response just by increasing agonist concentrations (increasing the size of the stimulus, if you like, to those platelets) whether *in vivo, in vitro*, or *ex vivo*.

Dr. Sherry: I wonder whether we're fascinated with the platelet because that is an easily isolated cell fragment in which to study the effect of sulfinpyrazone. Perhaps we're losing sight of a more major area, i.e., the interaction of cells with the vessel wall. We may not be dealing just with platelets, but with granulocytes as well. Something is eluding us (perhaps Harker is pointing to it in his studies) which needs further elaboration for a true understanding of the mechanism of action of sulfin-pyrazone.

Dr. Butler: I would like to make two points. First, with arachidonic acid experiments *in vivo*, Vargaftig showed that this is not a platelet-dependent reaction in that death of the animals follows arachidonic acid infusion even if the animals are made thrombocytopenic. However, in that situation, sulfin-pyrazone still protects against the death of the animal, and consequently it isn't a platelet-mediated event, as such. The second point is that Henson showed a long time ago that leukocytes will augment either the platelet aggregation or release reaction, and this must always be considered in models where there is leukocyte involvement. Even if the leukocyte response is not fully inhibited the leukocyte-platelet interaction may still be affected.

Dr. McDonald: In separating effects which may be due to inhibition of prostaglandin or thromboxane synthesis from those which are not, clearly those effects which seem to be inhibited by all the nonsteroidal, anti-inflammatory drugs are probably due to inhibition of prostaglandin synthesis. Those effects in which, indomethacin, let us say, (it being about the most potent inhibitor) has no effect, are pretty clearly not due to inhibition of prostaglandin synthesis. Some effects which have been thought to fall into the latter category on closer scrutiny are found to be due to inhibition of thromboxane or prostaglandin synthesis. Consequently, we should perhaps work from the known to the unknown. Although sulfinpyrazone can be shown to have some effects that appear to be unrelated to prostaglandin or thromboxane inhibition, they are not neces-sarily involved in the clinical effect that is observed, that is to say, prevention of sudden death. If clinical trials of aspirin or indomethacin showed effects similar to the Anturane trial, that might be strong evidence that sulfinpyrazone worked by the mechanism of prostaglandin inhibition; if they didn't show similar effects, it would perhaps be evidence that sulfinpyrazone was working by another mechanism.

Dr. Domenet: In the same model sulfinpyrazone inhibits thromboxane formation and prostacyclin to a lesser extent, and this all occurs at the cyclooxygenase level; is that possible?

Dr. McDonald: Different tissue sources were used in the tests of the two effects and the tissues differed in sensitivity to the effect of the drug. While measurements are made only in the plasma, the source of material in the plasma can be platelets, leukocytes, vascular tissues, and so on.

Dr. Mustard: In regard to Dr. Cooper's ADP experiments, the simplest explanation for the results with the sheep blood is that when you take blood into citrate, you get the same effect as you do with human blood when you depress ionized calcium. When you do that and stimulate the platelets with large quantities of ADP, phospholipase A_2 is activated and the platelets will undergo a release reaction. The simple way to determine if this is happening is to label the platelets with some ^{14}C-serotonin and see if it is released during ADP-induced aggregation. Of course, when phospholipase A_2 is activated, the arachidonic pathway comes into operation, and aspirin and sulfinpyrazone will inhibit the conversion of arachidonate to thromboxane A_2 and prevent the release reaction. Rabbit platelets taken into citrate do not show this phenomenon, that is, activation of the arachidonate pathway during ADP-induced aggregation. Dr. Cooper showed a striking difference in the platelet response in the sheep versus the rabbit, and there may be an interesting species difference in the ease of phospholipase A_2 activation.

Dr. Cooper: I assume that there was some sort of species difference since we could show maximum activation of the complement system in the rabbit without producing the pulmonary response. But in our sheep model, where we infuse the activated plasma, does the mere fact that there is no change in platelet numbers or, in fact, platelet responsiveness to a crude ADP stimulation test give any assurance that the pulmonary response is not platelet-mediated? What type of information would you want to have, to be certain of this?

Dr. Mustard: I would do as you have done and concentrate on the leukocytes. The evidence that you've presented is fairly convincing that that is the direction to pursue.

Dr. Oliver: In regard to species differences, there are fundamental differences concerning the availability of arachidonic acid. For example, the cat species cannot transfer γ-linoleic acid or γ-linolenic acid into arachidonic acid. It has to absorb its arachidonic acid through meat that it eats. There may well be other quite important controlling mechanisms concerning the availability and the transfer of certain of the essential fatty acids. If transfer of dihomo-γ-linolenic acid to the eicosapentanoic pathway is favored, it will be to the detriment of the arachidonic acid pathway. We should not assume that all tissues or all species have the same concentration of available arachidonic acid. Nor should we assume that different tissues within the same species can release arachidonic acid at the same speed, even if the same concentration of phospholipase A_2 is present.

Dr. Mustard: Concerning Dr. McDonald's comments about PGI_2, if you inhibit PGI_2 production by the vessel wall by exposing it to aspirin *in vivo*, platelets do not accumulate on it. It is possible to show that PGI_2 production has been prevented if the vessel is removed and exposed to sodium arachidonate and the reaction mixture assayed for PGI_2-like activity. In other words, the thesis that PGI_2 production prevents platelets from adhering to the endothelium is not viable under these test conditions, nor is it viable when you test it *in vitro*. However, Jack Hirsh and his colleagues have been carrying out a very interesting study in which they cause experimental thrombosis by damaging the vessel wall under conditions in which extensive thrombin formation would be expected to occur. Under those circumstances the administration of high doses of aspirin leads to very marked platelet accumulation. In circumstances where little thrombin forms and stasis does not occur, high doses of aspirin do not have that effect. The explanation may be that the thrombin formation is a very potent stimulus to increased PGI_2 production, which tends to diminish the extent of thrombus formation; when PGI_2 production is blocked by high doses of aspirin, thrombosis is augmented. This suggests that the PGI_2 — vessel wall situation is much more complicated than the simple story which has been presented to us so far.

Effect on Platelet Function: Chairman's Summary

J. Fraser Mustard, M.D., Ph.D.

The principal points set out in the presentations in this section include evidence that sulfinpyrazone has effects in addition to those of aspirin and that sulfinpyrazone forms metabolites *in vivo*. One of these metabolites appears able to inhibit the platelet cyclooxygenase and may account for the longer duration of the sulfinpyrazone effect on platelet cyclooxygenase in some species. Evidence for the existence of this metabolite was first demonstrated by Buchanan and his co-workers [1]. The evidence presented by Wallis and his colleagues indicates that a thioether metabolite of sulfinpyrazone (G 25671) is one of the active metabolites. It appears to inhibit the platelet cyclooxygenase (and presumably other cyclooxygenases) and thereby inhibits the platelet aggregation and release response that is dependent upon the formation of thromboxane A_2 from arachidonic acid. The amount of the metabolite formed varies from species to species. Much less appears to be formed in man than in the experimental animals used.

There are some indications that sulfinpyrazone has effects *in vivo* in addition to its effect on cyclooxygenase. For example, sulfinpyrazone prolongs shortened platelet survival [2, 3], whereas aspirin has not been shown to have this effect [4]. To date there has been no explanation for this difference in the effect of these two drugs. The experimental studies reported by White further emphasize the difference between the effects of aspirin and sulfinpyrazone. In the Forssman reaction, sulfin-

---

J. Fraser Mustard, M.D., Ph.D., Dean, Faculty of Health Sciences, McMaster University, Hamilton, Ont., Canada.

pyrazone prevents the development of thrombocytopenia, whereas aspirin has no effect. In the Arthus reaction, however, both aspirin and sulfinpyrazone protect against the development of thrombocytopenia. The thioether metabolite of sulfinpyrazone does not protect the guinea pigs against the thrombocytopenia induced by the Forssman reaction. In contrast, in the Arthus reaction sulfinpyrazone, the thioether metabolite, aspirin, and indomethacin all inhibit the fall in platelet count. Since sulfinpyrazone, but not the thioether metabolite, inhibits the thrombocytopenia induced by the Forssman reaction, it may be that the action of sulfinpyrazone is not due directly to its ability to inhibit the platelet cyclooxygenase. The Forssman reaction is likely a complement-mediated reaction since it does not occur in animals that have been depleted of complement. Possibly some aspect of the response involving complement is inhibited by sulfinpyrazone.

In Cooper's experimental work with sheep, the leukopenia produced by infusion of activated complement, possibly C5a, is not inhibited by the prior administration of sulfinpyrazone. However, sulfinpyrazone treatment prevents the rise in pulmonary arterial pressure that is caused by activation of C5a. Administration of activated complement to rabbits did not cause the rise in pulmonary arterial pressure, although it did cause a fall in leukocyte count. The results of these experiments of Cooper, when taken together with those of Craddock and associates [5, 6], indicate that sulfinpyrazone may be inhibiting a mechanism that is involved in causing increased pulmonary resistance as a result of C5a activation. In addition, in sheep on cardiopulmonary bypass, sulfinpyrazone prevents the rise in pulmonary artery pressure and the development of thrombocytopenia. This latter effect may be related to the action of sulfinpyrazone on platelet accumulation on artificial surfaces. All this evidence is in keeping with there being another action of sulfinpyrazone in addition to its inhibitory effect on cyclooxygenase. It has been reported that this drug diminishes the extent of endothelial cell injury [7].

McDonald and his collaborators have shown that sulfinpyrazone is a competitive inhibitor of the platelet cyclooxygenase. Sulfinpyrazone will therefore antagonize the inhibition of cyclooxygenase produced by aspirin. Presumably sulfinpyrazone occupies a site on the cyclooxygenase that can be acetylated by aspirin. One of the points discussed in relation to McDonald's paper was the ability of aspirin and sulfinpyrazone to block PGI_2 production by the vessel wall. It appears that sulfinpyrazone may not have as strong an inhibitory effect as aspirin. This could be important since in some experimental situations inhibition of PGI_2 formation by the vessel wall has been shown to cause enhanced thrombosis [8].

References

1. Buchanan, M.R., Rosenfeld, J. and Hirsh, J.: The prolonged effect of sulfinpyrazone on collagen-induced platelet aggregation *in vivo*. Thromb. Res. 13: 883-892, 1978.
2. Smythe, H.A., Ogryzlo, M.A., Murphy, E.A. and Mustard, J.F.: The effect of sulfinpyrazone (Anturan) on platelet economy and blood coagulation in man. Can. Med. Assoc. J. 92: 818-821, 1965.
3. Steele, P., Battock, D. and Genton, E.: Effects of clofibrate and sulfinpyrazone on platelet survival times in coronary artery disease. Circulation 52: 473-476, 1975.
4. Harker, L.A. and Slichter, S.J.: Platelet and fibrinogen consumption in man. New Engl. J. Med. 287: 999-1005, 1972.
5. Craddock, P.R., Fehr, J., Dalmasso, A.P., Brigham, K.L. and Jacob, H.S.: Hemodialysis leukopenia. Pulmonary vascular leukostasis resulting from complement activation by dialyzer cellophane membranes. J. Clin. Invest. 59: 879-888, 1977.
6. Craddock, P.R., Hammerschmidt, D., White, J.G., Dalmasso, A.P. and Jacob, H.S.: Complement (C5a)-induced granulocyte aggregation *in vitro*. A possible mechanism of complement-mediated leukostasis and leukopenia. J. Clin. Invest. 60: 260-264, 1977.
7. Harker, L.A., Wall, R.T., Harlan, J.M. and Ross, R.: Sulfinpyrazone prevention of homocysteine-induced endothelial cell injury and arteriosclerosis. Clin. Res. 26: 554A, 1978.
8. Kelton, J.G., Hirsh, J., Carter, C.J. and Buchanan, M.R.: Thrombogenic effect of high-dose aspirin in rabbits. Relationship to inhibition of vessel wall synthesis of prostaglandin I_2-like activity. J. Clin. Invest. 62: 892-895, 1978.

Platelet-Vessel Wall Interaction

Sulfinpyrazone in Primate Models of Vascular Disease

Laurence A. Harker, M.D.

Endothelial Injury

Endothelial cells form a continuous luminal monolayer that comprises a thrombo-resistant barrier between blood and the vascular tree. Some form of altered or "injured" endothelium is central to most contemporary hypotheses that attempt to explain atherogenesis [1, 2]. Cellular and molecular studies have permitted characterization of: (a) endothelium in maintaining the nonthrombogenic character of the artery and in acting as a barrier to the passage of constitutents of the plasma into the artery wall; (b) platelets in mediating intimal proliferation and vascular thrombotic occlusive complications; and (c) the role of the smooth muscle cells as the principal proliferative component of the lesions of atherosclerosis [1, 2]. Since most of the lipid that accumulates in the lesions of atherosclerosis is derived from the plasma, the critical role of the endothelium as a protective barrier between the artery wall and the circulation is evident.

Endothelial "injury" can be defined in a number of different ways as a result of examining different stimuli used to induce "injury." Alterations in the endothelium may be subtle and manifest themselves simply as functional changes, such as disturbances in the permeability characteristics of the cells. At the other extreme, endothelial injury may lead to endothelial disruption or detachment of the endothelial cells into the blood

Laurence A. Harker, M.D., Department of Medicine (Hematology) and the Regional Primate Center, University of Washington School of Medicine, Seattle, Wash.

Supported by research grants (HL-11775, HL-18645, and RR-00166) from the U.S. Public Health Service.

stream. Three types of injury are operationally defined at present: (a) endothelial desquamation with residual denudation; (b) compensated endothelial desquamation (increased endothelial cell turnover as determined by autoradiography but without measurable denudation); and (c) nondesquamative injury, manifest as altered endothelial function. Each of these manifestations of endothelial injury can be observed in vivo; in each instance "injury" to the endothelium precedes the intimal smooth muscle proliferative response.

Experimentally, endothelial desquamation has been induced mechanically by surgery [3], a chronic indwelling catheter [4], or an intraarterial balloon catheter [5], chemically by chronic homocystinemia [6, 7], immunologically by humoral or cell-mediated mechanisms [8], or nutritionally by diet-induced chronic hyperlipidemia [9]. A number of other factors are also considered to be injurious to the endothelium: bacteria and products such as endotoxin [10, 11], viruses [12], products associated with smoking such as hypoxia, carbon monoxide and tobacco proteins [13-15], antigen-antibody complexes [16, 17], and hemodynamic forces [18]. Altered flow patterns may concentrate substances and formed blood elements that are injurious to the endothelium at certain sites [19, 20]. A number of factors can influence the endothelium, such as bradykinin, angiotensin, cationic protein from leukocytes, platelets, and thrombin [21-23].

Recently it has been shown that endothelial cells synthesize PGI_2, which causes relaxation of arterial smooth muscle and inhibits platelet adhesion and aggregation [24, 25]. Exposure of the endothelium to arachidonic acid, trypsin, thrombin, and possibly other factors increases the rate of PGI_2 synthesis by cultured endothelial cells [26]. Production of thrombin at a site of vascular injury could, by increasing the production of PGI_2 by endothelial cells adjacent to the injury, localize thrombus formation. Moreover, enhanced PGI_2 synthesis might serve as an indicator of sublethal endothelial injury. There are a number of components of the blood that may modify the response of the vessel to endothelial injury: hormones, such as insulin; vasoactive peptides; substances released by formed elements, such as platelets and leukocytes; products derived from blood coagulation; and plasma lipoproteins [27].

Endothelial denudation permits interaction between platelets from the circulation and the connective tissue of the subendothelium, resulting in platelet adherence, aggregation, and release of platelet products at local sites of exposed subendothelium. At the same time, plasma constituents, such as lipoproteins, have access to the underlying artery wall, since the permeability barrier has been altered.

In some cases of endothelial denudation, survival of isotopically labeled, autologous platelets is measurably shortened. The interaction of material released from the platelets with plasma components leads to migration of medial smooth muscle cells into the intima and proliferation of smooth muscle cells within the intima, allows formation of new connective tissue by these cells, and in the case of injury resulting from chronic hyperlipoproteinemia, leads to deposition of lipids within the cells and in the extracellular material. If the injury is a single event, the lesions may be reversible and regress. On the other hand, if the injury is chronic and continues for long periods, the lesions may become progressive and eventually lead to clinical sequelae. Thrombocytopenia [28] and defective platelet function, due to hereditary defects, such as von Willebrand's disease [29], or to the use of pharmacologic inhibitors of platelet function, such as dipyridamole [7] or sulfinpyrazone [30], have been shown to inhibit the intimal smooth muscle proliferative response. These observations suggest that intact platelet function is necessary for development of the intimal smooth muscle proliferative lesions of experimentally induced atherosclerosis.

In steady-state chronic endothelial cell desquamation the amount of denudation is the summation of: (a) the rate of desquamation, (b) endothelial cell migration, and (c) endothelial cell regeneration. Since these three processes are not easily separable *in vivo*, endothelial cell cultures have been useful in characterizing each process independently. Several laboratories have demonstrated that endothelial cells grown in culture form confluent monolayers and retain phenotypically differentiated properties, including the presence of Weibel-Palade bodies and factor VIII antigen, and the synthesis of basement membrane collagen [31, 32]. Investigators have utilized cells derived from the human umbilical vein, as well as bovine and porcine aortae [33].

The relative roles of blood cell products and plasma factors on endothelial cell proliferation have been evaluated by studying the proliferative response of human umbilical vein endothelial cells to cell-free plasma-derived serum, whole blood serum, platelet releasate, fibroblast growth factor, and macrophage-conditioned medium *in vitro* [34]. These studies show that endothelial cell proliferation is directly related to the concentrations of whole blood serum or cell-free plasma-derived serum. Growth rate in whole blood serum is marginally greater than that observed in cell-free plasma-derived serum, but the addition of platelet releasate does not further stimulate endothelial cell proliferation in cell-free plasma-derived serum. In contrast, smooth muscle cells are quiescent in cell-free plasma-derived serum, even with increasing concentrations, but proliferate actively in the presence of platelet releasate. Both human macrophage-conditioned medium and fibroblast growth factor increase endothelial cell and smooth muscle cell proliferation significantly when added to cell-free plasma-derived serum. Hence it is apparent that human endothelial cell proliferation in preconfluent cultures is dependent upon plasma factors, while human vascular smooth muscle cells require a platelet constituent to proliferate. In addition, a mitogenic substance in macrophages may have an important role in endothelial cell proliferation *in vivo*.

In vitro studies of cell migration with agarose plate technique [35] have also been carried out with cultured endothelial cells [36]. The results indicate that migration of endothelial cells at the margin of de-endothelialized areas represents an important initial process of covering exposed subendothelial structures. Migration from adjacent intact endothelial cells appears to be of particular importance in maintaining endothelialization in association with widespread patchy injury, such as that observed with the chemical injury of homocystinemia. Endothelial cell migration is enhanced by platelet factor(s) but inhibited by type IIa familial hypercholesterolemic sera.

The role of direct cytoxicity to endothelial cells has also been studied recently *in vitro* in cultured human vessel-wall cells [37]. In these studies endothelial cell injury was measured in confluent human umbilical vein endothelial cells labeled with radiochromium and incubated with test material. Heterologous antihuman endothelial cell antibody produces endothelial cell injury, as seen by trypan blue exclusion and phase microscopy. A clear dose response relationship between ^{51}Cr-specific release and antibody titer is observed. In the radiochromium-specific release test, homocysteine or 2-mercaptoethanol induces dose response release with concentrations as low as 0.1 mM (the level observed in homocystinuric patients evidencing moderately severe vascular disease).

When platelets are stimulated to undergo the release reaction, they release a platelet-derived growth factor (PDGF) that is mitogenic for smooth muscle cells, fibroblasts, glial cells, and 3T3 cells, but not endothelial cells [2, 34]. The growth factor does not appear to be present in plasma in any significant amounts, unless the platelets have undergone the release reaction. Thus, the localized release of this material when platelets adhere to subendothelial connective tissue may be an important factor in localized smooth muscle cell migration and proliferation in response to endothelial injury [2-9]. The platelet is not the only source of mitogens that may mediate smooth muscle cell proliferation; it is known that other mitogens are found in plasma, such as epithelial growth factor (and perhaps fibroblast growth factor), as well as in macrophages. Thrombin, however, apparently does not stimulate smooth muscle cell proliferation [39, 40]. Even more relevant is the recent observation by several different investigators that endothelial cell conditioned medium is mitogenic for smooth muscle cells or 3T3 cells [41, 42]. These initial observations suggest that the endothelium may directly stimulate the underlying smooth muscle cells to proliferate in the absence of endothelial denudation (Fig. 1). This might explain the observation that the area of maximal lesion formation in the balloon injury model is in the intima below the edge of the regenerating endothelial sheet [43].

Recent studies have shown that in primates the response of circulating platelets to nonendothelialized surfaces can be detected *in vivo* by at least four different approaches: (a) localized accumulation at the site of vascular injury determined by ^{111}In-platelet imaging [44, 45]; (b) platelet consumption measured by means of isotopically labeled platelets [6, 7, 46,

L. A. HARKER

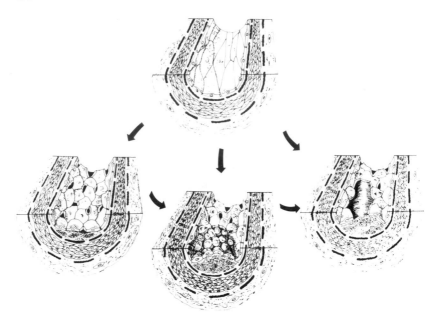

FIG. 1. Response to injury hypothesis. The normal blood vessel (upper panel) comprises the endothelial lining (luminal to the internal elastic lamina), the media of smooth muscle cells (SMC), and the outer adventitia of fibroblasts and connective tissue matrix. Endothelial injury may consist of (a) nonlethal functional alterations, possibly including the stimulated synthesis of endothelial derived mitogen (left lower panel); (b) compensated desquamation without measurable denudation (central lower panel); and (c) desquamation with denudation (right lower panel). Platelet adhesion and release of platelet-derived growth factor at sites of endothelial denudation is postulated to mediate the migration of SMC from media to the intima and to stimulate the proliferation of intimal SMC. With repeated chronic injury, intimal lesion formation is progressive and involves lipid accumulation, ultimately resulting in atherosclerotic disease.

47]; (c) release of constituents from platelet-dense bodies determined by simultaneous ^{14}C-serotonin and ^{51}Cr-platelet disappearance studies [48]; and (d) the detection in plasma of platelet-specific proteins from platelet alpha granules, i.e., PF4, BTG, or PDGF [49-51]. Constituents from dense bodies and alpha granules are of interest because the release of granular constituents may occur without platelet destruction [52], and they would therefore be expected to be more sensitive yet relevant indicators of platelet activation *in vivo*.

Three drugs, dipyridamole, sulfinpyrazone, and aspirin, have been shown to have clinical usefulness that has been attributed to their modifying effects on platelet behavior. While aspirin acts pharmacologically as a potent noncompetitive inhibitor of platelet cyclooxygenase through permanent acetylation [53], its lack of effect on collagen-induced platelet thrombus formation is apparently due to its inability to modify platelet adhesion and prevent degranulation of adherent platelets [54]. Dipyridamole increases platelet cyclic AMP (cAMP) levels by inhibiting platelet phosphodiesterase and thus appears to have increased efficacy *in vivo* through synergy with PGI_2, which increases platelet cAMP by stimulating platelet adenylcyclase [70]. Since high doses of aspirin inhibit PGI_2 production [55, 56], the combination of aspirin and dipyridamole requires an optimal dose combination [55, 57]. *In vitro* evidence indicates that sulfinpyrazone is a modestly potent inhibitor of platelet adhesion and platelet release through its action as a competitive inhibitor of platelet prostaglandin synthesis [58, 59]. Sulfinpyrazone's protective action on endothelium is an important additional effect in models that involve injury to the endothelium, such as homocystinemia [60].

Homocystinemic Baboon Model

The arteriosclerotic mechanism of homocystinemia has been studied by measuring endothelial cell loss and regeneration, platelet consumption, and intimal lesion formation in a primate model [6, 7]. Four groups of baboons have been studied: (a) 8 control animals; (b) 15 animals after 3 months of continuous homocystinemia; (c) 11 animals after 3 months of combined homocystinemia and oral treatment with dipyridamole; and (d) 7 animals after 3 months of combined homocystinemia and oral treatment with sulfinpyrazone.

Experimental homocystinemia caused patchy endothelial desquamation comprising about 10% of the aortic surface despite a 25-fold increase in endothelial cell regeneration. Neither endothelial cell loss nor regeneration was changed significantly by dipyridamole (60 μmol/kg body weight per day). Homocystine-induced vascular de-endothelialization produced a threefold increase in platelet consumption that was interrupted by dipyridamole inhibition of platelet function.

All homocystinemic animals developed typical arterio-sclerotic or preatherosclerotic intimal lesions composed of proliferating smooth muscle cells, averaging 10 to 15 cell layers and surrounded by large amounts of collagen, elastic fibers, glycosaminoglycons, and sometimes lipid. Intimal lesion formation was prevented by dipyridamole therapy. In summary, homocystine-induced endothelial cell injury results in arterio-sclerosis through platelet-mediated intimal proliferation of smooth muscle cells that can be prevented by drug-induced dysfunction.

The capacity of pharmacological agents to protect endo-thelium from injury has been studied *in vitro* with a cyto-toxicity assay of cultured ^{51}Cr-labeled endothelial cells and *in vivo* with a primate model of arteriosclerosis. *In vitro* specific release of ^{51}Cr from prelabeled confluent human umbilical vein endothelial cells was induced by rabbit antibody prepared against human endothelial cells or homocysteine in a dose-dependent manner. Sulfinpyrazone reduced specific ^{51}Cr-release induced by either immune or sulfhydryl-mediated endo-thelial injury in a concentration-related fashion between 10^{-4} and 10^{-6} M. Dipyridamole and aspirin did not measurably modify specific ^{51}Cr-release induced immunologically or chem-ically.

Oral sulfinpyrazone (250 μmol/kg body weight per day in three divided doses) in seven homocystinemic animals (0.14 mM ± 0.04) decreased markedly the extent of aortic endothelial desquamation, normalized platelet survival measurements, and prevented intimal lesion formation when compared with the effects in 15 untreated homocystinemic animals. Oral dipyrid-amole had no measurable protective effect on endothelial integrity in this model. We conclude from these studies that endothelial cell protection by sulfinpyrazone from injury *in vitro* predicts *in vivo* prevention of endothelial cell desquama-tion and its consequences and that pharmacologic protection of the endothelium may be therapeutically important in the prevention of arteriosclerotic vascular disease.

Diet-Induced Hyperlipidemic Monkey Model

Despite the established importance of lipids in athero-genesis, the mechanism whereby hyperlipidemia induces atherosclerosis remains unclear [1, 2, 61, 62]. While alterations in endothelial cell permeability and endocytosis per se have been implicated [62-64], the possibility that some type of underlying endothelial cell "injury" is involved has become increasingly attractive [65-70].

Numerous studies of the role of endothelial injury in atherogenesis have been carried out. In our own laboratory [9] we used pigtail monkeys (*Macaca nemestrina*), made hyperlipidemic by maintenance on a cholesterol-rich diet. The hyperlipidemic monkeys were subjected to a single balloon-catheter de-endothelialization of one iliac artery and of the abdominal aorta. This procedure resulted in the removal of virtually all the endothelium in the ballooned segment. The animals remained hyperlipidemic until they were sacrificed at 1 month, 3 months, 6 months, 9 months, and 1 year after the operation. The contralateral iliac artery served as a noninjured control for the vascular effects of chronic hyperlipidemia.

At 6 weeks to 3 months after balloon injury to the iliac artery and abdominal aorta, the chronically hyperlipidemic animals displayed a markedly thickened intima containing numerous smooth muscle cells with lipid inclusions. Between 3 months and 1 year, the catheter-induced lesions of the chronically hyperlipidemic animals showed a persistence of the lipid-laden cells with no evidence of the regression observed in normolipidemic animals. Indeed, after 6 to 18 months, the lesions in the injured vessels were somewhat larger than those seen 3 months after injury in the chronic hyperlipidemic animals.

In the animals on the lipid-rich diet, there were very few alterations in the nonballooned vessels after 1.5 months. An occasional lipid-laden cell was present in the still thin intima of the noninjured artery. Four months after initiation of the diet (i.e., 3 months after the contralateral artery was ballooned), the intima of the noninjured iliac was slightly increased in thickness and contained one to two layers of lipid-laden smooth muscle cells. Within 10 months after initiation of diet, there were no significant differences between the injured and noninjured iliac arteries. Both contained 10 to 15 layers of lipid-laden smooth muscle cells surrounded by extracellular lipid and large quantities of newly formed connective tissue matrix.

Chronically hyperlipidemic animals without mechanical injury were assessed for endothelial integrity by examination of the entire aorta and iliac arteries after pressure perfusion *in vivo* with glutaraldehyde. While there were occasional areas of focal endothelial loss, greater than 99% of the endothelium was intact, albeit abnormal. The endothelial cells were altered in shape, appeared to have lost their characteristic longitudinal orientation, demonstrated areas of increased cell density and showed the appearance of punctuate accumulation of silver at the site of junctional complexes. Many endothelial cells were polyhedral or round, suggesting abnormal endothelial regeneration.

Although a number of studies by scanning electron microscopy have reported that endothelial denudation is found in association with hyperlipidemia [9, 64-70], more recent studies using carefully controlled conditions of fixation have not shown significant endothelial denudation until after intimal lesions had already developed [71]. Endothelial cell turnover, however, is reported to be increased within 3 days of the onset of hyperlipidemia in swine fed an atherogenic diet [72], suggesting that compensated desquamation develops early in hyperlipidemia.

Hyperlipidemic monkeys treated with sulfinpyrazone (250 mg/kg per day) showed markedly reduced lesion formation compared with hyperlipidemic untreated controls.

References

1. Arteriosclerosis: A report by the National Heart and Lung Institute Task Force on Arteriosclerosis. [DHEW Publication No. (NIH) 72-219] Vol. 2. Washington, D.C.: Government Printing Office, 1971.
2. Ross, R. and Glomset, J.: The pathogenesis of atherosclerosis. N. Engl. J. Med. 295: 369-377, 420-425, 1976.
3. Bjorkerud, S. and Bondjers, G.: Arterial repair and atherosclerosis after mechanical injury. I. Permeability and light microscopic characteristics of endothelium in non-atherosclerotic and atherosclerotic lesions. Atherosclerosis 13: 355-363, 1971.
4. Moore, S.: Thromboatherosclerosis in normolipemic rabbits: A result of continued endothelial damage. Lab. Invest. 29: 478-487, 1973.
5. Stemerman, M.B. and Ross, R.: Experimental arteriosclerosis. I. Fibrous plaque formation in primates, an electron microscope study. J. Exp. Med. 136: 769-789, 1972.

6. Harker, L., Slichter, S., Scott, C.R. and Ross, R.: Homocystinemia: Vascular injury and arterial thrombosis. N. Engl. J. Med. 291: 537-543, 1974.

7. Harker, L., Ross, R., Slichter, S. and Scott, C.: Homocystine-induced arteriosclerosis: The role of endothelial cell injury and platelet response in its genesis. J. Clin. Invest. 58: 731-741, 1976.

8. Minick, C.R. and Murphy, G.E.: Experimental induction of athero-arteriosclerosis by the synergy of allergic injury to arteries and lipid rich diet. II. Effect of repeatedly injected foreign protein in rabbits fed a lipid-rich, cholesterol-poor diet. Am. J. Pathol. 73: 265-300, 1973.

9. Ross, R. and Harker, L.: Hyperlipidemia and atherosclerosis. Science 193: 1094-1100, 1976.

10. Gaynor, E., Bouvier, C. and Spaet, T.H.: Vascular lesions: Possible pathogenetic basis of the generalized reaction. Science 170: 986, 1970.

11. Gerrity, R.G., Richardson, M., Caplan, B.A., Cade, J.F., Hirsh, J. and Schwartz, C.J.: Endotoxin-induced vascular injury and repair. Exp. Mol. Pathol. 24: 59-69, 1976.

12. Turpie, A.G.G., Chernesky, M.A., Larke, R.P.B., Moore, S., Regoeczi, E. and Mustard, J.F.: Thrombocytopenia and vasculitis induced in rabbits by Newcastle disease virus. Proc. III Congr. Intl. Soc. Thromb. Haemostas., Washington, D.C., 1972, p. 344.

13. Kjeldson, K. and Thomsen, H.K.: The effect of hypoxia on the fine structure of the aortic intima in rabbits. Lab. Invest. 33: 533-543, 1975.

14. Thomsen, H.K.: Carbon monoxide-induced atherosclerosis in primates. Atherosclerosis 20: 233-240, 1974.

15. Becker, C.G., Dubin, T. and Wiedemann, H.P.: Hypersensitivity to tobacco antigen. Proc. Natl. Acad. Sci. U.S.A. 73: 1712-1716, 1976.

16. Henson, D.M.: In: Bayer Symposium VI. Experimental Models of Chronic Inflammatory Diseases. Berlin: Springer-Verlag, 1977, pp. 94-106.

17. Hirschberg, H., Thorsby, E. and Rolstad, B.: Antibody-induced cell-mediated damage to human endothelial cells in vitro. Nature 255: 62-64, 1975.

18. Fry, D.L.: Responses of the artieral wall to certain physical factors. In: Atherogenesis: Initiating Factors. Ciba Foundation Symposium 12 (new series). New York: Associated Scientific Publishers, 1972, pp. 93-125.

19. Caro, C.G. and Nerem, R.M.: Transport of ^{14}C-4-cholesterol between serum and wall in the perfused dog, common carotid artery. Circ. Res. 32: 187-205, 1973.

20. Goldsmith, H.L.: The flow of model particles and blood cells and its relation to thrombogenesis. In Spaet, T.H. (ed.): Progress in Hemostasis and Thrombosis, Vol. 1. New York: Grune and Stratton, 1972, pp. 97-139.

21. Ryan, U.S., Ryan, J.W., Smith, D.S. and Winkler, H.: Fenestrated endothelium of the adrenal gland: Freeze-fracture studies. Tissue Cell 7: 181-190, 1975.

22. Movat, H.Z., Uriuhara, T., Macmorine, D.L. and Burke, J.S.: A permeability factor released from leukocytes after phagocytosis of immune complexes and its possible role in the Arthus reaction. Life Sci. 3: 1025-1032, 1964.

23. Nachman, R.L., Weksler, B. and Ferris, B.: Characterization of human platelet vascular permeability-enhancing activity. J. Clin. Invest. 51: 549-556, 1972.

24. Weksler, B.B., Marcus, A.J. and Jaffe, E.A.: Synthesis of prostaglandin I_2 (prostacyclin) by cultured human and bovine endothelial cells. Proc. Natl. Acad. Sci. U.S.A. 74: 3922-3926, 1977.

25. Harker, L.A., Ross, R. and Glomset, J.A.: The role of endothelial cell injury and platelet response in atherogenesis. Thromb. Haemostas. 39: 312-321, 1978.

26. Weksler, B.B., Ley, C.W. and Jaffe, E.A.: Stimulation of endothelial cell prostacyclin production by thrombin, trypsin, and ionophore A 23187. J. Clin. Invest. 62: 923-930, 1978.

27. Mustard, J.F., Packham, M.A. and Kinlough-Rathbone, R.: Platelets, thrombosis and atherogenesis. Adv. Exp. Med. Biol. 104: 127-144, 1978.

28. Friedman, R.J., Stemerman, M.B., Wenz, B. et al.: The effect of thrombocytopenia on experimental arteriosclerotic lesion formation in rabbits. Smooth muscle cell proliferation and reendothelialization. J. Clin. Invest. 60: 1191-1201, 1977.

29. Fuster, V., Bowie, E.J., Lewis, J.C., Fass, D.N. and Owen, C.A., Jr.: Resistance to arteriosclerosis in pigs with von Willebrand's disease. Spontaneous and high cholesterol diet-induced arteriosclerosis. J. Clin. Invest. 61: 722-730, 1978.

30. Baumgartner, H.R. and Studer, A.: Platelet factors and the proliferation of vascular smooth muscle cells. In: Atherosclerosis IV. Proceedings of the IVth International Symposium on Atherosclerosis, Tokyo, 1976. Berlin: Springer, 1977.

31. Jaffe, E.A., Nachman, R.L., Becker, C.G. and Minick, C.R.: Culture of human endothelial cells derived from umbilical veins: Identification by morphologic and immunologic criteria. J. Clin. Invest. 52: 2745-2756, 1973.

32. Gimbrone, M.A., Jr., Cotran, R.S. and Folkman, J.: Human vascular endothelial cells in culture: Growth and DNA synthesis. J. Cell. Biol. 60: 673, 1974.

33. Booyse, F.M., Sedlak, B.J. and Rafelson, M.E., Jr.: Culture of arterial endothelial cells. Characterization and growth of bovine aortic cells. Thrombos. Diath. Haemorrh. 34: 825-839, 1975.

34. Wall, R.T., Harker, L.A., Quadracci, L.J. and Striker, G.E.: Factors influencing endothelial cell proliferation in vitro. J. Cell. Physiol. 96: 203-214, 1978.

35. Nelson, R.D., Quie, P.G. and Simmons, R.L.: Chemotaxis under agarose: A new and simple method for measuring chemotaxis and

spontaneous migration of human polymorphonuclear leukocytes and monocytes. J. Immunol. 115: 1650-1656, 1975.

36. Wall, R.T., Harker, L.A. and Striker, G.E.: Human endothelial cell migration: stimulation by a thrombin released platelet factor. Lab. Invest. 39: 523-529, 1978.

37. Wall, R.T., Harlan, J.M., Harker, L.A. and Striker, G.E.: Homocystine-induced endothelial cell injury in vitro. Thromb. Res., in press.

38. Leibovich, S. and Ross, R.: A macrophage-dependent factor that stimulates the proliferation of fibroblasts *in vitro*. Am. J. Pathol. 84: 501-513, 1976.

39. Nemerson, Y. and Pitlick, F.A.: The tissue factor pathway of blood coagulation. *In*: Spaet, T.H. (ed.): Progress in Hemostasis and Thrombosis, Vol. 1. New York: Grune and Stratton, 1972, pp. 1-37.

40. Rutherford, R.B. and Ross, R.: Platelet factors stimulate fibroblasts and smooth muscle cells quiescent in plasma serum to proliferate. J. Cell Biol. 69: 196-203, 1976.

41. Fass, D.N., Downing, M.R., Meyers, P. et al.: A mitogenic factor from porcine arterial cells (Abst.). *In*: Abstracts, 32nd Annual Meeting, Council on Arteriosclerosis, American Society for the Study of Arteriosclerosis, November 13-15, 1978, Dallas, p. 11.

42. Gajdusek, C., Schwartz, S., DiCorleto, P. and Ross, R.: Endothelial cell derived mitogenic activity (Abst.). Fed. Proc. 38 (part II): 1075, 1979.

43. Minick, C.R., Stemerman, M.B. and Insull, W., Jr.: Effect of regenerated endothelium on lipid accumulation in the arterial wall. Proc. Natl. Acad. Sci. U.S.A. 74: 1724-1728, 1977.

44. Thakur, M.L., Welsh, M., Joist, J.H. et al.: Indium-111 labeled platelets: Studies on preparation and evaluation of *in vitro* and *in vivo* functions. Thromb. Res. 9: 345-357, 1976.

45. Goodwin, D.A., Buchberg, J.T. and Doherty, P.W.: ^{111}In-labeled autologous platelets for localization of vascular thrombi in humans. J. Nucl. Med. 19: 623, 1978.

46. Harker, L.A.: Platelet survival time: Its measurement and use. *In*: Spaet, T.H. (ed.): Progress in Hemostasis and Thrombosis, Vol IV. New York: Grune and Stratton, 1978, pp. 321-347.

47. Harker, L.A. and Hanson, S.R.: Experimental arterial thromboembolism in baboons: Mechanism, quantitation and pharmacologic preparation. J. Clin. Invest., in press.

48. Hanson, S. and Harker, L.A.: Simultaneous [51]Cr- and ^{14}C-serotonin platelet survival measurements. Thromb. Haemostas. 38: 140, 1977.

49. Witte, L.D., Kaplan, K.L., Nossel, H.L., et al.: Studies of the release from human platelets of the growth factor for cultured human arterial smooth muscle cells. Circ. Res. 42: 402-409, 1978.

50. Kaplan, K.L., Drillings, M. and Nossel, H.L.: Radioimmunoassay of thromboglobulin (BTG) and platelet factor 4 (PF4). *In* Day, J.H., Zudker, M.B. and Holmsen, H., (eds.): The Significance of Platelet Function Tests in the Evaluation of Hemostatic and Thrombotic Tendencies. Workshop on Platelets, Philadelphia, 1978. DHEW, National Institutes of Health, pp. 78-108.

51. Bolton, A.E., Ludlam, C.A., Petter, D.S. et al.: A radioimmunoassay for platelet factor 4. Thromb. Res. 8: 51-58, 1976.
52. Reimers, H.J., Cazenave, J.P., Senyi, A.F. et al.: *In vitro* and *in vivo* functions of thrombi-treated platelets. Thromb. Haemostas. 35: 151-166, 1976.
53. Roth, G.J. and Majerus, P.W.: The mechanism of the effects of aspirin on human platelets. I. Acetylation of a particulate fraction protein. J. Clin. Invest. 56: 624-632, 1975.
54. Weiss, H.J., Tschopp, T.B. and Baumgartner, H.R.: Impaired interaction (adhesion-aggregation) of platelets with the subendothelium in storage-pool disease and after aspirin ingestion. A comparison with von Willebrand's disease. N. Engl. J. Med. 293: 619-623, 1975.
55. Moncada, S. and Korbut, R.: Dipyridamole and other phosphodiesterase inhibitors act as antithrombotic agents by potentiating endogenous prostacyclin. Lancet 1: 1286-1289, 1978.
56. Roth, G.J. and Majerus, P.W.: Acetylation of prostaglandin synthetase by aspirin. Proc. Natl. Acad. Sci. U.S.A. 72: 3073-3076, 1975.
57. Kelton, J.G., Hirsh, J., Carter, C.J. and Buchanan, M.R.: Thrombogenic effect of high-dose aspirin in rabbits. Relationship to inhibition of vessel wall synthesis of prostaglandin I_2-like activity. J. Clin. Invest. 62: 892-895, 1978.
58. Cazenave, J.P., Packham, M.A., Guccione, M.A. and Mustard, J.F.: Inhibition of platelet adherence to a collagen coated surface by nonsteroidal antiinflammatory drugs, pyrimido-pyrimidine and tricyclic compounds and lidocaine. J. Lab. Clin. Med. 83: 797-806, 1974.
59. Ali, M. and McDonald, J.W.D.: Effects of sulfinpyrazone on platelet prostaglandin synthesis and platelet release of serotonin. J. Lab. Clin. Med. 89: 868-875, 1975.
60. Harker, L.A. and Ross, R.: Prevention of homocysteine-induced arteriosclerosis: Sulphinpyrazone endothelial protection. *In* Abe, T. and Sherry, S. (eds.): A New Approach to Reduction of Cardiac Death. Vienna: Hans Huber Publishers, 1978, pp. 59-72.
61. More, R.H.: Significance of the smooth muscle cell in atherogenesis. *In* Jones, R.J. (ed.): Evolution of the Atherosclerotic Plaque. Chicago: University of Chicago Press, 1963, p. 51.
62. French, J.E.: Atherosclerosis in relation to the structure and function of the arterial intima, with special reference to the endothelium. *In* Rickter, G.W. and Epstein, M.A. (eds.): International Review of Experimental Pathology, Vol. 5. New York: Academic Press, 1966, p. 253.
63. Bell, F.P., Day, A.J., Gent, M. and Schwartz, C.J.: Differing patterns of cholesterol accumulation and ^{3}H-cholesterol of influx in areas of the cholesterol-fed pig aorta identified by Evans blue dye. Exp. Mol. Pathol. 22: 366-375, 1975.
64. Davies, P.F. and Ross, R.: Mediation of pinocytosis in cultured arterial smooth-muscle and endothelial cells by platelet-derived growth factor. J. Cell Biol. 79: 663-671, 1978.

65. Still, W.I.S.: The topography of cholesterol-induced fatty streaks. Exp. Mol. Pathol. 20: 374-386, 1974.
66. Weber, G., Fabbrini, P. and Resi, L.: Scanning and transmission electron microscopy observations on the surface lining of aortic plaques in rabbits on a hypercholesterolic diet. Virchows Arch. [Pathol. Anat.] 364: 325-331, 1974.
67. Nelson, E., Gertz, S.D., Forbes, M.S. et al.: Endothelial lesions in the aorta of egg yolk-fed miniature swine. Exp. Mol. Pathol. 25: 208-220, 1976.
68. Svendsen, E. and Jorgensen, L.: Loss of endothelial cells in rabbit aorta following short-term cholesterol feeding (Abst.). In Schetteler, G., Hata, Y., Klose, G. and Goto, Y. (eds.): IV International Symposium on Atherosclerosis, Aug. 24-28, 1976, Tokyo, Japan. Berlin: Springer-Verlag, 1976, Abst. F-81.
69. Silkworth, J.B.: The effect of hypercholesterolemia on aortic endothelium studied en face. Atherosclerosis 22: 335, 1975.
70. Lewis, J.C. and Kottke, B.A.: Endothelial damage and thrombocyte adhesion in pigeon atherosclerosis. Science 196: 1007-1009, 1977.
71. Davies, P.F., Reidy, M.A., Goode, T.B. and Bowyer, D.E.: Scanning electron microscopy in the evaluation of endothelial integrity of the fatty lesion in atherosclerosis. Atherosclerosis 25: 125-130, 1976.
72. Florentin, R.A., Nam, S.C., Lee, K.T. and Thomas, W.A.: Increased ^{3}H-thymidine incorporation into endothelial cells of swine fed cholesterol for 3 days. Exp. Mol. Pathol. 10: 250-255, 1969.

Discussion

Dr. Clopath: In the case of homocystinemic baboons you nicely showed desquamation. Why was there no adhesion of platelets, and in those cases in which there were platelets, why were there no pseudopods? Secondly, did you ever try to use vitamin B_6 to prevent intimal lesions in baboons, inasmuch as it is common practice to treat homocystinemic patients in this way?

Dr. Harker: In homocystinemic patients the B_6 actually modifies the metabolic pathways to reduce homocystine. Since we have been interested in producing endothelial injury, we have never tried giving B_6. Our hypothesis is not that all atherogenesis is mediated through homocysteine, but rather that this is merely one model of injury.

After glutaraldehyde fixation scanning electron micrographs did show platelets at focal sites of desquamation. After preparation with the silver stain perfusion technique, however, platelets were usually not seen at the sites of desquamation.

There are several possible explanations. First, adherent platelets might have been removed by the preparation technique. Secondly, relatively few platelets may remain at areas exposed to circulating blood for a long period of time. Thirdly, there may be a component of endothelium lost *in vitro* as an artifact of the technique.

Dr. Folts: Have you made any acute denudations or damage to the endothelium and then applied sulfinpyrazone to see how soon it might have an effect on the endothelium?

Dr. Harker: In regard to balloon desquamation, Dr. Hans Baumgartner has found no effect of sulfinpyrazone, aspirin, or dipyridamole on acute adhesion and platelet thrombus formation.

Dr. Folts: When we've produced narrowing and some intimal damage, we can see the flow declining because platelets are accumulating; within 2 to 5 min after infusion of sulfinpyrazone, the platelet aggregation disappears. It actually clears out the lumen and flow is restored to a higher level, as if it somehow either caused all the platelets collected there to deaggregate or had some direct effect on the endothelium to prevent further aggregation.

Dr. Harker: There is a significant distinction between adherence and aggregation with the formation of platelet and thrombus. Flow modifies only the accumulation of aggregated platelets after the adherence of single-layer platelets on the surface.

Dr. Folts: Are there any data to show that sulfinpyrazone causes deaggregation of already aggregated platelets?

Dr. Wallis: In an *in vitro* experiment we have added ADP to platelet-rich plasma and, when aggregation was complete, added the test substance to determine the deaggregation rate. In this particular case, sulfinpyrazone had no effect, whereas PGE_1 and PGI_2 had a very strong effect.

Dr. Harker: Aspirin also has been reported to enhance deaggregation.

Dr. Wallis: Since aspirin inhibits aggregation, if it is added beforehand, it would have an effect, but not when the test substance is added after aggregation is complete.

Dr. Harker: As reported by Davis et al., aspirin enhanced the rate of deaggregation.

Dr. Wallis: Really? We haven't found that.

Dr. McDonald: Dr. Harker, were any of the differences in platelet survival in various groups of hyperlipidemic patients statistically significantly different from controls? In groups such as the type IV group, where some of the individual patients appeared to have shortened platelet survival, did they differ from other members of the group in having disease or complications of atherosclerosis?

Dr. Harker: Statistically significant differences were seen in type III and type IV-V. In that subset there was no characteristic identified showing shortened platelet survival that we could measure in terms of lipid levels.

Dr. Oliver: Could you explain what sulfinpyrazone might be doing to the type II monkey, in whom regression of the xanthomata seems to occur? Is there any significant difference in platelet survival in type IV-V compared with II?

Dr. Harker: In the absence of significant denudation in those animals, we hypothesize, on the basis of platelet survival studies, that a similar intactness of the endothelium is likely to be present for most of the surface. It has been suggested that endothelium-derived growth factor might be increased by the hyperlipidemia in a manner similar to PGI_2.

Dr. Sherry: Are these effects that you've demonstrated *in vivo* independent of any serum uric acid changes?

Dr. Harker: We have no uric acid measurements in these animals.

Dr. Clopath: I have measured serum uric acid concentration in rabbits and there was simply no uric acid in the plasma; I would think that in this case it would be the same.

Dr. Gordon: I noticed, Dr. Harker, that when you added homocysteine to endothelial cells *in vitro*, you expressed the results as a percentage of specific release, which is always 100% in controls. Am I right in assuming that that is the difference between the release you get in the presence of homocysteine and in the absence? If so, could you tell us what the absolute values were?

Dr. Harker: The calculation of specific release involves the subtraction of background. The background can be considerable, depending upon how the experiment is carried out. In 4 h, about 10% nonspecific release is observed, and at 24 h, as much as 30%.

Dr. Gordon: In the presence of the homocysteine, what would be the augmented release over that 10% or 30%?

Dr. Harker: Up to 100%, if the concentration is increased to 10 mM.

Dr. Mustard: Did sulfinpyrazone treatment of your lipid-fed monkeys actually diminish the amount of atherosclerosis?

Dr. Harker: Yes, sulfinpyrazone diminished the amount of intimal lesion formation.

Dr. Mustard: In your first experiments in the monkeys you reported that platelet survival was shortened. After the animals have been on the diet for a long period of time, as in your current experiments, is platelet survival still shortened?

Dr. Harker: Yes, there is some shortening of platelet survival in those animals.

Dr. Mustard: Does sulfinpyrazone lengthen the shortened platelet survival in the lipid-fed animals?

Dr. Harker: Yes, there is a measurable prolongation of the platelet survival by sulfinpyrazone.

Dr. Mustard: I think your dipyridamole/sulfinpyrazone data are interesting when contrasted to Baumgartner's studies in the rabbit. My colleagues Kinlough-Rathbone and Groves have looked at *in vivo* adhesion of the platelets to the surface of the denuded aorta and found dipyridamole to be a good inhibitor of platelet adherence to the subendothelium of the aorta. This is in good agreement with your results with the monkey. Sulfinpyrazone had little effect on platelet adherence to the subendothelium and it did not inhibit the release reaction of platelets adherent to the wall, which, I think, explains why sulfinpyrazone is not a good inhibitor of smooth muscle cell proliferation when the endothelium is removed from an artery.

Microscopic Observation of Small Blood Vessels in Sulfinpyrazone-Treated Animals

Mary P. Wiedeman, Ph.D.

Introduction

Numerous studies, in both clinical and laboratory settings, have supplied evidence that sulfinpyrazone has effective anti-thrombotic properties. The studies have included *in vitro*, *in vivo*, and *ex vivo* methods in man and animals. A comprehensive and well-documented review by Mustard and Packham in 1975 [1] covers the various investigations of the nonsteroidal anti-inflammatory drugs which demonstrate their ability to inhibit certain platelet functions. Sulfinpyrazone, although not specifically classified as an anti-inflammatory drug, is included in this category. Several of the studies deserve some elaboration to aid in the identification of the effects, if not the mechanisms, whereby sulfinpyrazone acts in a protective manner to modify platelet behavior.

Packham et al. [2], using rabbits as the experimental animal, demonstrated an inhibition of collagen-induced aggregation in platelet-rich plasma (PRP) prepared from the blood of animals infused with various doses of sulfinpyrazone. Suppression of aggregation was greatest (88% of a preinfusion sample) with the highest dose of sulfinpyrazone used. The investigators concluded that platelet aggregation induced by collagen could be blocked by sulfinpyrazone and that the

Mary P. Wiedeman, Ph.D., Department of Physiology, Temple University School of Medicine, Philadelphia, Pa.

This work was supported in part by a reserach grant (HL-20563) from the National Institutes of Health and by a grant from the CIBA-GEIGY Corporation.

99

mechanism did not appear to be a direct inhibition of the action of ADP. They suggested that the drug may interfere with the adherence to surfaces or with reactions which might occur at the platelet membrane. Because the drug did not block the action of ADP or thrombin, it was suggested that the inhibition shown was due to a decreased response of platelets to surface stimuli with a subsequent reduction in ADP and serotonin release.

Later, Ali and McDonald [3] presented supportive evidence showing that sulfinpyrazone added to PRP inhibited the release of serotonin induced by collagen and also found that the release of serotonin from PRP of patients treated with sulfinpyrazone was inhibited. They also showed sulfinpyrazone was a potent inhibitor of platelet prostaglandin synthesis.

Weily and Genton [4] studied the effect of sulfinpyrazone treatment in patients with prosthetic mitral valves and reported a reduction in platelet adhesiveness to glass bead columns when platelets from patients treated with sulfinpyrazone were used. No change in the aggregating properties of platelets from untreated patients was noted.

Essien and Mustard [5] used isolated aortic strips from rabbits to study platelet adherence to damaged endothelium of the vessel. They found that platelet adherence to the damaged area of aorta was significantly reduced when sulfinpyrazone was present in the solution used to perfuse an injured aortic strip.

From these studies it is seen that in various experimental methods, primarily *in vitro* or *ex vivo*, sulfinpyrazone can affect platelet behavior in such a way that it reduces the adherence of platelets to certain surfaces and inhibits aggregation induced by collagen, the release of serotonin, and the synthesis of platelet prostaglandin. Except for a study in which Lewis and Westwick [6] demonstrated that orally administered sulfinpyrazone reduced the number of thrombi that appeared during platelet aggregation production by iontophoresis, the effects of sulfinpyrazone on platelet behavior in the living animal have yet to be studied.

In an attempt to demonstrate the influence of sulfinpyrazone on platelet aggregates in peripheral vessels in the living animal, microscopic observation of vessels after exposure to sulfinpyrazone offered the most direct approach. Any effect of the drug on vascular smooth muscle, blood cellular components, and hemodynamics could be revealed by this technique. Toward this end, the vessels in the cheek pouch of the anesthetized hamster and the wing of the unanesthetized bat were monitored after the introduction of sulfinpyrazone by various routes. Platelet aggregates, artificially induced by a single-pulse ruby-red laser and by mechanical injury, were compared in treated and untreated animals. Comparisons were also made to see if the drug affected velocity of blood flow, vessel diameters, and adherence of leukocytes.

Methods

The hamster cheek pouch was prepared for visualization through the microscope according to the method of Duling [7]. The hamster is anesthetized by an intraperitoneal injection of sodium pentobarbital, 6 mg/100 g. The animal is then secured on a plastic board in a supine position and a tracheostomy and a femoral vein cannulation are performed. The cannulated femoral vein permits rapid administration of additional anesthesia and the administration of other materials when required by the experiment. The cheek pouch from the left side is everted with a cotton applicator and anchored by its tip to the outer margin of a circular opening in the plastic board. The pouch is then spread across the entire surface of the opening and pinned to an encircling rubber ring. This double layer of tissue is sectioned through the middle of the upper layer and the tissue reflected to the sides and pinned to the rubber ring. The remaining, thin, single layer of tissue is then cleared of connective tissue by careful dissection, a circular cover slip is placed on top, and the bed is ready for study. These vessels are usually observed at a magnification of 900×.

Preparation of the bat wing for observation is a relatively simple procedure in which the dormant bat is taken from the refrigerator, tucked gently into a plastic container, and secured to a large microscope slide which has a plastic border surrounding the glass, as previously described [8]. One wing is then extended over the glass plate and held in position with spring clips which are held by screws in the plastic border. A drop of mineral oil placed between the wing and the glass slide increases visibility and assures a flat field. For some procedures, the top layer of epithelial tissue is removed by gentle dissection and the exposed area is covered with physiological saline. Two slivers of glass, one on each side of the denuded area, support a coverslip which makes a small saline-filled chamber.

In both preparations small arteries can be cannulated with glass capillary tubes drawn to a fine point, attached to plastic tubing, which is in turn attached to a 1-ml syringe. Intraarterial injections are then made retrograde to arterial flow, permitting any injected material to be carried in the regular arterial distribution of flow from side branches of the cannulated artery.

Velocity flow measurements are made by projecting the image of the vessel under observation onto a viewing screen by means of a right-angle prism inserted into the trinocular barrel of a microscope. Two matched phototransistors in small slits of the viewing screen are positioned in the center of the vessel aligned parallel to its axis. The electrical signals from the sensors represent the optical density at the two sites. On-line velocity determinations are made by cross-correlating the up- and downstream optical signals with an IBM velocitometer. Output voltage from the velocitometer represents the red blood cell velocity and is recorded on a Brush recorder.

Diameters are measured with an eyepiece micrometer, which is calibrated with a stage micrometer. The inside diameters of vessels are measured, beginning with first-order arteries and then successive branches down to the fourth-order vessels.

Platelet aggregates are produced by the output from a single-pulse ruby-red laser. The laser, mounted on the trinocular head of a microscope, produces a discrete local thermal injury, when activated. By trial it was determined that an input of 170 to 180 J was sufficient to produce an immediate aggregate that adhered to the vessel wall. It was previously established that ADP released from injured red blood cells, lysed by the heat, was responsible for the formation of this aggregate [9]. The growth, embolization, and subsequent cessation of any platelet adherence around the cluster of red blood cells was timed and expressed as duration of activity. In control animals, after 5 or 6 min platelets from the flowing blood were no longer attracted to the initial clump of cells, emboli no longer broke off, and the reaction was considered to be over.

A second method of producing platelet aggregates is to deform or puncture an arterial vessel with a sharp metal probe attached to a micromanipulator. Damage by the probe to the vessel wall produces a platelet aggregate, presumably at the site where collagen is exposed.

Sulfinpyrazone is prepared for injection by dissolving 100 mg of powder in 5 to 6 ml of Normosol-R (Abbott Laboratories, Chicago). Five to six drops of 2N NaOH is added to the solution, which is then stirred with a magnetic stirring bar to complete the dissolution. The pH is adjusted to 7.5 by adding 1 M HCl. Additional Normosol is added to bring the total volume to 10 ml. The final concentration is 10 mg/ml.

Results

Vascular Diameter

Before other vascular or cellular responses to sulfinpyrazone could be considered, it was necessary to establish whether the drug had any vasoactive properties that would affect the peripheral vascular beds. In 24 measurements of arterial diameters in ten hamster cheek pouch preparations, no significant changes were seen in vessel diameters following the IV injection of sulfinpyrazone, 50 mg/kg of body weight. Similar measurements in arterial vessels in the bat wing also showed these vessels to be unaffected by intraarterial injections of sulfinpyrazone. So that the overall effects of the drug on the cardiovascular system could be tested, mongrel dogs were given IV injections of sulfinpyrazone (50 mg/kg) and systemic blood pressure and electrical activity of the heart were monitored. A carotid artery cannula attached to a pressure transducer recorded the systemic pressure on an Electronics for Medicine direct writer, and lead II of the electrocardiogram (ECG) was simultaneously recorded. No change in either the ECG or systemic blood pressure was seen following IV injection of the drug. It was concluded that sulfinpyrazone had no effect on vascular smooth muscle of hamster cheek pouch vessels or bat wing vessels and produced no changes in blood pressure, heart rate, or cardiac muscle.

Velocity of Blood Flow

Considering that a change in blood flow velocity with a subsequent change in shear rate might affect platelet aggregates and leukocyte adherence to the vessel wall, velocity measurements were made in arterial vessels in the bat wing before and after an IV injection of sulfinpyrazone, 50 mg/kg of body weight. In eight trials in four animals, average control values for velocity were found to be 0.37 cm sec^{-1} with a calculated shear rate of 384 sec^{-1}. At 10 min after an IV injection of sulfinpyrazone, the velocity was 34 cm sec^{-1} and the shear rate was calculated to be 358 sec^{-1}. These very minimal changes were not statistically significant. Similar studies in hamster cheek pouch vessels also showed no significant velocity changes. It was concluded that an IV injection of sulfinpyrazone of this magnitude does not alter the cardiovascular system in any way that results in a change in the velocity of blood flow in peripheral vessels. Therefore, any change in adherence of platelet aggregates and leukocytes to the vessel wall cannot be attributed to changes in the velocity of blood flow (Table 1).

Platelet Aggregate Activity and Adherence

Two methods were used to administer sulfinpyrazone to the experimental animals so that the effect of the drug on artificially induced platelet aggregates in arterial vessels could be tested. In one case, a dose of 50 mg/kg of sulfinpyrazone was injected IV 1 h before aggregate production in both bats and

Table 1. Effects of Sulfinpyrazone on the Cardiovascular System

Animal	Observation	Response
Hamster	Arterial Diameter	No Change
Bat	Arterial Diameter	No Change
Dog	Blood Pressure	No Change
Dog	Electrocardiogram	No Change
Hamster	Flow Velocity	No Change
Bat	Flow Velocity	No Change
Bat	Shear Rate	No Change

Control values were determined as described, and measurements were repeated after an IV injection of sulfinpyrazone, 50 mg/kg. Shear rate was calculated from velocity and diameter measurements.

hamsters, and in the other, IP injections were administered daily to a group of hamsters, for as long as 5 days. The latter were observed at different periods of time—from 2 to 5 days following initiation of daily IP injections. The duration of platelet activity around a laser-induced aggregate was determined in hamsters and bats 1 h after IV injection. A double-blind study with 32 trials in eight hamsters showed a 47% reduction in activity in the sulfinpyrazone-treated animals. Although no inhibition of the production of the initial ADP-induced aggregate was seen, the continued adherence of platelets to the aggregate and the adherence of the aggregate to the wall was reduced in time. In 22 trials in four bats, a reduction of 18% in adherence was demonstrated if the bats were tested immediately after the injection. If the tests were begun 1 h later, the reduction of platelet activity was 58.8%.

In 22 hamsters, IP injections of sulfinpyrazone also inhibited the duration of platelet adherence to the initial ADP laser-induced aggregate and the adherence of the aggregate to the vessel wall. The greatest reduction in timed activity was seen in hamsters receiving five injections. There was a marked reduction, however, after two injections (Table 2).

It was concluded from these studies that the presence of sulfinpyrazone in the blood stream reduces the adhesiveness of platelets to one another, as well as to the endothelial lining of an arterial vessel in the living animal.

Collagen-induced aggregates are assumed to result from direct injury to a blood vessel. This type of injury was achieved mechanically by deforming or puncturing the arterial vessel wall with a sharp probe. After duration of activity of platelets at the site of injury in a hamster was established, the procedure was repeated on the same vessel 1 h after an IV injection of sulfinpyrazone, 50 mg/kg. The duration of platelet activity following injury from the microprobe was reduced by 44.9%. It would appear from these results that sulfinpyrazone can also affect collagen-induced aggregates in the same way that it affects the ADP-induced aggregate (Table 2).

Adherence of Leukocytes

The appearance of leukocytes moving slowly along the wall of arteries and veins in preparations *in vivo* is considered a sign of injury or an inflammatory response [10]. Although the

Table 2. Platelet Aggregating Activity after Sulfinpyrazone Treatment*

Method of Inducing Aggregation	Animal	Route of Sulfinpyrazone Injection	Time of Test	Duration of Platelet Aggregate Activity (min)		Change (%)
				Control	Postinjection	
Laser (ADP)	Bat	IV	1 min	4.47	3.64	−18.5
	Hamster	IV	1 h	6.07	2.5	−58.8
	Hamster	IV	1 h	5.28	2.8	−47.0
Probe (Collagen)	Hamster	IV	1 h	6.92	3.81	−44.9
Laser (ADP)	Hamster	IP	2 days	5.75	2.77	−51.8
			3 days		2.55	−55.6
			4 days		2.89	−49.7
			5 days		2.40	−58.3

*The duration of activity of platelets around an aggregate produced by a laser beam in bats and hamsters or by mechanical injury in hamsters was determined for control periods and after administration of sulfinpyrazone in a single IV dose of 50 mg/kg or after daily IP doses of 50 mg/kg for 2 to 5 days (in hamsters).

mechanism is not understood, most investigators using the techniques consider that the slow-moving leukocytes appear in instances when the vessels have been exposed to conditions incompatible with the normal internal milieu, after direct mechanical injury to a vessel, exposure to cold, or the release of abnormal amounts of endogenous materials. Adhering leukocytes are frequently seen in the arterial vessels in the bat wing preparation, in which the top layer of epithelium has been removed for better visualization. Although the denuded vessels are covered with physiological saline, the teasing-away of their protective cover induces leukocyte adhesion initially. As a test of the possibility that sulfinpyrazone might have a protective effect, the number of leukocytes passing through a short segment of an exposed artery was counted for 1 min. Sulfinpyrazone was then injected intraarterially several times as a bolus so the observed vessel was completely filled with the solution (1 mg/ml) for 1 to 2 sec. A second section of the arterial vessel was then denuded and the observations were repeated. In most instances, no leukocytes were seen in the section of the vessel which was exposed after being perfused with sulfinpyrazone, although in some experiments two or three rapidly moving leukocytes were seen. Further studies are required to assess this finding, but it is apparent that the drug reduced the adhesiveness of leukocytes to the vessel wall. This could be an effect of sulfinpyrazone on the endothelial lining of the vessel or on the surface of the leukocyte.

Summary

In these studies of the effects of sulfinpyrazone in peripheral vascular beds of living animal, both anesthetized and unanesthetized, sulfinpyrazone has no demonstrable effect on cardiovascular parameters such as vascular diameter, velocity of blood flow, heart rate, or systemic blood pressure. Therefore, it is concluded that the drug is not vasoactive nor does it have an inotropic effect on cardiac muscle. Furthermore, while sulfinpyrazone does not inhibit aggregation induced artificially, either by ADP released from red blood cells or by exposure to collagen, it does reduce the adhesiveness of platelets to one another and also the ability of a cluster of aggregated platelets to adhere to the endothelial lining of a blood vessel. Sulfinpyrazone also reduces the adherence of leukocytes to the arterial vessel wall.

Acknowledgments

The author gratefully acknowledges the assistance of Dr. R. F. Tuma for the velocity and shear rate determinations and the technical assistance of Lynn Heinel and Scott Zane.

References

1. Mustard, J.F. and Packham, M.A.: Platelets, thrombosis and drugs. Drugs 9: 19-76, 1975.
2. Packham, M.A., Warrior, E.S., Glynn, M.F., Senyi, A.S. and Mustard, J.F.: Alteration of the response of platelets to surface stimuli by pyrazole compounds. J. Exp. Med. 126: 171-188, 1967.
3. Ali, M. and McDonald, J.W.D.: Effects of sulfinpyrazone on platelet prostaglandin synthesis and platelet release of serotonin. J. Lab. Clin. Med. 89: 868-875, 1977.
4. Weily, H.S. and Genton, E.: Altered platelet function in patients with prosthetic mitral valves. Circulation 42: 967-972, 1970.
5. Essien, E.M. and Mustard, J.F.: Inhibition of platelet adhesion to rabbit aorta by sulfinpyrazone and acetylsalicylic acid. Atherosclerosis 27: 89-95, 1977.
6. Lewis, G.P. and Westwick, J.: The effect of sulfinpyrazone, sodium aspirin and oxprenolol on the formation of arterial platelet thrombi. Br. J. Pharmacol. 55 (2): 255P-256P, 1975.
7. Duling, B.R.: The preparation and use of the hamster cheek pouch for studies of the microcirculation. Microvasc. Res. 5: 423-429, 1973.
8. Wiedeman, M.P.: Vascular reactions to laser in vivo. Microvasc. Res. 8: 132-138, 1974.
9. Wiedeman, M.P.: Preparation of the bat wing for in vivo microscopy. Microvasc. Res. 5: 417-422, 1973.
10. Grant, L.: The sticking and emigration of white blood cells in inflammation. In Zweifach, B.W., Grant, L. and McCluskey, T.R. (eds.): The Inflammatory Process, Vol. 2. New York: Academic Press, 1973, pp. 205-244.

Discussion

Dr. Margulies: We've heard from Professor Harker that sulfinpyrazone apparently has the capacity of protecting the endothelium. I know there are methods whereby one can measure vascular fragility in microcirculatory preparations. Have you done any studies to measure vascular fragility in response to pretreatment with Anturane, and if not, do you know of any studies that have been done?

Dr. Wiedeman: No, we haven't, and I don't know of any studies that have been done. We tried to measure changes in permeability of the blood vessels, but we haven't found a good technique for that. We tried histamine with fluorescein injections, but that gave an "all-or-nothing" type of response, and we tried tween 80 as a somewhat nonspecific permeability changer. We hope to be able to measure permeability changes, and we also could do vascular fragility studies, I would think, very easily.

Dr. McGregor: Was the dosage, the concentration used, in the same range as in Dr. Harker's experiments?

Dr. Wiedeman: When we injected intraarterially, in actual contact with the vessel wall, we used a dose of 1 mg/kg of body weight. A great many dilutions are needed for a bat that weighs only 10 g.

Dr. Minick: You suggested that the effect of the laser was on the platelets actually within the lumen or on erythrocyte release of ADP as it then acted on the platelets. Have you actually examined the structure of the wall at these sites to see if there are changes in the blood?

Dr. Wiedeman: Yes, and Arfors in Sweden did similar studies. Other investigators have introduced iron filings, carbon black, or something else to cause the heat of the laser to really injure the vessel wall. But electron micrographs done by Dr. Stewart at our Thrombosis Center, and information from Dr. Arfors in Sweden, showed no real removal of the lining of the blood vessel. There may be some slight change. In an extensive study in our laboratory, we found that if we perfused a homolysate and zapped it while it was going through the blood vessel, we could still get a platelet aggregate. If we dialyzed the homolysate until there was no ADP left in it and zapped that, we didn't get an aggregate. Consequently we felt that we were really dealing with an ADP-induced aggregate when we dealt with the laser injury.

Dr. Minick: Can you induce similar lesions in larger vessels by these techniques?

Dr. Wiedeman: Yes, but we refer to these as "microvessels" somewhat erroneously. The large vessel that comes into the bat's wing is only small because the bat is small; as far as the number of its muscle layers and its function in the arterial bed, it's the same as my brachial artery or an elephant's. They just happen to be different sizes because the animal is a different size. It's actually very difficult to make a platelet aggregate in a microvessel, that is, in a vessel that we consider to be in the terminal vascular bed; it either ruptures it or makes no aggregate at all.

Dr. McGregor: Are we to understand that the laser did not damage endothelium, that the laser beam was shooting a red blood cell which then released ADP, and that's the cause of the aggregate in the laser damage?

Dr. Wiedeman: That's what we believe.

Dr. McGregor: Why does the aggregate stay where it is then? It appears to be stuck to a place in the vessel wall.

Dr. Wiedeman: The heat of the laser lyses a cluster of red blood cells; we've demonstrated this not just in the blood vessel, but also on a microscope slide. It makes a little cluster of these damaged red blood cells. Why it sticks just to that area, I don't know, but if it doesn't stay for at least 20 sec, it never rebuilds. We have tried to investigate the interaction between the aggregate and the vessel wall by attempting to measure changes in electrical potential at the site. Dr. Mayrovitz who was pursuing those studies moved away and they haven't been continued. We are aware that we need some explanation of why the aggregate stays at that site, if there is no real disruption of the vascular wall.

Dr. White: Have you seen any effects in your preparation which you might regard as unique to sulfinpyrazone, that is, which would not be seen if you were to pretreat with, say, aspirin?

Dr. Wiedeman: We used aspirin without any success. At first it puzzled me, but we reported that the laser aggregate is not inhibited by aspirin. If aspirin is only really effective on collagen-induced aggregates, then we wouldn't expect it to be as effective on our ADP-induced aggregate. We have used other materials, but for a different reason, testing vasoactive drugs (both vasoconstrictors and vasodilators) to see what sort of changes they made. We've used a number of agents, including dipyridamole, but for the inhibition of the aggregates — and

certainly for the duration of activity around the aggregate —
sulfinpyrazone was effective.

Dr. White: Have you tested chlorpromazine, a classical
membrane stabilizer?

Dr. Wiedeman: No.

Dr. White: It would be interesting to do that.

Dr. Folts: What is the largest vessel you've been able to
observe these effects in?

Dr. Wiedeman: The arterial diameters are probably about 60
μm in the bat; in the hamster, they would be closer to 100 to
110 μm. The hamster arterial vessels are, of course, larger than
the bat arterial vessels; the same kind of response occurs in
both.

Dr. Folts: What is the largest?

Dr. Wiedeman: From 100 to 120 or 130 μm.

Dr. Mustard: I would like to return to the mechanism of
action that occurs at the laser injury site. It seems that the
initial aggregates are formed by the ADP released from the red
blood cells. However, when the initial platelet aggregate breaks
up, a new one forms. That must mean that there is some
stimulus from the wall that is not due to released ADP. It's
interesting that sulfinpyrazone does not appear to prevent the
initial mass from forming; this is compatible with the well-
established experimental evidence showing that primary ADP-
induced platelet aggregation is not inhibited by sulfinpyrazone.
However, the effect of sulfinpyrazone preventing the subsequent formation of platelet aggregates could be related to
Harker's observation of the effect of sulfinpyrazone on the
endothelium. It would be interesting if you could determine
whether there are changes in the endothelium at that site that
act as a subsequent stimulus for platelet aggregate formation
and whether sulfinpyrazone prevents the endothelial changes.

Dr. Wiedeman: In an earlier study we demonstrated that in
the bat wing over a period of 30 min, the distance upstream
from the initial platelet aggregation at which platelets adhered
increased tremendously, from just locally at the injury to about
50 μm upstream. Therefore it can't be anything that is being
delivered downstream that changes the endothelium. We suggested that there was certainly a change in the endothelial wall
that was self-propagating from one area upstream to the next by

an unknown mechanism. It may be that if sulfinpyrazone inhibits that mechanism, then we could say, yes, it's certainly making a change in the endothelial wall.

Dr. Robson: Thromboxane causes platelets to aggregate and it also causes vasoconstriction. When you measured the diameter of these small vessels, during the process of damage, whether caused by the laser beam or the probe, were you able to detect any vasoconstriction?

Dr. Wiedeman: No. The laser sometimes produces vasoconstriction just from the heat and so does the probe, but if the injection of sulfinpyrazone does anything, it enhances the blood flow, possibly through some slight vasodilation.

Dr. Robson: Supposing, in the process of aggregation, the platelets release thromboxane.

Dr. Wiedeman: Any vasoconstriction that occurred after the laser zap we equated with the heat from the laser.

Dr. Cooper: Do leukocytes participate in the platelet aggregation and is there a difference in the degree of participation with and without sulfinpyrazone?

Dr. Wiedeman: We haven't made any quantitative determinations about that; there are so few white cells ordinarily that we don't pay much attention to them.

Lack of Protective Effect
of Sulfinpyrazone
on Endothelial Cells from Pig
Aorta in Culture

Klaus R. Müller, Ph.D.

Introduction

Patients with the rare genetic disorder of homocystinemia tend to develop progressive arteriosclerosis early in their life [1]. Experiments with baboons have demonstrated that plasma homocystine concentrations above 0.1 mM, induced by continuous infusion of homocysteine, cause patchy endothelial desquamation and formation of atherosclerotic lesions in the aorta [2]. Simultaneous treatment with sulfinpyrazone protected these homocystinemic baboons against endothelial cell loss and atherosclerotic lesion formation [3]. These findings *in vivo* have been supported by results from studies *in vitro*: endothelial cells from human umbilical vein in culture were found to become damaged when homocysteine was added to the medium, and cell damage was significantly reduced by the presence of 10^{-8} to 10^{-6} M sulfinpyrazone [3]. Cell damage was assessed in these experiments by labeling the cells with ^{51}Cr and measuring its release into the medium.

In view of these findings we tried to demonstrate this protective effect of sulfinpyrazone on endothelium in an *in vitro* system using endothelial cells from pig aorta, that is, from an artery which is known to be susceptible to the development

Klaus R. Müller, Ph.D., Research Department, Pharmaceuticals Division, CIBA-GEIGY Limited, Basle, Switzerland.

of spontaneous and experimentally induced atherosclerosis. Cell damage was assessed by measuring the rate of ^{3}H-adenine uptake [4].

Methods

Cell Isolation and Conditions of Culture

Endothelial cells were obtained from the thoracic aorta of pigs aged 3 to 6 months. The cell culture method was based on that described by de Bono [5] and Pearson et al. [6]. The aorta was opened longitudinally and the luminal surface was thoroughly rinsed with phosphate-buffered (3 mM) Hanks' balanced salt solution (HBSS) containing 50 IU penicillin per ml and 50 μg streptomycin per ml. The aorta was spread on a metal block with the intima upward, and a sterile metal frame was pressed on top of it so that the endothelium formed the bottom of a trough measuring 15 $\times$ 2 cm. The endothelial cells were loosened by filling the trough with a 0.1% mixture of collagenase/dispase (Boehringer Mannheim) in HBSS and incubating for 15 min at 37°C. The endothelial cells were removed by gently passing a polyester fiber-tipped wood applicator (Falcon) across the intimal surface and dipping it into culture medium.

The cells were centrifuged, washed once with fresh culture medium and then plated into 25 cm^2 tissue-culture flasks (Corning). One thoracic aorta yielded cells for two 25-cm^2 flasks. The culture medium consisted of Waymouth's medium MB 752/1 (Gibco), 20% heat-inactivated fetal calf serum (Gibco), 50 IU penicillin per ml and 50 μg streptomycin per ml.

The cells were subcultured at a 1:2 split after the first 24 h and then every 3 to 4 days when they had reached confluency. Culture medium was not changed in between. For subculturing, the cultures were treated with a mixture of 0.05% trypsin and 0.25% viokase (Gibco) for 2 min at 37°C and the cells were washed twice with Waymouth's medium containing 40% fetal calf serum. At the third or fourth passage, the cells were seeded into 96-well microtest II plates (Falcon) at the nearly confluent density of 3 $\times$ 10^4 cells/well. Experiments were started 2 to 3 days later with a monolayer of quiescent cells.

Cytotoxicity Tests

The ^{51}Cr release assay was performed essentially as described by Harker and Ross [3]. The cells were labeled by adding 5 μCi ^{51}Cr-sodium chromate in 0.1 ml culture medium per well, incubating for 90 min at 37°C, and washing three times with 0.2 ml HBSS. The labeled cells were incubated with 0.2 ml fresh culture medium containing homocysteine thiolactone as appropriate. Release of ^{51}Cr into the medium was measured after different periods of incubation and calculated as a percentage of the maximum release. The latter was determined after twice freezing and thawing the cells. All determinations were done in quadruplicate.

^{3}H-adenine uptake was assayed according to the method of de Bono et al. [4]. The cells in the microwells were incubated for up to 48 h with 0.2 ml culture medium containing homocysteine thiolactone and sulfinpyrazone as appropriate. Fresh medium containing the test compounds was added after 24 h if the cells were incubated for 48 h. After incubation, the cells were washed twice with HBSS. Then 0.1 ml of a mixture containing 0.33 μM adenine, 0.032 μCi 8-^{3}H-adenine, 20 mM glucose and 0.5% bovine serum albumin in HBSS was added, and incubation was continued for 30 min at 37°C. After three washes with HBSS the cells were digested with 0.2 ml 1N NaOH and the radioactivity was determined. All determinations were done in triplicate.

Results

Homocysteine-Induced Cell Damage

In the cytotoxicity test based on the release of ^{51}Cr from prelabeled endothelial cells into the medium, it was found that the addition of homocysteine thiolactone to the culture medium had no effect during the first 6 h of incubation. Incubation with 10 mM homocysteine thiolactone for 24 h was necessary to increase ^{51}Cr release clearly above background (Table 1). Thus, cell damage caused by homocysteine was a rather slow process.

The ^{51}Cr release assay appeared to be not well suited for measuring this process of cell damage, due to a high spon-

Table 1. Homocysteine-Induced Cell Damage
Assessed by ^{51}Cr Release Assay

Homocysteine Thiolactone (mM)	Specific ^{51}Cr Release (%) at			
	2 h	4 h	6 h	24 h
0	5.1 ± 1.6	11.5 ± 0.8	17.3 ± 1.8	61.8 ± 1.9
0.4	7.0 ± 0.6	14.4 ± 0.7	18.3 ± 1.2	66.3 ± 2.6
2	9.2 ± 1.5	15.3 ± 0.6	18.1 ± 1.1	63.3 ± 3.0
10	8.5 ± 1.3	16.2 ± 1.0	22.2 ± 1.4	87.8 ± 2.7

Values are mean ± SE of quadruplicate determinations.

taneous ^{51}Cr leakage, amounting to 60% to 70% within 24 h. Attempts to reduce this spontaneous leakage by replacing fetal calf serum with pig or human serum, or by increasing the concentration of these sera up to 100%, failed. The method of ^{51}Cr release as cytotoxicity test was therefore abandoned and replaced by an assay consisting of measurement of the rate of ^3H-adenine uptake at the end of the incubation period. This latter assay was developed for endothelial cells of pig aorta and has been shown to be well suited to quantify processes of cell damage requiring incubation times of 24 h or more [4].

In the ^3H-adenine uptake assay a time- and concentration-dependent damage of pig endothelial cells by homocysteine thiolactone could be demonstrated (Fig. 1). A concentration of 30 mM homocysteine thiolactone was necessary to reduce adenine uptake significantly within 4 h of incubation. The minimal effective concentration of homocysteine thiolactone decreased to 1 mM when the cells were incubated for 24 h, and it dropped further to 0.1 mM if the incubation period was prolonged to 48 h. Incubation for 24 h with 10 mM homocysteine thiolactone abolished ^3H-adenine uptake almost completely and extensive visible cell rupture occurred.

Effect of Sulfinpyrazone

Except for a slight inhibition at the highest concentration, exposure of the culture to 5×10^{-7} to 5×10^{-4} M sulfinpyrazone alone for 24 h had no effect on ^3H-adenine uptake. Cell damage induced by the presence of homocysteine thiolactone in concentrations between 1 and 10 mM for 24 h was not prevented by 5×10^{-5} or 5×10^{-4} M sulfinpyrazone, and

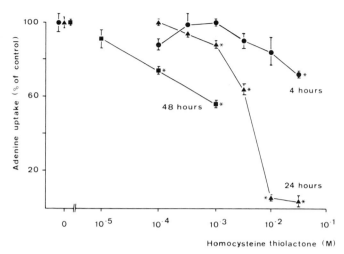

FIG. 1. Homocysteine-induced damage of endothelial cells from pig aorta, as assessed by ^{3}H-adenine uptake. Effect of different incubation periods and different concentrations of homocysteine thiolactone. Points represent means ± SEM of triplicate determinations. *p< 0.05 vs. control.

the slight damage induced by 0.2 to 0.8 mM homocysteine thiolactone within 48 h was not reduced, either by 5×10^{-7} or 5×10^{-6} M sulfinpyrazone (Table 2). Thus, no protection by sulfinpyrazone against homocysteine-induced cell damage could be demonstrated in this *in vitro* system using endothelial cells from pig aorta and ^{3}H-adenine uptake as the cytotoxicity test.

Discussion

The damaging effect of homocysteine on endothelial cells could also be demonstrated with endothelial cells from pig aorta in culture. The concentration range of 1 to 10 mM homocysteine thiolactone that effectively caused cell damage within 24 h was the same as that described by Harker and Ross [3] for endothelial cells from human umbilical vein. Hence, the endothelial cells from both sources show a similar sensitivity towards homocysteine thiolactone *in vitro*.

The finding that sulfinpyrazone in the range of therapeutic concentrations did not protect the pig aorta cells against homocysteine-induced cell damage is at variance with the results of the study with cells from human umbilical vein. No

Table 2. Effect of Sulfinpyrazone on Homocysteine-Induced Cell Damage

Duration of Incubation (h)	Homocysteine Thiolactone (mM)	³H-adenine Uptake (% of Control) Concentration of Sulfinpyrazone (M)				
		0	5×10^{-7}	5×10^{-6}	5×10^{-5}	5×10^{-4}
24	0	100.0 ± 2.8	96.1 ± 1.5	94.8 ± 3.3	97.9 ± 1.6	85.4 ± 0.1
24	1	98.5 ± 4.3			90.2 ± 5.0	
	2	88.0 ± 4.2			80.7 ± 8.4	
	4	70.8 ± 6.3			69.5 ± 7.3	
	8	32.5 ± 2.4			27.4 ± 2.1	
24	2.5	88.0 ± 2.2			92.8 ± 5.6	85.6 ± 4.3
	5	75.5 ± 2.9			69.0 ± 7.8	62.2 ± 4.0
	10	6.4 ± 0.8			8.5 ± 0.7	7.4 ± 0.4
48	0.2	94.1 ± 0.8	93.0 ± 2.5	94.5 ± 1.1		
	0.4	87.7 ± 3.3	86.4 ± 2.3	85.5 ± 3.0		
	0.8	85.2 ± 5.8	87.9 ± 2.4	80.8 ± 2.1		

Values are mean ± SE of triplicate determinations.

explanation for this discrepancy can be given so far. Several possibilities may be considered, as the two *in vitro* systems differ in many respects. In the first place, the cells stem from different species, man and pig. Sulfinpyrazone has proved to be ineffective in a model of atherosclerosis in pigs, whereas antiatherosclerotic activity has been established in rats [7], rabbits [8], and baboons [3]. Thus, species differences may be implicated, and pig endothelium may be insensitive to sulfinpyrazone. Secondly, the cells stem from different kinds of vessels: umbilical vein and thoracic aorta. Furthermore, the pig endothelial cells differ ultrastructurally from the human umbilical vein cells in their total, or almost total, lack of Weibel-Palade bodies [J.L. Gordon, personal communication; 9]. The high rate of spontaneous leakage of ^{51}Cr from pig cells as compared with human cells under similar conditions represents a further difference between these two kinds of cells. Finally, ^{3}H-adenine uptake instead of ^{51}Cr release had to be used as cytotoxocity test, and the possibility cannot be excluded that the two test systems detect different forms of cell damage that are not equally affected by sulfinpyrazone.

The results with the cells from human umbilical vein *in vitro* correlated with the protective effect of sulfinpyrazone in homocystinemic baboons, indicating that the *in vitro* system with human cells might reflect the situation *in vivo* more closely than the system with porcine cells. However, elucidation of the reasons underlying the discrepancy between the two *in vitro* systems may afford a better understanding of the effect of sulfinpyrazone on the endothelium.

References

1. McCully, K.S.: Vascular pathology of homocysteinemia: implications for the pathogenesis of arteriosclerosis. Am. J. Pathol. 56: 111-128, 1969.
2. Harker, L.A., Ross, R., Slichter, S.J. and Scott, C.R.: Homocystine-induced arteriosclerosis: The role of endothelial cell injury and platelet response in its genesis. J. Clin. Invest. 58: 731-741, 1976.
3. Harker, L.A. and Ross, R.: Prevention of homocysteine-induced arteriosclerosis: Sulphinpyrazone endothelial protection. *In* Abe, T. and Sherry, S. (eds.): A New Approach to Reduction of Cardiac Death. Bern: H. Huber, 1979, pp. 59-71.
4. De Bono, D.P., MacIntyre, D.E., White, D.J.G. and Gordon, J.L.: Endothelial adenine uptake as an assay for cell- or complement-mediated cytotoxicity. Immunology 32: 221-226, 1977.

5. De Bono, D.: Effects of cytotoxic sera on endothelium *in vitro*. Nature 252: 83-84, 1974.
6. Pearson, J.D., Olversman, H.J. and Gordon, J.L.: Transport of 5-hydroxytryptamine by endothelial cells. Biochem. Soc. Trans. 5: 1181-1183, 1977.
7. Clopath, P., Horsch, A.K. and Dieterle, W.: Effect of sulfinpyrazone on development of atherosclerosis in various animal models. This volume.
8. Baumgartner, H.R. and Studer, A.: Platelet factors and the proliferation of vascular smooth muscle cells. *In* Schettler, G., Goto, Y., Hata, Y. and Klose, G. (eds.): Atherosclerosis IV. Proc. 4th Int. Symp. Atherosclerosis, Tokyo, 1976. Berlin: Springer-Verlag, 1977, pp. 605-609.
9. Slater, D.N. and Sloan, J.M.: The porcine endothelial cell in tissue culture. Atherosclerosis 21: 259-272, 1975.

Discussion

Dr. McGregor: Dr. Harker, would you like to comment on the discrepancy between your results and those of Dr. Müller?

Dr. Harker: The most obvious concern is to be aware of the difficulties in looking at cells derived from different species. Certainly this has become increasingly apparent in the field of endothelium; bovine endothelial cells behave very differently from human umbilical cells, which are likewise different from porcine and rabbit cells. These differences appear to be quite confusing. For example, there is a difference in sensitivity to endotoxin; bovine endothelial cells are exquisitely sensitive to nanogram amounts, whereas human umbilical-vein endothelial cells resist milligram amounts. Differences in techniques are similarly troublesome.

Dr. McGregor: Do you see any other cause for differences?

Dr. Harker: It would be very difficult to know. Perhaps an exchange of materials would help to clarify the issues.

Mr. Povalski: Have you tried any other pharmacologic interventions in this preparation?

Dr. Müller: No, nothing.

Dr. Mustard: Have you or Dr. Harker tried to use the fluorescein isocyanate method for measuring endothelial injury? Harry Jacobs' group in Minneapolis has used that, and it corroborates the ^{51}Cr-derived data. It would be a useful technique for both of you to use to determine whether you are measuring the same degree of endothelial injury in your respective experiments.

Effect of Sulfinpyrazone on Development of Atherosclerosis in Various Animal Models

P. Clopath, D.Sc., A. K. Horsch, M.D.
and W. Dieterle, Ph.D.

Introduction

The role of platelets during atherogenesis has not been precisely elucidated, but increasing evidence supports the thrombogenic or incrustation hypothesis of atherogenesis [1]. Platelets initiate thrombosis by aggregating at the site of previous vascular injury, and during the process of clotting a factor released from the platelets (PDGF: platelet-derived growth factor) stimulates the proliferation *in vitro* of smooth-muscle cells, the principal cells accumulating in atherosclerotic lesions [2-4].

It has been shown in experimental animals that reduction in platelet count or inhibition of platelet function suppresses the development of atherosclerosis [5-7]. Pigs with von Willebrand's disease, in which platelets cannot adhere effectively to subendothelial surfaces and show decreased retention in glass-bead columns, appear to be protected from the development of atherosclerosis [8]. Moore and co-workers also showed that the full range of atherosclerotic lesions, provoked in rabbits by intraarterial balloon catheterization, can be markedly inhibited or prevented by inducing thrombocytopenia with antiplatelet serum [5, 6]. Similarly, Pick and co-workers recently reported

P. Clopath, D.Sc. and W. Dieterle, Ph.D., Research Department, Pharmacueticals Division, CIBA-GEIGY Limited, Basle, Switzerland; and A. K. Horsch, M.D., Department of Medicine, University of Heidelberg, Heidelberg, Germany.

that aspirin inhibits the development of coronary atherosclerosis in cynomolgus monkeys fed an atherogenic diet [7].

These results suggest that substances which interfere with
platelet adhesion and aggregation might be expected to inhibit
or modify the response to injury and thrombosis [9]. Of
particular interest are the studies carried out with sulfinpyrazone, a well-known platelet-function regulator. It was
found that this drug was capable of inhibiting platelet thrombus
formation. Baumgartner and co-workers demonstrated in *ex-
vivo* flow systems that treatment of rabbits with 40 mg/kg of
sulfinpyrazone resulted in strong inhibition of mural thrombus
formation [10]. Butler and co-workers reported recently that
the thrombocytopenia observed in the Arthus reaction was also
markedly reduced by sulfinpyrazone [11]. In hamsters, Lewis
and Westwick reported that formation of platelet aggregates
produced in an arteriole of the cheek pouch was significantly
reduced by administration of 20 to 65 mg/kg of sulfinpyrazone [12]. These results appear to support a direct and rapid
inhibition of platelet aggregation by the drug.

The present paper summarizes studies of the effect of
sulfinpyrazone on the development of atherosclerotic lesions
carried out in rats, rabbits, and miniature swine. A brief account
is given of the results obtained by Baumgartner and Studer [13]
relating to the effects of treatment with antiplatelet agents on
the volume of the neointima which developed after balloon-
catheter injury in rabbits, and also of the effect of sulfinpyrazone on the development of injury-induced atherosclerotic
lesions in swine. In addition, preliminary observations on the
metabolism of sulfinpyrazone in rabbits and swine are reported,
in an attempt to find clues to the mode of action of the
substance and possible explanations for the species differences
noted.

Material and Methods

Studies in Rats:
Early Atherosclerotic Lesions
of the Rat Aorta

The effect of sulfinpyrazone on the development of early
atherosclerotic lesions of the rat aorta was studied in a group of

10 rats given 160 mg/kg of sulfinpyrazone PO once daily and compared with the results seen in a control group of rats given the vehicle only. Early atherosclerotic lesions were produced by a combination of cholesterol feeding and immunological injury [14]. Cholesterol feeding (4 g cholesterol, 2 g cholate in 100-g pellets) and immunization were started on the same day. For the first immunization an emulsion of equal volumes of horseradish peroxidase (HRP) in saline with Freund's complete adjuvant was injected into the footpads (0.5 mg horseradish peroxidase per animal). On day 52, all rats were immunized again with 0.5 mg HRP IV. Four days later, the rats were killed, blood samples collected, and aortas removed. Tissue sections were always taken from the same area of the aortic arch and lower third of the thoracic aorta. Histology and immuno-cytology were performed double-blind with hematoxylin-eosin, van Gieson, Mason-Galdner, periodic acid-Schiff, and sudan staining. Positive lesion involvement was counted for those vessels showing disruption of the endothelium, enlargement of the subendothelial space, and smooth-muscle cell proliferation. The concentration of anti-HRP antibodies in rat sera was determined by radial immunodiffusion with serial dilutions of rat sera in agarose gel containing different concentrations of HRP (5 to 100 μM HRP/gel) [15]. Total serum and tissue cholesterol concentrations were determined according to previously published methods [14]. Platelet counts were made at the end of the experiment with a Coulter counter. Serum sulfinpyrazone concentrations were determined by the method of Burns et al. [16].

Studies in Rabbits

The effects of sulfinpyrazone and of other platelet-function regulators on the development of the neointima produced by balloon-catheter injury have been described by Baumgartner and Studer [13]. In their studies, the endothelium of the iliac artery was abraded by passing a balloon catheter through the lumen. The volume of the neointima was measured morpho-metrically and expressed as a percentage of media. All dosages tested were given daily by stomach tube, starting on the day before balloon injury. Sulfinpyrazone was given in a daily dosage of 67 mg/kg, aspirin 30 mg/kg daily, and dipyridamole 50 mg/kg twice daily [13].

Studies in Miniature Swine

Sixteen male Göttingen miniature swine (Institut für Zucht-hygiene, Universität Zürich, Zürich, Switzerland) were used. Two groups of eight animals each were fed throughout the course of the drug treatment on a commercial minipig chow (NAFAG AG, Gossau, Switzerland). One group of animals received sulfinpyrazone in a dose of 30 mg/kg twice daily, given as a 0.24% admixture to the minipig chow. The other group received the minipig chow only. In all animals, the abdominal aortic endothelium was injured twice at an interval of 2 weeks according to the technique devised by Baumgartner and recently published by us [17, 18].

All the swine were killed with a captive-bolt gun 4 weeks after the first ballooning. At autopsy, the whole aorta was carefully freed from connective tissue and samples from three segments (aortic arch, thoracic and abdominal aorta) were taken for determination of total cholesterol, collagen, and elastin content, according to previously published methods [17, 18]. A 1.0-cm segment of the abdominal aorta, measured proximal to the trifurcation, was fixed in a 4% neutral formalin and embedded in paraffin. From each segment, ten longitudinal sections of 6-μm thickness were cut and stained with Verhoeff-van Gieson stain. The average intima/media coefficient was determined by means of a manual optical picture analysis system (MOP; Kontron AG, Zürich, Switzerland). The histological section was projected from a Leitz-Orthoplan microscope onto the MOP recording plate. Neointima and media were traced manually with an electronmagnetic pen. The tracing signals were transmitted to a microprocessor, which determined the area of both layers. From each segment the average intima/media (I/M) ratio was calculated, representing the average intimal thickening of the arterial wall.

Metabolic Studies

Single IV 100 mg/kg doses of ^{14}C-sulfinpyrazone were administered to male rabbits (New Zealand White, 2.0 to 2.4 kg) and Göttingen minipigs (18.4 to 20.4 kg). For excretion studies, two rabbits and two minipigs were used. Samples of urine and feces were collected at 24-h intervals over 3 (rabbit) and 4 (minipig) days. At various times up to 24 h after administration, blood was drawn from two additional rabbits and the two minipigs used in the excretion study. From each individual blood sample, plasma was prepared. Total radio-activity was measured in all samples of urine, feces, and plasma [19]. Unchanged sulfinpyrazone and the metabolites G 31442, G 32642, GP 52097 and CGP 17385 (for structures, see Fig. 1) were specifically determined in urine and plasma by means of multiple inverse isotope dilution analysis [19].

Results

Effects of Sulfinpyrazone on Early Atherosclerotic Lesions in Rats

Early atherosclerotic lesions were produced by synergy of immunological injury and cholesterol feeding. Five out of nine control rats had early aortic lesions whereas none of the 10 sulfinpyrazone-treated rats showed changes of the intima (Table 1). In rats given 160 mg of sulfinpyrazone/kg PO, a serum concentration of 140 μg/ml was reached 1 h after treatment.

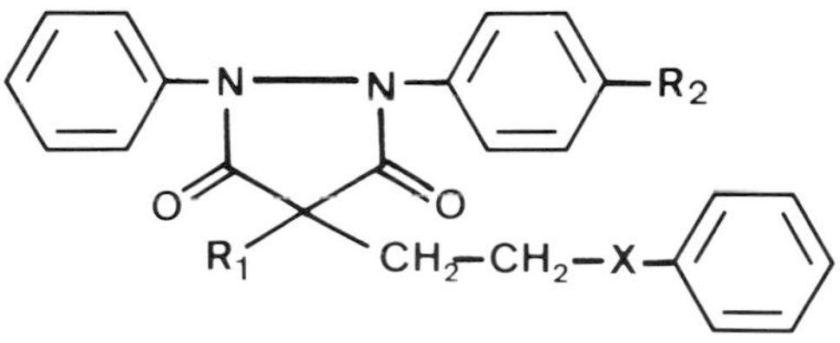

Compound	R_1	R_2	X
G 28 315 (Sulfinpyrazone)	H	H	SO
G 31 442	H	H	SO_2
G 32 642	H	OH	SO
GP 52 097	OH	H	SO
CGP 17385	H	OH	SO_2

FIG. 1. Sulfinpyrazone and known metabolites.

Table 1. Effect of Sulfinpyrazone on Development of Early Atherosclerotic Lesions of the Aorta, Body Weight, and Various Serum Parameters in Rats

Treatment Group	Day of Measurement	No. Rats with Aortic Lesions	Serum Cholesterol (mg/100 ml)	Aortic Cholesterol (µg/mg protein)	Body Weight (g)	Sulf. Serum Conc. (µg/ml)	Antibody Conc. (µg/10 ml)
Control (n = 9)	1		84 ± 15		256 ± 2		
	21		209 ± 45				
	51		179 ± 41				2.69 ± 0.72
	56	5/9	164 ± 41	4.43 ± 0.79	364 ± 15	0	9.77 ± 6.24
Sulfinpyrazone-treated (n = 10)	1		71 ± 13		250 ± 12		
	21		256 ± 103				
	51		149 ± 35				2.14 ± 0.48
	56	0/10	161 ± 42	4.54 ± 0.90	346 ± 38	144 ± 41	8.24 ± 3.12

Rats were given sulfinpyrazone 160 mg/kg daily. Results are mean ± SEM.

The drug did not affect the cholesterol concentration in the serum and aorta, nor were differences in the appearance of serum anti-HRP antibodies observable.

Effects of Sulfinpyrazone, Aspirin, and Dipyridamole on Intimal Thickening in Rabbits [13]

Intraarterial balloon catheterization caused intimal thickening of the iliac artery of rabbits. The effects of sulfinpyrazone, aspirin, and dipyridamole on the volume of neointima (as percentage of media) 14 days after ballooning of the iliac artery are summarized in Table 2. Sulfinpyrazone, in a daily dosage of 67 mg/kg, caused a significant reduction of the neointima by approximately 30%, whereas neither aspirin nor dipyridamole influenced the development of atherosclerotic lesions in rabbits.

Effects of Sulfinpyrazone on Injury-Induced Atherosclerotic Lesions in Miniature Swine

Repeated ballooning of the abdominal aorta produced severe, progressive intimal lesions. The effect of sulfinpyrazone on the intima/media ratio is summarized in Table 3. Treatment

Table 2. Effect of Antiplatelet Agents on the Volume of the Neointima
Developing after Balloon Catheter Injury in
Rabbit Iliac Artery within 2 Weeks

	No. of Rabbits	Volume of Neointima (% of media)
All controls	18	68.0 ± 5.6
Control I	6	64.0 ± 7.9
Dipyridamole (50 mg/kg twice daily)	7	65.7 ± 7.6
Control II	5	76.9 ± 12.9
Aspirin (30 mg/kg daily)	3	97.1 ± 39.0
Control III	7	65.2 ± 9.5
Sulfinpyrazone (67 mg/kg daily)	9	40.6 ± 9.5*

Reprinted, with permission, from [13].
Drugs were fed daily by stomach tube, starting the day before balloon injury. Results are mean ± SEM. *Significantly different from corresponding control III ($p < 0.05$) and from all controls ($p < 0.01$; Student's t test).

Table 3. Effect of Sulfinpyrazone on Development of Atherosclerosis
in Miniature Swine: Intimal Thickening and Serum Cholesterol

Treatment Group	n	I/M Ratio*	Serum Cholesterol (mg/100 ml)
Control	8	0.22 ± 0.04	55.30 ± 2.86
Sulfinpyrazone	8	0.29 ± 0.09	49.81 ± 3.45

Swine were given sulfinpyrazone, 30 mg/kg twice daily. Results are mean ±
SEM. *I/M ratio = area of the neointima : area of the media.

of minipigs with 30 mg/kg of sulfinpyrazone twice daily caused
no reduction of the I/M ratio. It also had no effect on the
collagen, elastin, or cholesterol contents of the aortic arch and
thoracic and abdominal (ballooned) aorta (Table 4). In addition, the drug had no effect on the serum cholesterol
concentration of the minipigs (Table 3). Analysis of the
lipoprotein pattern revealed that none of the individual lipoprotein fractions, i.e., very-low-density, low-density, or high-
density lipoproteins, was significantly affected by the drug (K.
Müller and P. Clopath, unpublished results).

Metabolic Studies in Rabbits

Concentrations in Plasma. The plasma concentration of
total ^{14}C and of the individually determined metabolites after
IV administration of 100 mg/kg ^{14}C-sulfinpyrazone to rabbits
are given in Figure 2A as semilogarithmic plots (average of n =
2). Total radioactivity in plasma slowly decreased from 552
μg/ml (19 min) to 223 μg/ml (6 h), but rose again to 260 μg/ml
after 8 h. At 24 h after dosing, a level of 41 μg/ml was
measured. In contrast, the time course of the concentration of
unchanged sulfinpyrazone was characterized by a linear decay.
The plasma level declined at first from 532 μg/ml (19 min) to
178 μg/ml after 3 h with a half-life of 2 h, and thereafter with a
second half-life of 3.2 h to 2.3 μg/ml after 24 h. The sulfone
metabolite G 31 442 showed a concentration minimum of 8.7
μg/ml after 3 h and a maximum of 16.8 μg/ml at 6 h. For the
p-hydroxy metabolite G 32 642, the highest level was measured
after 30 min (15.2 μg/ml), then the concentration decreased to
0.9 μg/ml after 24 h. The metabolites GP 52 097 and CGP 17
385 were present at low levels not exceeding 2.8 μg/ml beyond

Table 4. Effect of Sulfinpyrazone on Development of Atherosclerosis
in Miniature Swine: Chemical Composition of the Aorta

Treatment Group	n	Collagen (% dry wt.)	Collagen ($\mu g/mm^2$)	Elastin (% dry wt.)	Elastin ($\mu g/mm^2$)	Cholesterol (% dry wt.)
Aortic Arch						
Control	8	14.46 ± 0.50	ND	50.04 ± 1.49	ND	0.29 ± 0.02
Sulfinpyrazone	8	14.40 ± 0.51	ND	49.31 ± 0.69	ND	0.24 ± 0.01
Thoracic Aorta						
Control	8	16.83 ± 0.38	62.04 ± 3.52	52.25 ± 1.68	191.70 ± 8.95	0.27 ± 0.01
Sulfinpyrazone	8	17.64 ± 0.78	61.38 ± 2.73	51.38 ± 0.73	186.78 ± 6.68	0.24 ± 0.02
Abdominal Aorta						
Control	6	42.88 ± 1.25	138.61 ± 10.72	19.03 ± 0.81	62.76 ± 5.57	0.44 ± 0.03
Sulfinpyrazone	8	35.57 ± 4.70	109.84 ± 19.19	20.59 ± 0.70	57.59 ± 6.79	0.42 ± 0.04

Swine were given sulfinpyrazone, 30 mg/kg twice daily. Results are mean ± SEM. ND = Not Determined.

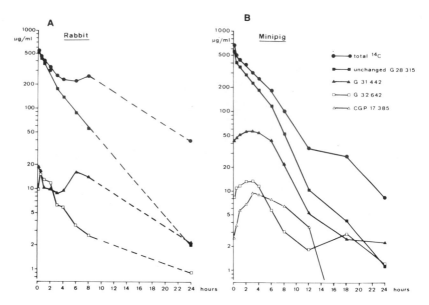

FIG. 2. Concentration of total radioactivity, of unchanged sulfinpyrazone (G 28 315), of the sulfone metabolite (G 31 442), of the p-hydroxy metabolite (G 32 642), and the p-hydroxy-sulfone metabolite (CGP 17 385) after IV dosing of 100 mg/kg ^{14}C-labeled sulfinpyrazone to rabbits (A) and minipigs (B) (n = 2) as semilogarithmic plots. The 4-hydroxy metabolite GP 52 097 was present at low levels not exceeding 4 μg/ml at times beyond 30 min and was therefore not included in the graph.

30 min. Judging from the area under the concentration-time curve (AUC, 0 to 24 h), these two compounds accounted for only 0.4% and 0.2% of total ^{14}C. The AUC values for sulfinpyrazone, the sulfone metabolite, and the p-hydroxy metabolite correspond to 42.6%, 5.0%, and 1.8%, respectively, leaving 50% of the plasma radioactivity unidentified (Fig. 3A).

   Compounds Excreted in Urine. Following intravenous administration of 100 mg/kg ^{14}C-sulfinpyrazone to the rabbit, on an average 96.3% of the dose was recovered in the excreta within 3 days. The renal excretion was predominant, since 70.0% was eliminated in the urine and 26.3% in the feces. Analysis of the pooled urine (0 to 48 h) for unchanged sulfinpyrazone and the metabolites showed that 65.0% of the urinary radioactivity was present as sulfinpyrazone, 6.9% as G 31 442, 3.4% as G 32 642, and 1.5% as CGP 17 385 (Fig. 3A).

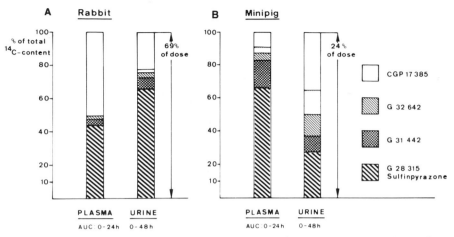

FIG. 3. Comparison of the quantities of sulfinpyrazone and individual sulfinpyrazone metabolites in plasma and urine of rabbits (A) and minipigs (B) following a single IV dose of 100 mg/kg ^{14}C-labeled sulfinpyrazone (n = 2).

Only 0.2% was accounted for by the 4-hydroxy compound GP 52 097. Thus, the sum of the specifically determined compounds covers 77.0% of total ^{14}C-substances in urine.

Metabolic Studies in Miniature Swine

Concentrations in Plasma. The plasma levels of total ^{14}C and of the individually determined compounds in minipigs after a 100 mg/kg dose IV are given in Figure 2B as semilogarithmic plots (average of n = 2). Total radioactivity in plasma declined from 662 μg/ml (10 min) to 8.4 μg/ml (24 h). The concentration of intact sulfinpyrazone rapidly decreased from 572 μg/ml after 10 min to 1.2 μg/ml after 24 h. An apparent half-life of about 3 h was calculated from the results, though the decay was not strictly linear (Fig. 3B). For the sulfone metabolite G 31 442, the p-hydroxy metabolite G 32 642, and the p-hydroxy-sulfone metabolite CGP 17 385, peak concentrations of 57.4 μg/ml, 13.4 μg/ml, and 9.7 μg/ml, respectively, were reached within 3 h. Only the p-hydroxy metabolite showed a second, flat maximum of 3.0 μg/ml after 18 h. For all three metabolites low levels (<2.5 μg/ml) were measured 24 h after dosing. The plasma AUC values for sulfinpyrazone and the sulfone metabolite corresponded to 65.8% and 16.9%, respectively, of that of total ^{14}C-substances; the values for the metabolites G 32 642 and CGP 17 385 accounted for 4.3% and 3.3%. The 4-hydroxy compound was present in low amounts; the AUC value was 0.6%. Totally, these specifically determined compounds cover 90.9% of the plasma radioactivity (Fig. 3B).

Compounds Excreted in Urine. Ater IV administration of ^{14}C-sulfinpyrazone (100 mg/kg) to the minipig, on an average 93.8% of the dose was recovered in the excreta within 4 days. The biliary excretion was favored, since 68.6% was eliminated in the feces and 25.2% in the urine. The results obtained by multiple inverse isotope dilution analysis of the pooled urine (0 to 48 h) showed that 27.1% of the total ^{14}C-content was present as unchanged sulfinpyrazone (Fig. 3B). Of the metabolites, G 31 442 corresponded to 9.7%, G 32 642 to 13.3%, and CGP 17 385 to 14.6%. The percentage of the 4-hydroxy compound was 0.7%. Thus, the sum of these compounds equals 65.4% of the radioactive substances excreted in urine (Fig. 3B).

Discussion

The present study was undertaken to determine whether sulfinpyrazone has any primary preventive effect on the development of atherosclerosis. The results indicate that although the substance does display antiatherosclerotic activity in rats and rabbits, it does not in swine.

In rats, sulfinpyrazone was effective in preventing early lesions induced by cholesterol feeding and immunization, as manifested by the decrease in number of aortas covered with early atherosclerotic plaques. These results are similar to those published by Vaessen and co-workers, who reported on the effect of sulfinpyrazone on the degree of vascular lesions and survival of cardiac allografts in rats [20]. They showed that treatment of rats with 160 mg/kg of sulfinpyrazone decreased the severity of intimal thickening in heart allografts and slightly prolonged the time before the grafts were rejected.

Sharma and co-workers reported that sulfinpyrazone was effective in preventing hyperacute rejection of kidney and heart allografts in dogs [21]. Vascular injury and platelet aggregation in the kidney were also markedly reduced. Sulfinpyrazone was also found to be effective in preventing endothelial cell injury and atherosclerosis [22]. In studies *in vitro* these authors showed that sulfinpyrazone in concentrations of 10^{-6} to 10^{-8} mM, incubated with ^{51}Cr-labeled human endothelial cells, reduced the ^{51}Cr release induced by 10 mM of homocysteine. *In vivo*, they found that baboons rendered homocysteinemic developed arteriosclerosis, and that treatment of these animals with sulfinpyrazone resulted in minimal loss of endothelium, normalization of the pathologically shortened platelet survival time, and a significant decrease in intimal lesion formation [22].

The studies in rabbits by Baumgartner and Studer showed sulfinpyrazone to be effective in preventing lesions caused by ballooning, whereas neither aspirin nor dipyridamole had any such effect [13]. In contrast, in our studies with minipigs sulfinpyrazone was found to be ineffective in preventing myointimal thickening following repeated arterial mechanical injury. Our metabolic studies showed that there are distinct differences as to the fate of sulfinpyrazone in rabbits and miniature swine. Determination of total radioactivity, unchanged sulfinpyrazone, and four known metabolites in plasma showed that in the minipig sulfinpyrazone was predominant among all radioactive compounds. In the rabbit, as can be deduced from the plasma concentration curves (Fig. 2A), unidentified metabolites appear, since the increase of total ^{14}C-substances cannot be explained by the concentrations of the specifically measured compounds. The plasma levels of the known metabolites were low in both species, with the exception of the sulfone metabolite G 31 442 in the minipig.

In fact, the sum of the plasma AUC values of sulfinpyrazone and the metabolites accounted for 50.0% of the plasma radioactivity in the rabbit. In the minipig, 90.9% of the AUC is covered by known compounds. This again demonstrates the occurrence of quantitatively important plasma metabolites in the rabbit. The unidentified metabolites may be responsible for the prolonged inhibition of prostaglandin synthesis-dependent platelet functions observed in the rabbit [23].

The different pathways of biotransformation of sulfinpyrazone in rabbits and minipigs are evident, too, from the renally excreted compounds. In the rabbit, unchanged sulfinpyrazone covered 65% of urinary radioactivity and the metabolites formed by oxidation processes (G 31 442, G 32 642, GP 52 097 and CGP 17 385) 12%, whereas in the minipig less sulfinpyrazone (27.1%) and more of these metabolites (38.2%) were found. Though the route of excretion was different in the two species (rabbit, mainly renal; minipig, mainly biliary), the results demonstrate that oxidative pathways are more important in the minipig than in the rabbit.

In summary, the results obtained suggest that the effectiveness of sulfinpyrazone in prevention of atherosclerosis may depend partly on its biotransformation and possibly on the appearance of yet unidentified metabolites. The identification of these metabolites is in progress. Data so far obtained indicate that the thioether analog of sulfinpyrazone (G 25 671) is a plasma metabolite in rabbits. The same metabolite was also isolated from guinea pig plasma [24]. Studies are now under way to ascertain whether G 25 671 itself has antiatherosclerotic activity.

Recently, Rüegg reported on the antithrombotic effect of sulfinpyrazone and its metabolites in rabbits. He found that preparation G 25 671 was about 30 times as potent as sulfinpyrazone in protection against arachidonate-induced pulmonary embolism [25].

Müller has reported that sulfinpyrazone has no protective effect against homocysteine-induced damage in cells from pig aorta [26], which is in contrast to the findings of Harker and Ross with endothelial cells from human umbilical veins [22]. Therefore, the usefulness of the miniature swine, as well as endothelial cells from pig aorta, for testing the efficacy of sulfinpyrazone in atherosclerosis needs further investigation.

Acknowledgments

We thank M. Erard, R. Bachmann, and K. Handloser for their technical assistance; Dr. G. Bullock for processing the tissue for histology; and Dr. S. Brechbühler for serum sulfinpyrazone analysis. The encouragement of Dr. P. A. Desaulles throughout this work is gratefully acknowledged. Particular thanks are due to Drs. Baumgartner and Studer for permission to reprint their findings.

References

1. Duguid, J.B.: The Dynamic of Atherosclerosis. Aberdeen: Aberdeen University Press, 1976.
2. Ross, R., Glomset, J., Kariya, B. and Harker, L.: A platelet-dependent serum factor that stimulates the proliferation of arterial smooth muscle cells in vitro. Proc. Natl. Acad. Sci. U.S.A. 71: 1207-1210, 1974.
3. Ross, R. and Glomset, J.A.: Atherosclerosis and the arterial smooth muscle cell. Science 1332-1339, 1973.
4. Haust, M.D.: The morphogenesis and fate of potential and early atherosclerotic lesions in man. Hum. Pathol. 2: 1-29, 1971.
5. Moore, S., Friedman, R.J., Singal, D.P., Gouldie, J. and Blajchman, M.A.: Inhibition of injury-induced thromboatherosclerotic lesions by anti-platelet serum in rabbits. Throm. Haemostas. 35: 70-81, 1976.
6. Friedman, R.J., Stemerman, M.B., Wenz, B., Morre, S., Gaudie, J., Gent, M., Tiell, M.C. and Spaet, T.H.: The effect of thrombocytopenia on experimental arteriosclerotic lesion formation in rabbits. J. Clin. Invest. 60: 1191-1201, 1977.
7. Pick, R., Chediak, J. and Glick, G.: Aspirin inhibits development of coronary atherosclerosis in cynomolgus monkey (*Macaca fascicularis*) fed an atherogenic diet. J. Clin. Invest. 63: 158-162, 1979.
8. Fuster, V., Bowie, E.J.W., Lewis, J.C., Fass, D.N., Owen, C.A. and Brown, A.L.: Resistance to arteriosclerosis in pigs with von Willebrand's disease. J. Clin. Invest. 61: 722-730, 1978.
9. Packham, M.A. and Mustard, J.F.: Clinical pharmacology of platelets. Blood 50: 555-573, 1977.
10. Baumgartner, H.R., Muggli, R., Tschopp, T.B. and Turitto, U.T.: Platelet adhesion, release and aggregation in flowing blood — Effects of surface properties and platelet function. Thromb. Haemostas. 35: 124-138, 1976.
11. Butler, K.D., Pay, G.F. and White, A.M.: A comparison between sulfinpyrazone and other drugs on the thrombocytopenia of the Arthus reaction in the guinea pig. Br. J. Pharmacol. 57: 411, 1976.
12. Lewis, G.P. and Westwick, J.: An *in vivo* model for studying arterial thrombosis. *In* Mitchell, J.R.A. and Domenet, J.G. (eds.): Thromboembolism — A New Approach to Therapy. New York: Academic Press, 1977, pp. 40-54.
13. Baumgartner, H.R. and Studer, A.: Platelet factors and the proliferation of vascular smooth muscle cells. *In* Schettler, G., Goto, Y., Hata, Y., Klose, G. (eds.): Atherosclerosis. IV. Proc. 4th Intl. Symp. Atheroscl., Tokyo, 1976. Berlin: Springer-Verlag, 1977, pp. 605-609.
14. Horsch, A.K., Kuhlman, W.D., Bleyl, U. and Salomon, J.C.: Early atherosclerotic lesions in rat aorta. Res. Exp. Med. (Berl.) 173: 251-259.
15. Mancini, G., Vaerman, J.P., Carbonara, A.V. and Haermans, J.F.: A single radial diffusion method for the immunological quantitation of proteins. *In* Peters, H. (ed.): Protides of Biological Fluids, Vol. II. London: Pergamon Press, 1964, p. 370.

16. Burns, J.J., Yü, T.F., Ritterbrand, A., Perel, J.M., Gutman, A.B. and Brodie, B.B.: A potent new uricosuric agent, the sulfonide metabolite of the phenylbutazone analog, G 25 671. J. Pharmacol. Exp. Ther. 119: 418-426.
17. Clopath, P.: Rapid production of advanced atherosclerosis in swine. Artery 3: 429-438, 1977.
18. Clopath, P.: Arteriosclerotic and atherosclerotic lesions induced in swine by single and repeated endothelial cell injury. Artery 4: 275-288, 1978.
19. Dieterle, W., Faigle, J.W., Mory, H., Richter, W.J. and Theobald, W.: Biotransformation and pharmacokinetics of sulfinpyrazone (Anturan®) in man. Eur. J. Clin. Pharmacol. 9: 135-145, 1975.
20. Vaessen, L.M.B., Benthuis, F., Hesse, C.J. and Lameizer, L.D.F.: Effect of sulfinpyrazone (Anturane) on degree of vascular lesions and survival of cardiac allograft in rats. Transplant. Proc. 9: 993-996, 1977.
21. Sharma, H.M., Moore, S., Merrick, H.W. and Smith, M.R.: Platelets in early hyperacute allograph rejection in kidneys and their modification by sulfinpyrazone therapy. Am. J. Pathol. 66: 445-460, 1972.
22. Harker, L.A. and Ross, R.: Prevention of homocysteine-induced arteriosclerosis: Sulphinpyrazone endothelial protection. In Abe, T. and Sherry, S. (eds.): A New Approach to Reduction of Cardiac Death. Bern: H. Huber, 1979, pp. 59-71.
23. Buchanan, M.R., Rosenfeld, J. and Hirsh, J.: The prolonged effect of sulfinpyrazone on collagen-induced platelet aggregation in vivo. Thromb. Res. 13: 883-892, 1978.
24. Butler, K.D., Dieterle, W., Maguire, E.D., Pay, G.F., Wallis, R.B. and White, A.M.: Sustained effects of sulfinpyrazone. This volume.
25. Rüegg, M.: Antithrombotic effects of sulfinpyrazone in animals: Influence on fibronolysis and sodium arachidonate-induced pulmonary embolism. Pharmacology 14: 522-536, 1976.
26. Müller, K.R.: Lack of protective effect of sulfinpyrazone on endothelial cells from pig aorta in culture. This volume.

Discussion

Dr. Robson: I recently heard a paper by Kornetsky, who was trying to induce atherosclerosis in rats by feeding them high-lipid diets and modifying thyroid function. To his surprise no atherosclerotic lesions occurred in the aorta at all; they were all restricted to the mesentery artery. You mentioned the study in the cynomulgus monkey, in which aspirin had a positive effect. Those investigators also found no effect of aspirin in the aorta; it was restricted to the coronary vessels. Is it conceivable that one could have missed a beneficial effect of Anturane merely by not looking at the coronary vessels? I'm not suggesting you use ballooning, but it's the coronary vessels, not the aorta, where the events occur in a heart attack.

Dr. Clopath: Yes, I certainly agree that other studies with other techniques should be done as well.

Dr. Cargill: We've been studying effects of sulfinpyrazone on the PGI_2 synthesis, and a difficult problem has been finding the best way to express PGI_2 production. We have avoided using weights of any description, because of variations in thickness of aortic tissue. Instead, we used surface area to determine linear production of PGI_2. Do you think the data on your animals would differ if you had used surface area to determine the amount of PGI_2 that was synthesized?

Dr. Clopath: In atherosclerotic tissue it was unwise to express prostacyclin generation per milligram of wet weight, but that is the method we used at first. Now we are punching out pieces of aorta of equal surface area. We have remeasured prostacyclin generation and again found a decrease with both drugs. In the thoracic aorta, where ballooning is not used, our measurement per milligram of wet weight is still valid; nonetheless we have reexpressed it per surface area. With both drugs prostacyclin generation is decreased; it's also decreased by 50% by simply ballooning.

Dr. McDonald: Your study of the sulfinpyrazone metabolites appears to tie in quite nicely with the differences in effects on atherogenesis, but have you any explanation for the species difference in the aspirin effect? In some of the experiments in which aspirin was without effect, was it given less often than twice in 24 h?

Dr. Clopath: Yes, in his study Dr. Baumgartner gave 30 mg/kg once daily, and in our study in pigs the animals were treated with 30 mg/kg twice daily.

Dr. McDonald: This could be an important difference.

Platelet–Vessel Wall Interaction: General Discussion

Maurice McGregor, M.D., Moderator

Dr. Oliver: I am troubled by the loose usage of the word "atherosclerosis." We have had discussion of antibody-induced lesions, cholesterol-induced lesions, balloon trauma, laser lesions, homocysteine lesions and others, but there is no common denominator between these different types of lesions. Moreover, we have had discussion of rats, rabbits, swine, dogs, and monkeys with various types of extrapolation to man. This is quite unjustified. In relation to experimental atherosclerosis in these species, the high density/low density lipoprotein (HDL/LDL) ratio is critical for the induction of cholesterol lesions in the intimal area. This was learned 20 years ago in terms of experimental atherosclerosis. For example, Pick and Stamler in Chicago were particularly interested in chicks in which they could produce atheroma rapidly with 1% of cholesterol in the diet, and these birds had virtually no HDL present. There are fundamental, well-recognized, well-described differences in lipoprotein metabolism among these species. Perhaps the findings of Drs. Harker, Müller, and Clopath do not differ greatly, if you consider that atherosclerosis, as described here, is the result of five or six different insults in five or six different species.

Aspirin has an effect on cholesterol synthesis, and sulfinpyrazone, so far as I know, does not. It was shown some 12 years ago that the incorporation of ^{14}C-mevalonic acid into cholesterol can be blocked by aspirin. Aspirin also has an antilipolytic effect, which is not dissimilar from that of nicotinic acid. I don't think that sulfinpyrazone has either of these two effects. We should bear in mind that aspirin and sulfinpyrazone have effects other than those on platelets.

Dr. Clopath: That's the reason I used the swine as my model of atherosclerosis. Normolipemic swine have a lipoprotein distribution very similar to man. In normolipemic animals treated with either aspirin or sulfinpyrazone, Dr. Müller and I measured all the individual lipoproteins, and we could not find significant differences in any of them. We do use various species, but perhaps that is necessary in atherosclerosis research. It's a difficult disease to understand, and perhaps by making a puzzle with various animal models we will finally find a clue. In addition, we should do regression studies. If we have an interesting lesion with histologic characteristics very similar to man, and we can bring it to regression with various drug treatments, we have a much better situation to study. This is a large undertaking, especially with swine; they're big animals, expensive, and difficult to handle. Regression studies with swine on a regular diet have taken me two years to complete, and an analysis of the results will take another three years.

Dr. McGregor: Would anybody else like to respond to Dr. Oliver's concern that we are calling the lesions we're causing "atherosclerosis"?

Dr. Minick: I would like to respond to that. One of the problems with atherosclerosis is that we tend to consider it as a disease process, and it isn't. It's a type of tissue change, and the fact that you can induce atherosclerosis by several different processes that result in a chronic scarred fat-containing artery really supports this. In man, also, atherosclerosis may indeed come about in many ways. In experiments with diet-induced atherosclerosis in nonhuman primates, very carefully done by a group at Bowman Gray School of Medicine, over a 3-year period the correlation of the extent of atherosclerosis with the serum cholesterol concentration in those animals is always somewhat less and sometimes much less than 0.4. This suggests that a large portion of the variation, even in those experiments, can be accounted for by factors other than serum cholesterol concentration. One could draw an analogy with the changes one sees in the kidney in glomerular nephritis. The end-stage kidney is reached through very many different pathways, yet to the pathologist all end-stage kidneys look alike.

Dr. Mustard: In regard to the proliferation of smooth muscle cells in the intima, the experiments of Baumgartner were done in the rabbit iliac artery. We did the experiments in the rabbit aorta, stripping off the endothelium with a balloon catheter after treating the animal with sulfinpyrazone. When we studied the animal in the acute phase, we could not demonstrate any effect of sulfinpyrazone on the amount of platelet material that accumulated on the wall. In *in vitro* experiments we could not demonstrate an effect of this drug on the release reaction of the platelets that adhered to the walls. Therefore the full effect of the mitogen should be felt on the wall despite treatment with sulfinpyrazone. We then did experiments with Sean Moore using morphometric methods, and indeed there was no difference in the amount of smooth muscle cell proliferation over 14 days between the sulfinpyrazone-treated and untreated animals. Thus our results differ from Baumgartner's and agree with those of Dr. Clopath's aortic experiments in pigs. The question that arises is whether in experiments in the iliac arteries, because the blood hits a bifurcation, the flow effects lead to a different result. There may well be more platelet accumulation following injury in the iliac vessels than on the aorta, where there is just a thin layer on the surface. Possibly in Baumgartner's experiments there were platelet aggregates on top of adherent platelets, and the sulfinpyrazone in those experiments was therefore diminishing the thrombus component and consequently the amount of mitogen. Have you tried experiments with the iliac vessels in the pig to see if a sulfinpyrazone effect occurs there?

Dr. Clopath: No, but I could still do them. As far as iliac arteries are concerned, regression occurs in rabbits after ballooning in iliac arteries but not in the aorta. I have measured collagen elastin after a single mechanical trauma in the aorta, and after 2 years I have not found any regression at all. In the iliac arteries, however, the lesions do regress. Different arteries of different origins behave differently. In Glick's study, which I mentioned before, the aspirin effect occurred in the coronary arteries but not in the aorta. Of course, it is more important to find it there than in the aorta, if we think of atherosclerosis as an underlying disease which could cause mortality and morbidity.

Dr. Sherry: I was impressed with your observations on the differences in biotransformation in the rabbit as compared to the swine. My question is, what is known about the biotransformation in man?

Dr. Clopath: I don't have the data on IV biotransformation in man because they are still being determined, but I do have unpublished results of biotransformation studies in various animals. We have determined the area under the curve at 24 h after injection of 100 mg/kg of ^{14}C-labeled sulfinpyrazone in plasma. In the rhesus monkey, a little more than 80% were identifiable metabolites and 20%, phantom metabolite; that's the system in which Dr. Harker finds that sulfinpyrazone prevents lesion formation in the homocystinemic baboon. In the minipig, 90% were identifiable metabolites and only 10% phantom metabolite; in this laboratory animal I found that sulfinpyrazone was ineffective in prevention of injury-induced atherosclerotic lesions. In beagle dogs, biotransformation of sulfinpyrazone is similar to that in man; to my knowledge, nobody has yet studied the effect of sulfinpyrazone in this laboratory animal. In rabbits, there were 50% identifiable metabolites, and 50% phantom metabolite. Preliminary results revealed that the phantom metabolite might be the thioether analog of sulfinpyrazone (G 25671). Moreover, Dr. Baumgartner's studies showed that sulfinpyrazone is most effective in preventing injury-induced lesions in rabbits — a finding which could be due to the transformation of sulfinpyrazone to G 25671. In guinea pigs, as we have heard this morning, sulfinpyrazone was a very effective platelet function regulator. We could identify the reduced compound in guinea pig plasma as being the thioether analog of sulfinpyrazone (G 25671). In rats this metabolite appears to about 15%. In the rat studies that we carried out, early lesions were induced by circulating immune complexes, and perhaps the appearance of 15% of an active metabolite is enough to prevent those lesion formations. Last but not least, in man, we have data only on kinetics of oral dosage, and it's not appropriate to compare them directly with kinetics obtained after IV administration of the drug. Those data were published by Dieterle and co-workers (Europ. J. Clin. Invest. 13: 257, 1975). He found 95% identifiable metabolites and 5% unidentifiable metabolite, which might be the G 25671.

In man one can assume that if 5% of the sulfinpyrazone is converted to G 25671 that might be enough to show the interesting effects seen after 8 months in the Anturane Reinfarction Trial study. All these biotransformation data were collected during the past month and they need to be verified.

Dr. McDonald: How would the effects of sulfinpyrazone or, in some cases, aspirin on these early lesions of atherosclerosis (or some kind of injury to the artery) relate to the apparent clinical effect on the prevention of sudden death?

Dr. Clopath: A very good question. One of our goals should be to find an animal model of sudden death, after first arriving at a complete understanding of the pathogenesis of the disease process; then we might be able to assess whether a drug acts to prevent sudden death independently of an eventual effect on the arterial wall.

Platelet-Vessel Wall Interaction: Chairman's Summary

Maurice McGregor, M.D.

We have met to review several new pieces of a fascinating jigsaw puzzle, and as we are presented with them, we frantically try to fit some of the new pieces together into a coherent pattern which might complement our existing knowledge. In this, I believe, we have not been very successful.

However, in doing a jigsaw puzzle there is a stage at which it helps to make a guess at what the final picture is going to be. Even if this is quite a wild guess, some idea of overall pattern helps you to look for missing bits — green grass here, blue sky there — and put them together more speedily. In this sense, let us spend a few minutes trying to guess something about the overall picture and what it may look like when we have more of the parts.

First of all, we should try to define more sharply some of our terms. The disease which we loosely call coronary atherosclerosis is a process consisting of several stages. We should distinguish clearly between two of them.

The first is atheroma. This is characterized by a thickening of the vessel wall, an increase in several elements including the muscle, and deposits of cholesterol. This disease is probably caused by several factors of which damage to vascular endothelium and the presence of high levels of low-density lipoprotein in the blood are clearly important. Three of the papers have told us how experimental atherosclerosis can be caused by artificial endothelial damage, and they have shown the extra-

Maurice McGregor, M.D., Physician-in-Chief, Royal Victoria Hospital; Professor of Medicine, McGill University, Montreal, Canada.

ordinary protective influence of sulfinpyrazone in some of these models.

In the coronary circulation the consequence of this thickening of the vessel wall is significant encroachment on the lumen. When coronary narrowing has become sufficiently severe, the patient experiences angina. This disease, "Heberden's angina" or "stable angina," is, at first, provoked only by stress. Angina does not occur at rest until the ischemic threshold has fallen so low that even the slightest effort precipitates an attack. Even then attacks are stress-induced. The mortality of this disease is around 3% per year.

Every now and then this fairly benign and predictable disease suddenly changes its nature, and the clinical syndrome of stable angina pectoris is replaced by the syndrome of unstable angina. This event, let us suppose, is the consequence of the rupture of an atheromatous plaque such that there is a breach in the endothelial surface.

Once the plaque ruptures, the normal clotting mechanisms come into action. Here too, we should distinguish between at least two stages in a many-stage process. The first is the interaction between the vessel wall and the circulating platelets which causes the latter to coalesce over the endothelial breach, and the second is the reaction between platelets which causes the plug to continue growing long after the breach in the endothelium has been covered. While the former is thought to be a consequence of the interaction between the exposed collagen and the platelet (although Born points out that the collagen-platelet reaction is too slow to account for this), the second is a consequence of release of thromboxane and ADP by those platelets which have already coalesced. Since there appear to be two distinct steps to this reaction, a vessel wall-platelet interaction and a platelet-platelet interaction, it is not too surprising that an intervention should affect one step only. The exhibition of sulfinpyrazone to the traumatized small vessels shown to us by Wiedeman appeared, to the eye of this observer, to be affecting primarily the platelet-platelet interaction, at least to a greater extent than the platelet-vessel wall reaction.

The pathophysiological events associated with rupture of an atherosclerotic plaque can then follow several potential routes.

Platelet plugs may build up over the rupture site and embolize to the peripheral coronary circulation causing arrhythmias, one of which may be fatal. Alternatively the platelet activation may initiate the whole clotting cascade, causing a coronary thrombosis and a myocardial infarction. Finally, with the passage of time the ruptured plaque site may again endothelialize. However, until this happens, unstable angina replaces the stable, relatively benign form of angina pectoris. In the absence of any form of stress, spontaneous anginal attacks occur at rest. Whether this is a consequence of coronary spasm initiated by thromboxane derived from the platelet plug as suggested by Masseri and his co-workers, or whether it is due to the intermittent formation and dislodgement of plugs along the lines of the model developed by Folts, I do not know. But the disease is characterized by spontaneous episodes of pain coming on at rest. It carries a high mortality, and the high risk of death persists whether myocardial infarction takes place or not.

Not only, then, does "coronary artery disease" have two distinct stages, the atheromatous stage and the platelet thrombotic stage, but, from the evidence presented herein, sulfinpyrazone seems to be the "right medicine" for both. Certainly, we've seen that it may protect the endothelium, and hence if endothelial damage is a precursor of atheroma, this may be an effective medicine. It would appear also, however, that it may be extremely effective in the second stage, the stage of platelet clumping around the breached endothelium.

Finally, let me add one further conjecture. From the results of the Anturane Reinfarction Trial, it appears that it is the *high* mortality associated with *recent* infarction which is lowered by sulfinpyrazone. The low mortality associated with stable angina pectoris did not appear to be influenced.

We, of course, do not know through what mechanism the high mortality of the postinfarction patient was lowered. It could be that sulfinpyrazone had specific antiarrhythmic effects, either direct or indirect, and that the patients were protected from the consequences of myocardial irritability in the postinfarction state. It is equally possible, however, that sulfinpyrazone was protecting patients from the consequences of platelet accumulation at the site of initial plaque rupture. If this were so, it would be effective whether infarction took place or not and hence might prove just as successful in the management of unstable angina. So far as I am aware, this has not yet been investigated.

It is with great interest that we will follow these developments to see whether the overall picture does start to fit together in the way I have suggested. Should it do so, the next therapeutic steps we should try out will be obvious. Should it not, the pieces which do not fit will be the clues to the errors in our overall pattern.

Experimental Animal Studies

Opening Comments

Michael F. Oliver, M.D.

In this section we will be considering the relationship of sulfinpyrazone, aspirin and perhaps other drugs, to ventricular arrhythmias. It might be helpful to make one or two very simple, basic electrophysiological points concerning ventricular arrhythmias. There are two major forms of arrhythmia which are quite distinct. There are reentrant arrhythmias (for example, ventricular fibrillation, which is effectively what we mean by sudden cardiac death) and there are arrhythmias arising from disturbance of intrinsic automaticity. In general, reentrant arrhythmias arise from ventricular muscle, and automatic arrhythmias arise from Purkinje tissue. Ventricular muscle has a different blood supply from that of Purkinje tissue, which is mostly derived from ventricular cavity blood and not from the coronary circulation. Ventricular muscle, on the other hand, is supplied by the coronary circulation. Myocardial ischemia is not likely (in the first few hours, at least) to involve Purkinje tissue and is not likely to produce automatic rhythms.

Myocardial ischemia leads primarily to reentrant arrhythmias. There are three major conditions that are required for reentry — one is conduction delay through the ischemic muscle, another is inhomogeneity of refractoriness so that the impulse cannot spread in a homogenous fashion through ventricular muscle, and the third is unidirectional blocks of different degrees. Reentrant arrhythmias can be regional in their occurrence and the left ventricle can be in ventricular fibrillation when the right ventricle is not, or even part of the left ventricle can be in ventricular fibrillation when the rest of it is not. This is a phenomenon which is familiar in electrophysiological laboratories.

Dogs are frequently used for these studies, as is the open-chest, coronary artery occlusion preparation, in which

151

Harris many years ago described phase I, II, and III arrhythmias. The Harris I arrhythmia, which occurs immediately after the induction of ischemia, is a reentrant arrhythmia. Harris phase II is the silent phase where arrhythmias are uncommon and lasts for several hours. Harris phase III occurs some hours after the induction of ischemia; this is usually a Purkinje-based, automatic arrhythmia.

Comparative Effects
of Sulfinpyrazone and Aspirin
in the Coronary Occlusion-
Reperfusion Dog Model

H. J. Povalski, M.S., R. Olson, M.S., S. Kopia, M.S.
and P. Furness, B.S.

Studies in our laboratory were initiated in an effort to establish preclinical evidence of a cardioprotective effect for sulfinpyrazone to correlate with the clinical finding [1] that this compound reduced the incidence of sudden death in patients having a history of myocardial infarction. Our previous investigations showed that repeated administration of sulfinpyrazone to conscious dogs caused a reduction in the electrocardiographic manifestations of myocardial ischemia induced by coronary occlusion. This amelioration consisted of decreases in ST-T wave elevations and ectopic beats observed early after coronary occlusion and in the frequency of dysrhythmias seen on the day following the ischemic insult. In the same experiment other indices of experimental cardiac ischemia, such as creatine phosphokinase (CPK) release and morphological estimation of infarct size, were not affected by sulfinpyrazone therapy.

To further explore this initial finding, we expanded our study to include an additional dog arrhythmia model. This preparation, involving occlusion and reperfusion of the left anterior descending (LAD) coronary artery of the anesthetized dog, elicits a high frequency of ventricular tachycardias,

Henry J. Povalski, M.S., R. Olson, M.S., S. Kopia, M.S. and P. Furness, B.S., Research Department, Pharmaceuticals Division, CIBA-GEIGY Corporation, Summit, N.J.

fibrillation, asystole and mortality. It was felt that the model might afford a closer representation of the cardiac events accompanying the clinical sudden death syndrome than did our earlier model.

We also examined aspirin in the coronary occlusion-reperfusion dysrhythmia preparation, since aspirin has been reported (although not conclusively) to have a protective effect in patients with ischemic heart disease. Our own studies, as well as a published report [2], have shown modest and marked, respectively, antidysrhythmic activity in ischemic cardiac dog experiments. Moreover, similarities exist between the effects of aspirin and sulfinpyrazone on prostaglandin synthesis and platelet regulation.

Results of our earlier exploratory studies on the effect of sulfinpyrazone in several cardiac ischemia and arrhythmia models are also presented for the sake of completeness.

Methodology

Myocardial Ischemia Model:
Coronary Artery-Occluded Conscious Dog

Mongrel dogs of either sex weighing 10 to 20 kg were anesthetized with sodium pentobarbital (30 mg/kg IV), intubated with a cuffed endotracheal cannula, and respired artificially with a Harvard positive pressure respirator. After a left thoracotomy the heart was exposed through a pericardial excision and a portion of the left circumflex (CFX) coronary artery was dissected free so that a snare ligature device could be placed around the artery. Cessation of coronary flow was accomplished by means of the snare ligature threaded through a silastic tubing which was exteriorized for coronary artery occlusion experiments after the animal had recovered from surgery.

Groups of seven dogs were given oral doses twice daily at 6-h intervals for 4 consecutive days of a capsule containing either sulfinpyrazone or lactose at a dose of 30 mg/kg. On the fifth day both groups were dosed once and 1.5 h later they were subjected to CFX occlusion. No drugs were given after coronary occlusion. Prior to permanent coronary occlusion, venous blood samples were drawn for control (predrug) total CPK analysis.

Serum CPK values in international units (IU) per liter were determined by the method of Rosalki [3]. Sustained occlusion of the CFX artery was maintained throughout the course of the experiment (24 h). Electrocardiogram (ECG) analysis, using lead II, was performed on all animals for evaluation of ST-T wave elevations at 2 and 15 min and for ectopic beat frequency at 0.5, 3, 6, and 24 h after CFX occlusion. Plasma CPK determinations were made at 3, 6 and 24 h post ligation. Morphological estimation of infarct size was also performed at 24 h after anesthetizing each dog, administering trypan blue dye, and then sacrificing by an overdose of sodium pento-barbital. Complete coronary occlusion was verified by necropsy, at which time the heart was removed and weighed. The left ventricle was isolated and cut into eight transverse sections. Dissection of the necrotic (unstained) tissue was made by gross visual examination. The ischemic tissue was weighed and expressed as a percentage of the weight of the total left ventricle.

Delayed Dysrhythmia Model:
Coronary Artery-Ligated Dog

Animals were prepared for coronary artery exposure as described above, except that a portion of the LAD coronary artery, 1.5 to 2.5 cm from its origin, was dissected free so that an occluding ligature could be inserted. The artery was occluded gradually (over 1 min), which prevented the occasional fibrillation found with abrupt ligation. Following closure of the thorax, the dogs were allowed to respire naturally and recover from anesthesia.

A lead II ECG was taken 24 h after coronary ligation surgery. At this time nearly all beats were of ventricular ectopic origin. Ectopic beats or premature ventricular contractions (PVC) were defined as those QRS complexes that were not clearly related to a preceding P wave. Data on drug effectiveness are expressed as a reduction in the incidence of ectopic beats in relation to normal beats.

Sulfinpyrazone and aspirin were given orally via gelatin capsule at a dose of 30 mg/kg for 3 consecutive days to separate groups of animals. Coronary occlusion surgery was performed on the next to last day of drug therapy. ECG analysis was

Table 2. Effect of Sulfinpyrazone Pretreatment on Heart Rate and
Ectopic Heart Beats Caused by CFX Coronary Artery Occlusion in Dogs

Time of Measurement	Control (Placebo)*		Sulfinpyrazone*	
	Heart Rate (beats/min)	Ectopics† (%)	Heart Rate (beats/min)	Ectopics† (%)
Preocclusion	109.6 ± 12.5		106.8 ± 9.6	
Postocclusion				
15 min	156.4 ± 13.8	29.0	121.9 ± 8.8	12.8
3 h	116.1 ± 11.7	18.7	116.9 ± 7.0	4.4
6 h	152.0 ± 16.8	71.1	151.4 ± 14.5	56.3
24 h‡	175.5 ± 12.3	85.0	168.7 ± 10.0	79.6

Values are mean ± SE. The treatment schedule is given in Table 1. *n = 7.
†Ectopics = ectopic beats. ‡n = 6.

high (90%) incidence of abnormal cardiac beats of a ventricular
ectopic origin (Table 4). In comparison to placebo controls,
pretreatment with sulfinpyrazone (30 mg/kg daily for 2 days)
significantly ($p < 0.05$) reduced the number of abnormal or
ectopic beats 24 h after the second daily drug administration
(90% in control versus 82% in sulfinpyrazone-treated dogs).
This antidysrhythmic effect was also observed 1.5 and 3 h,
respectively, after the final dose of sulfinpyrazone given on the
day of ECG recording (Table 4) when the incidence of
abnormal beats was 91% and 89% in the placebo-treated group
and 75% and 78% in the sulfinpyrazone-treated group. Statistical significance also reached the level of $p < 0.05$ for the
differences between groups at both these time periods. Heart
rate appeared to be essentially unaltered by sulfinpyrazone
treatment when comparisons were made with control animals;
however, a slight bradycardic trend was noted after acute drug
administration in the sulfinpyrazone-dosed group (Table 4).
Stability of the preparation was evident from the finding that
six of seven placebo-treated dogs showed either no change or
increases in ectopic beat frequency over the 4-h recording
session, while five of seven sulfinpyrazone-treated dogs showed
decreases in the number of ectopic beats during this same
period.

Compared to placebo-treated control animals, aspirin pretreatment (30 mg/kg PO daily for 3 days) caused a modest
(14%) but significant ($p < 0.05$) decrease in the incidence of

Table 3. Effect of Sulfinpyrazone Pretreatment on Serum CPK Levels Caused by CFX Coronary Artery Occlusion in Dogs

| | | | Serum CPK (IU/L) | | | |
| | | Preocclusion | Postocclusion | | | Maximum |
Treatment Group	n		3 h	6 h	24 h*	
Control (Placebo)	7	44.1 ± 7.0	302 ± 69	1705 ± 291	1064 ± 116	1745 ± 269
Sulfinpyrazone	7	71.3 ± 22.9	237 ± 59	1541 ± 269	1544 ± 202	1829 ± 257

Values are mean ± SE. The treatment schedule is given in Table 1. *n = 6.

Table 4. Effect of Sulfinpyrazone Pretreatment* on Heart Rate and Ectopic Beats Caused by 24-H Prior Occlusion of the LAD Coronary Artery in Dogs

| | Control (Placebo) | | | Sulfinpyrazone | | |
Time of Measurement	Heart Rate (beats/min)	Ectopics (beats/min)	(%)	Heart Rate (beats/min)	Ectopics (beats/min)	(%)
After dose 2						
24 h	178.0 ± 7.8	164.0 ± 5.7	90	187.0 ± 8.7	153.0 ± 8.3	82†
After dose 3						
1.5 h	177.0 ± 6.2	162.0 ± 7.4	91	170.0 ± 7.0	126.0 ± 10.6	75†
3 h	174.0 ± 5.9	155.0 ± 7.6	89	177.3 ± 8.7	137.2 ± 7.9	78†

Values are mean ± SE. *Conscious dogs, seven in each group, were given sulfinpyrazone or placebo, 30 mg/kg PO, daily for 3 days. ECG measurements were taken 24 h after coronary artery ligation, which was performed on day 2, and at 1.5 h and 3 h after the final dose on day 3. †p < 0.05, Student's t test for unpaired data.

abnormal or ectopic beats in this dysrhythmia model. The effect, however, was only observed at 3 h after the last dose of the drug. It was not seen at 24 h after the penultimate dose nor at 1.5 h after the final dose of aspirin (Table 5). Heart rate was not appreciably affected by aspirin treatment except for a moderate (28 beats/min) decrease which also accompanied the ameliorating action on ectopic beat frequency (i.e., at 3 h post treatment). This effect on heart rate was also statistically significant. Three of ten aspirin-treated dogs fibrillated and died within 30 min after coronary occlusion, whereas all the controls survived the ischemic insult.

Early Dysrhythmia Model:
Coronary Occluded-Reperfused Dog

Oral pretreatment with sulfinpyrazone at 30 mg/kg daily for 7 consecutive days caused an appreciable reduction in the incidence of fibrillation and mortality induced by coronary artery occlusion and reperfusion in anesthetized dogs when compared to control (lactose-treated) animals. The incidence of fibrillation and total deaths seen in the placebo-treated dogs was 58% (7/12) and 75% (9/12), respectively. A 17% (2/12) fibrillation rate and a 50% (6/12) mortality were observed in the sulfinpyrazone-treated group (Table 6). Conversely, aspirin appeared to elicit no protection against these ischemic myocardial events. A high (30 mg/kg per day) oral dose of aspirin given for 7 days was associated with a 67% (8/12) incidence of fibrillation and a total mortality of 83% (10/12). A lower dose of aspirin (10 mg/kg per day) given orally over a similar time span effected 50% (4/8) fibrillation and 75% (6/8) mortality rates, respectively (Table 6). The fibrillation and mortality incidences represent the total number of those events occurring over the 4 h and 20 min observation period. Deaths not resulting from fibrillation were due to ventricular asystole. Most of the fibrillation (and deaths) occurred during the 10-min reperfusion of the LAD coronary artery (Tables 6 and 7).

ST-T segment elevation, another index of myocardial ischemia, observed during the initial coronary artery occlusion was reduced by sulfinpyrazone pretreatment. Values for this parameter were 4.1 mm for the control group and 2.5, 4.6 and 4.2 mm for the sulfinpyrazone-, high-dose aspirin-, and low-dose aspirin-treated groups, respectively (Table 7).

Table 5. Effect of Aspirin Pretreatment* on Heart Rate and Ectopic Beats Caused by 24-H Prior Occlusion of the LAD Coronary Artery in Dogs

Time of Measurement	Control (Placebo)			Aspirin		
	Heart Rate (beats/min)	Ectopics (beats/min)	(%)	Heart Rate (beats/min)	Ectopics (beats/min)	(%)
After dose 2						
24 h	182 ± 10.5	163 ± 13.4	89	172 ± 9.9	156 ± 11.8	91
After dose 3						
1.5 h	177 ± 6.2	149 ± 9.0	84	164 ± 6.7	138 ± 13.6	83
3 h	179 ± 9.2	163 ± 10.9	91	151 ± 5.7†	117 ± 10.7	77†

Values are mean ± SE. *Conscious dogs, seven in each group, were given aspirin or placebo, 30 mg/kg PO, daily for 3 days. ECG measurements were taken 24 h after coronary artery ligation, which was performed on day 2. and at 1.5 h and 3 h after the final dose on day 3. †p< 0.05, Student's t test for unpaired data.

Table 6. Effect of Sulfinpyrazone or Aspirin Pretreatment* on Fibrillation, Asystole, and Mortality Caused by Coronary Artery Occlusion-Reperfusion-Occlusion in Anesthetized Dogs

Treatment Group	n	Fibrillation			Asystole		Mortality					
							Total			During Primary Occlusion and Reperfusion		
		(n)	(%)	(%Δ)	(n)	(%)	(n)	(%)	(%Δ)	(n)	(%)	(%Δ)
Control (Placebo)	12	7	58		2	17	9	75		7	58	
Sulfinpyrazone	12	2	17†	−71	4	33	6	50	−33	3	25	−57
Aspirin (High-Dose)	12	8	67	+16	2	17	10	83	+11	8	67	+16
Aspirin (Low-Dose)	8	4	50	−14	2	25	6	75	0	6	75	+29

*Animals were given placebo, sulfinpyrazone, or aspirin, 30 mg/kg PO, or aspirin, 10 mg/kg PO, daily for 7 days. Animals were anesthetized 1.5 h after the final dose. At 3 h after the final dose, the LAD coronary artery was occluded for 10 min, coronary blood flow was restored for 10 min, a permanent occlusion was then performed, and animals were observed for the following 4 h. †$p < 0.05$ vs control, Fisher's exact test.

Table 7. Effect of Sulfinpyrazone or Aspirin Pretreatment on ST-TΔ, Fibrillation, and Asystole Caused by Coronary Artery Occlusion-Reperfusion-Occlusion in Anesthetized Dogs

Treatment Group	n	ST-TΔ (mm)	Fibrillation			Asystole		
			Occl. 1	Reper.	Occl. 2	Occl. 1	Reper.	Occl. 2
Control (Placebo)	12	4.1	0	6	1	0	1	1
Sulfinpyrazone	12	2.5	0	2	0	0	1	3
Aspirin (High-Dose)	12	4.6	1	7	0	0	0	2
Aspirin (Low-Dose)	8	4.2	1	3	0	1	1	0

The protocol is given in Table 6. Occl. 1 = First Occlusion (10 min); Reper. = Reperfusion (10 min); Occl. 2 = Second Occlusion (4 h).

Heart rates were differentially affected by pretreatment with these agents. The control group baseline value was 152 ± 11 beats/min, whereas the corresponding rates for the sulfinpyrazone, high-dose aspirin, and low-dose aspirin groups were 134 ± 8, 159 ± 12, and 169 ± 9.4 beats/min, respectively. Baseline heart rate tended to be lower after sulfinpyrazone pretreatment and higher after aspirin therapy; however, these differences were not statistically significant. The increase in heart rate occurring during occlusion and the lowering of rate subsequent to reperfusion were not altered by any of the drugs (Table 8) if the baseline differences are taken into account.

The frequency of dysrhythmia (excluding fibrillation) observed during the 10-min primary occlusion period was also reduced by sulfinpyrazone and either exacerbated by high-dose aspirin or not affected by low-dose aspirin pretreatment (Table 8).

Discussion

On the basis of separate studies involving the production of myocardial ischemia via the interruption of a substantial part of myocardial blood flow, sulfinpyrazone appeared to have a slight but consistent effect in reducing the incidence of ventricle-initiated ectopic beats following coronary flow insufficiency.

This antidysrhythmic effect was noted in both the CFX and LAD artery-occluded dogs to a similar degree at 24 h post ligation. Activity did not appear to be limited to these late dysrhythmias, for in the conscious CFX artery-occluded animals the less frequent but early-evolving (15 min to 6 h) ectopic beats were also decreased in the group of dogs receiving sulfinpyrazone. Possibly due to variation in response, plus the limited number of animals used in these studies, statistical significance ($p < 0.05$) for these effects was limited to the difference in ectopy seen 24 h after ligation of the LAD artery, although subsequent dosing with sulfinpyrazone in these dogs produced an antidysrhythmic effect that was statistically significant ($p < 0.05$).

Three days of aspirin dosing to conscious dogs whose LAD coronary artery was ligated on the penultimate day of drug administration did result in some reduction in the occurrence of cardiac rhythm disturbances caused by this ischemic insult. The

Table 8. Effect of Sulfinpyrazone or Aspirin Pretreatment on Heart Rate and Prodromal Dysrhythmias Caused by Coronary Artery Occlusion and Reperfusion in Anesthetized Dogs

Treatment Group	Heart Rate (beats/min)			Dysrhythmias*			
	Preoccl.	Occl. 1	Reper.	Pre-occl. (%)	Occl. 1 mean (%)	max (%)	Incidence in Dogs (n)
Control (Placebo)	152 ± 11.0	165 ± 2.8	131 ± 4.5	0	3.1	10.5	6/12
Sulfinpyrazone	134 ± 8.0	146 ± 1.6	126 ± 3.3	0	2.1	6.8	5/12
Aspirin (High-Dose)	159 ± 12.0	176 ± 2.4	130 ± 4.4	0.1	9.9	15.2	7/12
Aspirin (Low-Dose)	169 ± 9.4	178 ± 2.3	151 ± 5.3	0	4.8	12.4	5/8

Values are mean ± SE. The protocol is given in Table 6. Preoccl. = Before first occlusion; Occl. 1 = First occlusion (10 min); Reper. = Reperfusion (10 min). *Includes ventricular beats, premature ventricular contractions, and ventricular tachycardia, but not fibrillation or asystole.

effect on these ectopic beats or arrhythmias appeared to be both delayed and relatively transient. No antiarrhythmic effect of aspirin was seen at either 1.5 or 24 h after dosing. The activity seen 3 h after drug administration may have been related to a modest but significant decrease in heart rate, which also occurred only at this time period.

Analysis of the enzymatic and morphological indices of myocardial ischemia in the CFX artery-occluded dogs revealed no clear-cut evidence of a cardioprotective nature, but it should be noted that morphological estimation of infarct size involves gross methodology. CPK estimation of infarct size revealed inconsistent results, although the slight-to-modest reductions in serum CPK noted early after coronary artery occlusion in the sulfinpyrazone-treated dogs could be regarded as a positive finding despite the lack of effect noted at 24 h.

Lastly, there also appeared to be a less intense elevation of the ST-T segment of the ECG in response to CFX coronary artery ligation in conscious dogs receiving sulfinpyrazone. While the absolute values between both placebo- and sulfinpyrazone-treated groups at the 2- and 15-min periods were not that different, the extent of decline of ST-T elevation from 2 to 15 min postocclusion was substantially greater in the sulfinpyrazone-treated than in the placebo-treated dogs.

Data from these experiments appear to provide supportive evidence for a cardioprotective property of sulfinpyrazone. The antifibrillatory activity in the coronary occlusion-reperfusion dog model might be relevant to the effect of sulfinpyrazone in preventing sudden death in patients with a history of myocardial infarction. This dog fibrillation model, with the seemingly paradoxical occurrence of enhanced fibrillation at a time when flow is abruptly restored to the underperfused ischemic heart tissue, is receiving wide investigational attention. Corbalan et al. [4] have shown experimentally that coronary artery flow restoration is preceded by an early hyperperfusion, which, in turn, results in a decrease in fibrillation threshold, possibly caused by a release of toxic agents. A sudden exposure of the myocardium to high potassium levels appears to be the prime candidate for this morbid event [5, 6]. Furthermore, Oliva and Beckinridge [7] have recently presented evidence for and emphasized the importance of vasospasm in acute myocardial ischemic syndromes. It is possible that temporary restriction of coronary arterial blood flow in patients might mimic the dysrhythmic phenomena which occur in the coronary occlusion and reperfusion technique used in our studies.

The antifibrillatory effect of sulfinpyrazone seen in this dog model appears to be indicative of a general antiarrhythmic property of the drug. Support for this can be accrued from the effectiveness of sulfinpyrazone in reducing the incidence of late-occurring ventricular ectopic beats observed in the 24-h prior coronary artery ligated dog model and from the decrease in the prodromal rhythmic disturbances seen during primary occlusion in the present study following sulfinpyrazone treatment.

The failure of aspirin to afford any cardioprotective action in our model was unexpected, especially since there is some clinical evidence pointing toward a cardioprotective effect in patients who might be expected to be at high risk of coronary disease. Nevertheless, convincing prospective clinical trials in support of a palliative role for aspirin have not been completed. Preclinical evidence for a cardioprotective property attributable to aspirin is equivocal. Moschos et al. [2] found an antifibrillatory effect of aspirin in their dog model, whereas Lefer and Ogletree [8] found it ineffective in their ischemic myocardial cat model. The former investigators found a highly significant decrease in the incidence of ventricular fibrillation following aspirin pretreatment in dogs subjected to permanent coronary artery occlusion. These authors found no evidence of platelet accumulation in either their untreated or aspirin-treated dogs, thereby indicating that microthrombi can be discounted as contributing to these differential effects. In light of these findings it is difficult to assess a mechanism for aspirin's antiarrhythmic activity, for one would like to ascribe an antithrombotic-antiarrhythmic effect for aspirin via the compound's inhibitory action on prostaglandin and platelet susceptibility to aggregation. Along these lines Folts et al. [9] have reported on the ability of aspirin to abolish the cyclical reduction in coronary flow in dogs whose coronary arteries were partially constricted. This effect was also accompanied by a reduced platelet aggregability in those animals which had shown cyclic flow reductions before aspirin therapy. Although it was not delineated in their results, it was noted in their summary that mortality was associated with this cyclical flow reduction pattern in untreated dogs, and one could assume that aspirin, by completely eliminating the aberrant flow pattern, would also abolish or reduce this mortality. This mortality, although not documented, might have been caused by fibrillation, and if so, would support Moschos' results and fit our evidence for an antiarrhythmic effect of aspirin on nonlethal cardiac rhythm disturbances, were it not for our finding that high-dose aspirin seemed to enhance the fibrillation tendency which accompanied coronary artery occlusion.

Several recent investigators have shown that asprin [10] and sulfinpyrazone [11] increased collateral blood flow to the ischemic myocardium following coronary artery occlusion in dogs. The same authors also reported that despite aspirin's ability to increase epicardial flow and to inhibit platelet aggregation, the drug failed to reduce infarct size [12]. Our studies also noted a lack of effect on infarct size after sulfinpyrazone treatment in a similar dog model of acute myocardial infarction. Indomethacin, a nonsteroidal, anti-inflammatory agent that shares many properties with aspirin, was found to increase infarct size without altering ischemic myocardial collateral flow in coronary artery-occluded dogs [13]. These disparate findings seem to rule out any simple mechanism for sulfinpyrazone's antidysrhythmic effect based on inhibition of prostaglandin synthesis or platelet aggregation alone.

Stockman et al. [14] demonstrated that nitroglycerin infusion decreased susceptibility to ventricular fibrillation during both acute myocardial ischemia and reperfusion. Furthermore, since nitroglycerin only increased the ventricular fibrillation threshold in the ischemic, but not the normally perfused, myocardium, the authors reasoned that the basis for this drug's beneficial electrophysiological action might be due to its effect on blood flow distribution to ischemic tissue rather than to a nonspecific cardiac membrane-stabilizing effect. Sulfinpyrazone might similarly elicit its antidysrhythmic action by its aforementioned ability to increase blood flow to ischemic tissue via an effect on platelet microthrombus and microemboli formation. The latter occurrence has been demonstrated clinically by Mehta and Mehta [15] and Frink et al. [16] in patients with acute myocardial infarction and implicated as causative influence in the pathology of sudden death by Haerem [17].

The two dose levels of aspirin used in this investigation reflected a concern for the effect aspirin has on prostaglandin-platelet interactions. It has been shown by Roth et al. [18] that aspirin is a powerful inhibitor of such end products of prostaglandin synthesis as thromboxane (vasoconstrictor and platelet proaggregatory) and prostacyclin (vasodilator and platelet antiaggregatory). These substances may play a modulating role in both normal and abnormal cardiophysiological states [19, 20]. High doses of aspirin can block synthesis of the potentially harmful, as well as the beneficial, substances. Low doses of aspirin seem to preferentially inhibit the platelet production of thromboxane while causing only slight or negligible inhibition of endothelial-derived prostacyclin [20]. Our results with the two doses of aspirin are in partial agreement with this hypothesis in that an enhanced fibrillatory tendency was observed in the high-dose but not in the low-dose aspirin-treated dogs. Nevertheless we were unable to show any protective effect for aspirin per se in this model.

Sulfinpyrazone also affects platelet function and the prostaglandin synthetic pathways [21]. Recent evidence by Gordon and Pearson [22] has shown that, *in vitro*, at therapeutic drug levels, sulfinpyrazone was about one hundred times less potent than aspirin in inhibiting the production of the potentially beneficial substance prostacyclin. If these different effects on the prostaglandin pathway are important in limiting the consequences of myocardial ischemia, it is possible that sulfinpyrazone could have a better overall net therapeutic activity than aspirin. Acknowledging the hazards in extrapolating animal studies to the clinical situation, the conjectural relation suggested in this hypothesis seems worthy of further experimental assessment.

References

1. Anturane Reinfarction Trial: Sulfinpyrazone in the prevention of cardiac death after myocardial infarction. N. Engl. J. Med. 289-295, 1978.

2. Moschos, C.B. et al.: Antiarrhythmic effects of aspirin during non-thrombotic coronary occlusion. Circulation 57: 681-684, 1978.
3. Rosalki, S.B.: An improved procedure for serum creatine phosphokinase determination. J. Lab. Clin. Med. 69: 696-705, 1967.
4. Corbalan, R., Verrier, R.L. and Lown, B.: Differing mechanisms for ventricular vulnerability during coronary artery occlusion and release. Am. Heart J. 92: 223-230, 1976.
5. Surawicz, B.: Ventricular fibrillation. Am. J. Cardiol. 28: 268-287, 1971.
6. Hearse, D.J.: Reperfusion of the ischemic myocardium. J. Mol. Cell Cardiol. 9: 607-616, 1977.
7. Oliva, P.B. and Beckinridge, J.C.: Arteriographic evidence of coronary arterial spasm in acute myocardial infarction. Circulation 56: 366-374, 1977.
8. Lefer, A.M. and Ogletree, M.L.: Influence of nonsteroidal anti-inflammatory agents on myocardial ischemia in the cat. J. Pharmacol. Exp. Ther. 197: 582-593, 1976.
9. Folts, J.D., Crowell, E.B. and Rowe, G.R.: Platelet aggregation in partially obstructed vessels and its elimination with aspirin. Circulation 54: 365-370, 1976.
10. Capurro, N.L. et al.: Aspirin-induced increase in collateral flow after acute coronary occlusion in dogs. Circulation 59: 744-747, 1979.
11. Davenport, N. et al.: Sulfinpyrazone increases collateral blood flow following acute coronary occlusion. Am. J. Cardiol. 43: 396A, 1979.
12. Bonow, R.O. et al.: Myocardial infarct size in the dog as a function of myocardium at risk: Influence of aspirin. Am. J. Cardiol. 43: 395A, 1979.
13. Jugdutt, B.I. et al.: Effect of indomethacin on collateral blood flow and infarct size in the conscious dog. Circulation 59: 734-743, 1979.
14. Stockman, M.B., Verrier, R.L. and Lown, B.: Effect of nitroglycerin on vulnerability to ventricular fibrillation during myocardial ischemia and reperfusion. Am. J. Cardiol. 43: 233-238, 1979.
15. Mehta, P. and Mehta, J.: Platelet function studies in coronary artery disease. Evidence for enhanced platelet microthrombus formation activity in acute myocardial infarction. Am. J. Cardiol. 43: 757-760, 1979.
16. Frink, J.R., Trowbridge, J.O. and Rooney, P.A.: Nonobstructive coronary thrombosis in sudden cardiac death. Am. J. Cardiol. 42: 48-51, 1978.
17. Haerem, J.W.: Sudden, unexpected coronary death. The occurrence of platelet aggregates in the epicardial and myocardial vessels of man. Acta Pathol. Microbiol. Scand. (A) 86 (Suppl. 265): 1-47, 1978.
18. Roth, G.J., Stanford, N. and Majerus, P.W.: Acetylation of prostaglandin synthetase by aspirin. Proc. Natl. Acad. Sci. U.S.A. 72: 3073-3076, 1975.
19. Lefer, A.M. et al.: Prostacyclin: A potentially valuable agent for preserving myocardial tissue in acute myocardial ischemia. Science 200: 52-54, 1978.

20. Moncada, S. and Vane, J.R.: The role of prostacyclin in vascular tissue. Fed. Proc. 38: 66-71, 1979.
21. Ali, M. and McDonald, J.W.D.: Effects of sulfinpyrazone on platelet prostaglandin synthesis and platelet release of serotonin. J. Lab. Clin. Med. 89: 868-875, 1977.
22. Gordon, J.L. and Pearson, J.D.: Effects of sulfinpyrazone and aspirin on prostaglandin I_2 (prostacyclin) synthesis by endothelial cells. Br. J. Pharmacol. 64: 481-483, 1978.

Discussion

Dr. Cooper: How many dogs died in the sulfinpyrazone-treated group and in the control group?

Mr. Povalski: Six out of 12 animals died, over the total 4 h and 20 min period, in the sulfinpyrazone-treated group versus 9 out of 12 in the placebo group. If enough animals were included in the placebo group so that there would be enough survivors past that crucial fibrillation period in the reperfusion period, animals entering the 4-h secondary occlusion period would eventually succumb through asystole in the same proportion as in the sulfinpyrazone-treated group. In this particular experiment there were fewer survivors in the placebo group progressing into that secondary 4-h occlusion period.

Dr. McGregor: How many dogs died in the first experiment in which you ligated the circumflex artery?

Mr. Povalski: One or two animals in each group.

Dr. McGregor: That's remarkable, isn't it?

Mr. Povalski: Yes. Fibrillations didn't occur frequently in straight occlusions in our anesthetized or conscious dog preparations. The deaths in those particular animals occurred 6 h or more after occlusion, not during the crucial hour after straight occlusion.

Dr. Oliver: Where was the occlusion and what was the extent of original ischemia produced by the occlusion? An occlusion can be made at many different places in the left circumflex artery. With massive ischemia, a high mortality would occur. This must be a very small area of ischemia.

Mr. Povalski: The ligatures were very high up. I would have expected a much greater incidence of fibrillation. In the literature, however, you find incidence of 0 to about 50% of straight fibrillation on coronary occlusion, even at the same site, very close to the bifurcation. It depends on the anesthesia used, and other conditions, which I can't explain.

Dr. Kelliher: It also depends upon the species; the dog is unique in giving an incidence of ventricular fibrillation of from 0 to 50%, depending upon where the left anterior descending artery is tied. The cat is perhaps a more reproducible model. My question is, do you know what blood levels you achieved with a dose of 30 mg/kg of sulfinpyrazone given orally, and did you measure either platelet function or prostaglandin synthesis?

Mr. Povalski: The answer to all those questions is "no." We were interested in finding the effects, per se, at the time we did the experiments.

Dr. Kelliher: On the basis of earlier presentations, it would seem that an oral dose of 30 mg/kg might give a very low blood level. Perhaps this explains why there wasn't a very dramatic effect on your acute occlusions. Have you thought about the difference between aspirin and sulfinpyrazone? It seemed to be quite striking.

Mr. Povalski: Of course, we thought about it; I really expected to see some protective effect with aspirin. There are a number of explanations, but they are all hypothetical. One is the differential effect of these two drugs on the prostacyclin-thromboxane situation. There is evidence that prostacyclin is reduced by the action of the two drugs on the cyclooxygenase system, but far less so by sulfinpyrazone. That's one reason I used a lower dose of aspirin. Certain investigators have shown that 10 mg/kg of aspirin does not obliterate the prostacyclin production. I also ran experiments on the time course of the aspirin-treated animals in which I allowed a 24-h carry-over period to elapse before the last dosing. There have been reports that the effect of aspirin on thromboxane in platelets is rather protracted, on the order of days rather than hours, while aspirin's effects on prostacyclin in the endothelial lining last only a few hours. I thought that perhaps I would be able to achieve a cardioprotective antifibrillatory effect with aspirin by letting 24 h elapse before the final dose, but I wasn't able to.

Dr. Clopath: Concerning the question about blood levels, the concentration of sulfinpyrazone in plasma is 16 μg/ml in swine after a 30 mg/kg dose. I don't know what it is in dogs.

Dr. Oliver: Would it be reasonable to say that there is marginal evidence that there might be an effect of sulfinpyrazone on some of these arrhythmia preparations, and not much more than that?

Mr. Povalski: I would agree, except for the fibrillation results. Certainly, the 17% incidence of fibrillation with sulfinpyrazone versus 58% with lactose or 67% with high-dose aspirin is not a marginal difference.

Dr. Oliver: I would like to underscore two points. One is that sulfinpyrazone appeared to be effective in the first series of experiments, when the basic heart rate was lower, and, of course, fewer ventricular arrhythmias occur with a lower heart rate. The other is that in the second series of experiments, the incremental change (or the delta) of ST was also lower in the sulfinpyrazone-treated group, so that for some reason there was less ischemia in the experimental preparation.

Effects of Sulfinpyrazone on Ischemic Myocardium

C. B. Moschos, M.D., A. J. Escobinas
and O. B. Jorgensen, Jr.

Because of their ability to interfere with platelet function, anti-inflammatory agents became a part of the investigational effort in recent years into the identification of means to limit the adverse effects of undue thrombogenesis. Among the compounds labeled as antiplatelet agents, sulfinpyrazone was studied in the early 1960's by Smythe et al. [1], who determined its ability to decrease platelet turnover rate, an observation felt to be of importance in the interaction of platelets with the vascular wall, the process underlying the initiation of thrombus formation. In the light of recent developments regarding the effects of anti-inflammatory agents upon prostaglandin metabolism, as well as upon mediators, enzymes, and cell membranes [2, 3], the mechanism by which they might affect the process of thrombogenesis remains obscure, rendering their characterization as antiplatelet agents pathophysiologically limited. The recently reported protective effect of sulfinpyrazone in patients with coronary artery disease [4] prompted us to study its effects on ischemic myocardium, using an animal model with nonthrombotic coronary occlusion, which allowed us to study the effects of sulfinpyrazone in the absence of evident platelet thrombosis.

C. B. Moschos, M.D., A. J. Escobinas and O. B. Jorgensen, Jr., The College of Medicine and Dentistry of New Jersey — New Jersey Medical School, Newark, N.J.

This work was supported in part by a research grant (HL 13036) from the National Institutes of Health and by a grant from the CIBA-GEIGY Corporation.

175

Methods

A total of 50, apparently healthy, male mongrel dogs weighing 22 to 27 kg were divided into four groups. Groups I and II, each consisting of 11 animals, received by mouth 300 mg of sulfinpyrazone per day for seven consecutive days. The experiment took place for Group I on day 7 after morning treatment and for Group II on day 8 without treatment on the day of the experiment. Group III, consisting of nine dogs, received 300 mg of sulfinpyrazone on the day of the experiment intravenously, dispersed in 150 ml of distilled water and infused over a period of 3 h starting 0.5 h before coronary occlusion (see below). The control group consisted of 19 untreated animals.

After an 18-h fast all animals on the day of the experiment were anesthetized with morphine sulfate (3 mg/kg IM) and sodium pentobarbital (20 mg/kg IV) and placed on a respiratory pump for adequate ventilation. The left jugular vein and left and right carotid arteries were exposed through small skin incisions, and catheters were passed under fluoroscopic control into the left ventricle via the right carotid artery and into the root of the aorta via the femoral artery. Left ventricular and aortic pressures were recorded by means of Statham strain gauge transducers with an Electronics for Medicine DR-8 amplifier recorder. Cardiac output was determined by a thermodilution technique, with the thermodilution catheter placed in the main pulmonary artery via the jugular vein [5]. All animals were under continuous electrocardiographic monitoring and frequent pH determinations were performed.

Myocardial ischemia was induced as described before [6] by means of a double-lumen, balloon-tipped catheter inserted through the left carotid artery and positioned under fluoroscopic control in the left anterior descending coronary artery approximately 2.5 cm from its origin. Control hemodynamic parameters were determined before induction of ischemia, and the balloon was then inflated with 1 ml of air. Peripheral coronary pressure was monitored with a Statham strain gauge; complete coronary occlusion was evident by reduction of mean peripheral coronary pressure to approximately 30 mm Hg and the appearance of an injury potential on standard lead 1.

No traditional antiarrhythmic drug was used, and animals that fibrillated within the initial 15-min high-risk period were excluded from the study. Thus, four animals of the control group, one from Group I, and two animals each from Groups II and III were excluded from the study.

During a 4-h period of observation the hemodynamic parameters and electrocardiogram were continuously monitored and recorded intermittently, along with cardiac output. The size of the ischemic area was estimated during the 4-h period from 20 precordial electrocardiographic leads which determined the number of ST elevations (N-ST) and the sum of the ST elevation (ΣST), using an electrical calibration of 0.1 mV [7]. Serial arterial blood samples were taken from all groups for plasma free-fatty-acid determination [8]: increments of the latter are thought to be related to arrhythmias during acute ischemia.

At the conclusion of the studies, the thorax was incised and the heart rate was rapidly arrested with iced Ringer's solution. The ischemic area of left ventricle was excised parallel to, and 1 mm lateral to, the anterior descending artery, beginning 1 cm below the obstruction site, down to the apex and then perpendicular to the anterior descending artery across to the termination of the most inferior diagonal branch (or an imaginary extension when this branch terminated short of the apical level). The outer margin was formed at the termination of the main epicardial segment of the other diagonal branches. This formed an approximately triangular sample, with the base at the cardiac apex and the peak just below the obstruction site. In previous studies we have observed that injection of Evans blue dye distal to the obstruction site at diastolic pressure levels stains this area, except where there is aberrant vessel distribution [9]. Such animals were excluded from this study. A similar size segment approximately 12 g was taken from the non-ischemic posterior wall.

In view of the potential heterogeneity of the myocardial metabolic response, the ventricle was divided into inner and outer layers; the tip of the papillary muscle was excluded and the epicardial adipose tissue removed. For analysis of sodium and potassium concentrations, samples were homogenized and extracted for 48 to 72 h in distilled water, a sufficient time for complete extraction. Potassium and sodium concentrations were determined in duplicate on an Auto Analyzer system with flame attachment. Water content was determined by drying samples in an oven at 100°C to constant weight.

In the evaluation of our results, the study was blind in regard to tissue analysis of electrolytes and water and free fatty acid levels, as well as precordial ECG mapping. Statistical analysis was done with paired and nonpaired observations, as appropriate. Mortality rates were assessed by the Chi square formula.

Results

The groups studied, number of animals, procedures, and the dose used for assessment of the effect of sulfinpyrazone pretreatment upon nonthrombotic coronary occlusion of 4-h duration, are shown in Table 1. The parameters used to assess ventricular function during coronary occlusion failed to reveal overall consistent changes which could be related to the dose of sulfinpyrazone used or the day that the experiment was carried out (Fig. 1). The only statistically significant change observed was lower aortic pressure throughout the experimental period in the animals pretreated for seven days with sulfinpyrazone ($p < 0.01$). The rest of the changes were sporadic, indicating a significant drop in stroke volume at 4 h in the untreated group ($p < 0.01$) and to a lesser extent in Group I ($p = 0.015$). The extent of ischemia, as judged by electrocardiographic mapping, is shown in Table 2. The changes observed in Group I were

Table 1. Treatment Groups and Number Evaluated for Various Parameters

Group*	Total	No. of Animals Hemodynamics	ECG Mapping	Tissue Electrolytes	Plasma Free Fatty Acids
Control	19	8	9	9	8
I	11	11	11	11	10
II	11	8	8	8	8
III	9	4	5	3	5

*Treatment: Group I, 300 mg sulfinpyrazone/day for 7 days; Group II, 300 mg sulfinpyrazone/day for 7 days, no drug on day 8; Group III, 300 mg sulfinpyrazone IV (single dose); Control, untreated.

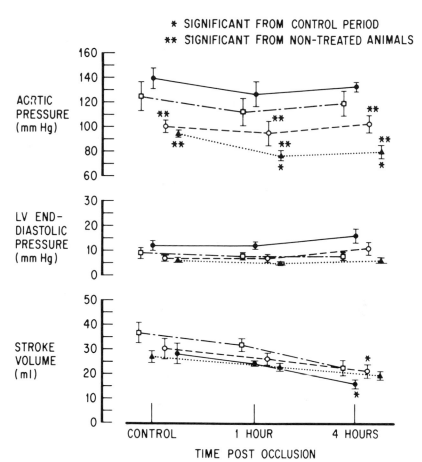

FIG. 1. Hemodynamic parameters in untreated and sulfinpyrazone-treated animals. Untreated, n = 8 (●————●); Group I, n = 11 (○-----○); Group II, n = 8 (▲·········▲); Group III, n = 4 (□—·—·□).

significant when compared to the control group (p=0.02). Although not significantly different from either of the above two groups, the extent of ischemia in Groups II and III showed a trend similar to that of the untreated group.

Figure 2 shows the results of the analysis of water and electrolyte composition in the ischemic and nonischemic tissue of the different groups. Compared to untreated animals, all groups receiving sulfinpyrazone showed significantly less increase in intracellular water in the myocardium supplied by the

Table 2. Electrocardiographic Mapping

Group*	n	N-ST Elevations at			ΣST Elevation at		
		15 min	1 h	4 h	15 min	1 h	4 h
Control	9	14.00 ± 1.1	12.77 ± 1.23	13.53 ± 1.25	4.41 ± 0.74	4.21 ± 0.52	4.53 ± 0.73
I	11	7.73 ± 1.46†	8.55 ± 1.72	7.46 ± 1.64†	2.08 ± 0.96	1.72 ± 0.79†	1.59 ± 0.87
II	8	10.75 ± 1.80	11.62 ± 1.76	11.25 ± 1.70	3.96 ± 1.50	4.32 ± 1.60	2.61 ± 0.60
III	5	13.40 ± 2.32	13.00 ± 3.03	11.60 ± 3.59	4.01 ± 1.29	3.36 ± 1.08	3.18 ± 1.34

*Treatment: Group I, 300 mg sulfinpyrazone/day for 7 days; Group II, 300 mg sulfinpyrazone/day for 7 days, no drug on day 8; Group III, 300 mg sulfinpyrazone IV (single dose); Control, untreated. †$p > 0.004 < 0.02$ vs. control.

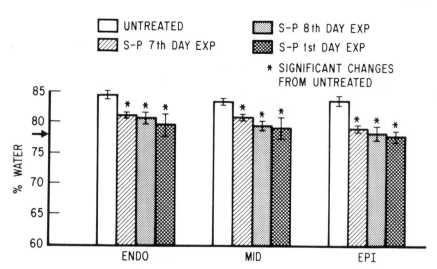

FIG. 2. Left ventricular water after 4 h of ischemia.

occluded coronary artery ($p < 0.001$). The changes in sodium
(Fig. 3) were of lower magnitude in the day 7 group ($p < 0.04$),
with less accumulation of intracellular sodium in at least two
layers, as contrasted to only the epicardial layer in the day 8
group ($p = 0.02$). The changes in Group III, although in the same
direction as in the other treated groups, did not reach a level of
statistical significance as compared to the untreated group.
Intracellular loss of potassium was of lesser degree in all layers
of Group I ($p < 0.019$).

Regarding the plasma free-fatty-acid levels (Table 3), the
expected increase occurred in the untreated group following the
4-h period of ischemia. In contrast, in the pretreated groups
changes in free fatty acids from control were not significant,
with the exception of Group II where the initial unusually high
level in the control period decreased rather than increased.
When mortality among the various groups is compared, it can be
seen that there was no death in Group I (Table 4), a difference
that was statistically significant from the group of the untreated
animals. Mortality in Groups II and III was 27% and 33%,
respectively. However, it was not statistically significantly different from either Group I or the untreated group.

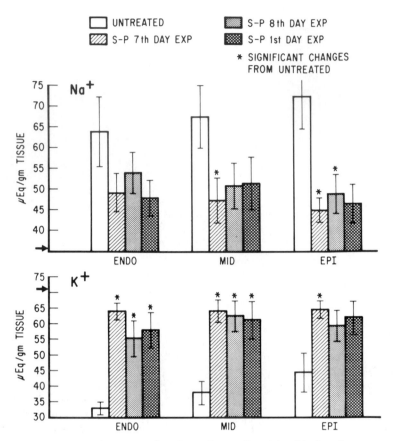

FIG. 3. Left ventricular electrolytes after 4 h of ischemia.

Table 3. Plasma Free Fatty Acid Levels

| | | Levels (μEq/L) | | |
Group*	n	Before Treatment	At 4 h	p
Control	8	197 $\pm$ 35.1	627 $\pm$ 22.4	0.037
I	10	199 $\pm$ 47.4	319 $\pm$ 97.6	NS
II	8	725 $\pm$ 97.1	566 $\pm$ 85.2	0.05
III	5	427 $\pm$ 79.9	478 $\pm$ 151.6	NS

*Treatment: Group I, 300 mg sulfinpyrazone/day for 7 days; Group II, 300 mg sulfinpyrazone/day for 7 days, no drug on day 8; Group III, 300 mg sulfinpyrazone IV (single dose); Control, untreated. NS = Not significant.

Table 4. Effect of Sulfinpyrazone on Mortality

Group*	n	Deaths n	%	p
Control	19	8	39	
I	11	0		0.025
II	11	3	27	NS†
III	9	3	33	NS†

*Treatment: Group I, 300 mg sulfinpyrazone/day for 7 days; Group II, 300 mg sulfinpyrazone/day for 7 days, no drug on day 8; Group III, 300 mg sulfinpyrazone IV (single dose); Control, untreated. †NS = Not significant vs. Group I and controls.

Discussion

The results of this study suggest that in the absence of a thrombotic process pretreatment with sulfinpyrazone significantly reduces the mortality associated with balloon obstruction of the coronary artery. Analysis of the data indicates that there was less myocardial injury following balloon occlusion in sulfinpyrazone-treated animals, particularly in those receiving the anti-inflammatory agent on the day of the experiment. Water and cation changes during the 4-h period appeared to be less extensive in the treated group, suggesting a possible mechanism for the higher incidence of fatal arrhythmias associated with more intensive ischemia in the groups that displayed more extensive swelling [10, 11].

The difference in mortality between the Groups I and II suggests a definite trend, whose statistical significance is limited by virtue of the small number of animals involved in each group. The even higher mortality in Group III, the one with the smallest number of animals, although not statistically significant, enhances the impression that daily, long-term administration of the drug is probably important. The explanation for the differences in mortality between the treated groups might lie in the fact that sulfinpyrazone levels in Group II were 100 times lower than the levels found in Group I (Table 5). Since the inhibitory effect of sulfinpyrazone has been characterized as competitive [12], a continuous effective level of the drug, whose half-life is less than 3 h [13], might be necessary for the manifestation of its beneficial effect. Thus, significantly reduced plasma levels of sulfinpyrazone would be unable to counteract the effects associated with the induced myocardial

Table 5. Sulfinpyrazone Levels in Plasma

Group*	n	Levels ($\mu g/ml$)
Control	3	0
I	3	20.3
II	11	0.244
III	4	9.85

*Treatment: Group I, 300 mg sulfinpyrazone/day for 7 days; Group II, 300 mg sulfinpyrazone/day for 7 days, no drug on day 8; Group III, 300 mg sulfinpyrazone IV (single dose); Control, untreated.

ischemia. Even the presence of an active metabolite [14] would not be effective more than 18 h, as indicated by its effect upon platelet function.

There is now evidence in regard to their inhibitory activity upon prostaglandin synthesis that anti-inflammatory agents exhibit tissue specificity in which dosage, degree of binding to albumin, chemical structure, and time of exposure are important determinants [3, 15, 16]. Such a variable effect of the anti-inflammatory agents results in preferential, weaker, or more potent inhibition of the prostaglandin system stored in both the platelets and the vascular endothelium. Thus, the studies of Korbut and Moncada [16] showed the distinct difference between small doses of aspirin, preferentially blocking platelet cyclooxygenase, and large doses of aspirin, blocking both platelet and endothelial prostaglandin. Our own studies, with relatively low doses of aspirin and the same animal model as in the present study, supported this concept, since we observed significantly decreased mortality comparable to that obtained with sulfinpyrazone [6]. Furthermore, the studies by Baenzinger et al. [17], Ali and McDonald [12], and Gordon and Pearson [18] determined that compared to aspirin, sulfinpyrazone appears to be a substantially weaker inhibitor of endothelial prostacyclin, but a potent inhibitor of platelet prostaglandin synthesis. On the basis of such a mode of action, one could postulate on the favorable effects of unopposed endothelial prostacyclin which, by virtue of its vasodilating and platelet anti-aggregating properties, counteracts the adverse effect of induced ischemia, leading to fewer fatal arrhythmias.

Another factor possibly contributing to the favorable effects observed with sulfinpyrazone is the absolute levels of blood pressure which were significantly lower in treated animals (Groups I and II) than in the other groups, making decreased mechanical demands on the myocardium. The aborted rise in free fatty acids in all treated groups, irrespective of incidence of mortality, suggested that changes in that parameter cannot be used to explain mortality differences in various groups of treated and untreated animals. In our previous studies with aspirin and indomethacin, we found that the expected free fatty acid rise in myocardial ischemia was aborted by these agents ([6]; unpublished observations).

In order to determine the presence of microcirculatory thrombosis in our model, in previous studies we used ^{51}Cr-labeled [6, 19] or ^{111}In-labeled (unpublished observations) platelets that were infused into the animals before coronary occlusion by thrombus or balloon. Microcirculatory thrombosis was expressed as the radioactivity ratio of multiple tissue samples taken from the obstructed and unobstructed areas. Only when thrombus was obstructing the left anterior descending coronary artery did a significant accumulation of platelets in the microcirculation occur, expressed as an increased ratio, whereas with balloon obstruction there were no significant differences. Therefore, microcirculatory thrombosis did not appear to be a feature of this model.

At present the mode of action of sulfinpyrazone in ischemic myocardium is not clear. Evidence to date suggests that preferential prostaglandin inhibition, favoring the manifestation of a net effect characterized by the properties ascribed to endothelial prostacyclin, is probably one of the modes of action. While microcirculatory thrombosis does not appear to be a part of this model, lower levels of blood pressure in the treated group, along with less tissue swelling as a direct or indirect effect of the anti-inflammatory agent through prosta-glandin activity upon cellular membrane [2, 3, 20-22], could account for the observed lesser incidence of fatal arrhythmias in the treated group.

References

1. Smythe, H.A., Ogryzlo, M.A., Murphy, E.A. et al.: The effect of sulfinpyrazone (Anturan) on platelet economy and blood coagulation in man. Canad. Med. Assoc. J. 92: 818-821, 1965.

2. Shen, T.Y.: Perspectives in non-steroidal and inflammatory agents. Angew Chem. Intl. Edit II (6): 460-472, 1972.
3. Flower, R.J.: Drugs which inhibit prostaglandin biosynthesis. Pharmacol. Rev. 26: 33-67, 1974.
4. The Anturane Reinfarction Trial Research Group: Sulfinpyrazone in the prevention of cardiac death after myocardial infarction. New Engl. J. Med. 298: 289-295, 1978.
5. Ganz, W., Donoso, R., Marcus, H. et al.: A new technique for measurement of cardiac output by thermodilution in man. Am. J. Cardiol. 27: 392-396, 1971.
6. Moschos, C.B., Haider, B., DeLaCruz, C. et al.: Anti-arrhythmic effects of aspirin during non-thrombotic coronary occlusion. Circulation 57: 681-684, 1978.
7. Maroko, P., Kyershus, J., Sobel, B. et al.: Factors influencing infarct size following experimental coronary occlusion. Circulation 43: 67-82, 1971.
8. Kelley, T.F.: Improved method of microtitration of fatty acids. Anal. Chem. 37: 1078-1079, 1965.
9. Regan, T.J., Harman, M.A., Lehan, P.H., et al.: Ventricular arrhythmias and K^+ transfer during myocardial ischemia and intervention with procainamide, insulin or glucose solution. J. Clin. Invest. 46: 1657-1662, 1967.
10. Leaf, A.: Editorial: Cell swelling, a factor in ischemic tissue injury. Circulation 48: 455-458, 1973.
11. Regan, T.J., Markov, A., Khan, M.I., et al.: Myocardial ion and lipid changes during ischemia and catecholamine induced necrosis: Relation to regional blood flow. Myocardiology 1: 656-663, 1972.
12. Ali, M. and McDonald, J.W.D.: Effects of sulfinpyrazone on platelet prostaglandin synthesis and platelet release of serotonin. J. Lab. Clin. Med. 89: 868-875, 1977.
13. Dieterle, W., Faigle, J.W., Mory, H. et al.: Biotransformation and pharmacokinetics of sulfinpyrazone (Anturan) in man. Eur. J. Clin. Pharmacol. 9: 135-145, 1975.
14. Buchanan, M.R., Rosenfeld, J. and Hirsh, J.: The prolonged effects of sulfinpyrazone on collagen-induced platelet aggregation in vivo. Thromb. Res. 13: 883-892, 1978.
15. Ali, M. and McDonald, J.W.D.: Reversible and irreversible inhibition of platelet cyclo-oxygenase and serotonin release by non-steroidal anti-inflammatory drugs. Thromb. Res. 13: 1057-1065, 1978.
16. Korbut, R. and Moncada, S.: Prostacyclin (PGI_2) and thromboxane A_2 interaction in vivo. Regulation by aspirin and relationship with anti-thrombotic therapy. Thromb. Res. 13: 489-500, 1978.
17. Baenziger, N.L., Dillinger, M.J. and Majerus, P.W.: Cultured human skin fibroblasts and arterial cells produce a labile platelet inhibitory prostaglandin. Biochem. Biophys. Res. Comm. 78: 294-301, 1977.
18. Gordon, J.L. and Pearson, J.D.: Effects of sulfinpyrazone and aspirin on prostaglandin I_2 (Prostacyclin) synthesis by endothelial cells. Br. J. Pharmacol. 64: 481-483, 1978.

19. Moschos, C.B., Lahiri, K., Lyons, M.M. et al.: Relation of micro-circulatory thrombosis to thrombus in the proximal coronary artery: Effects of aspirin, dipyridamole and thrombolysis. Am. Heart J. 86: 61-68, 1973.
20. Rennick, R.B.: Renal tubular transport of prostaglandins: Inhibition by probenecid and indomethacin. Am. J. Phsyiol. 233: F133-F137, 1977.
21. Wiley, J.S., Chesterman, C.N., Morgan, F.J. et al.: The effect of sulfinpyrazone on the aggregation and release reactions of human platelets. Thromb. Res. 14: 23-33, 1979.
22. Ogletree, M.L. and Lefer, A.M.: Prostaglandin-induced preservation of the ischemic myocardium. Circ. Res. 42: 218-224, 1978.

Discussion

Dr. White: There are a number of points I would like to make. First of all, at the end of the 4-h occlusion period, you say that there are no platelets present, as evidenced by the absence of ^{51}Cr or ^{111}In, but presumably you couldn't rule out the possibility that during that time platelet secretion products might be around. Do you have any measure of that?

Dr. Moschos: No.

Dr. White: That brings me to the second point. In your final conclusion, bringing out the possible differences between sulfinpyrazone and aspirin with respect to prostaglandin synthesis, are you suggesting that the effects could be due to continued maintenance of prostacyclin production in the presence of sulfinpyrazone, but not in the case of aspirin?

Dr. Moschos: I don't have personal knowledge of it, but sulfinpyrazone was found by Gordon and Pearson to be one hundred times weaker than aspirin in its effect upon production of endothelial prostacyclin. If sulfinpyrazone is indeed a stronger inhibitor of platelet thromboxane than of endothelial prostacyclin, then in this model with ischemia sulfinpyrazone might have a beneficial effect capable of minimizing the adverse effects of vasoconstriction and whatever results from platelet aggregation, if aggregation is involved at all.

Dr. White: You seem to be saying that there are no platelets, but at the same time, you seem to be invoking a platelet mechanism.

Dr. Moschos: Yes. In our model we don't see platelets in terms of mechanical occlusion. Platelets trapped in the area distal to the occlusion might release their content which, due to sulfinpyrazone treatment, should be deficient in thromboxane, thereby canceling an adverse effect regionally, since aggregation will not occur and the endothelial prostacyclin, which is weakly affected by sulfinpyrazone, will not be counteracted. We consider that action rather humoral at the prostacyclin—thromboxane level, independent of mechanical occlusion. When I mention platelets and studies with ^{51}Cr-labeled platelets, I actually mean mechanical obstruction. In our previous studies with thrombotic occlusion of the coronaries we found that the microcirculation was full of microthrombi. In the present model with balloon obstruction, we don't have this evidence at the end of 4 h. This is a distinct difference in our experience.

Dr. White: Have you ever tried infusing the product of platelet secretion induced by thrombin to see what would happen?

Dr. Oliver: May I reformulate Dr. White's question another way. Do you believe that there is a prostaglandin component in arrhythmogenesis which has nothing whatsoever to do with platelet aggregation?

Dr. Moschos: With my own concept as a cardiologist, I wanted to see something with obstruction at the microcirculatory level and evaluate its importance, and I don't see that. I don't know about circulating platelets and the extent to which they are functionally affected. I have to take the information that biochemists and scientists in other disciplines give about the effects of prostaglandins and the effects of sulfinpyrazone on platelets and try to explain my results by what I know from the literature. When I mention platelet microcirculatory thrombosis, I am speaking in terms of obstruction. I am comparing two basic models, one with obstruction by thrombus, and the other with obstruction by balloon. In the latter case we haven't yet found thrombosis (platelet aggregation) in more than 100 animals, treated or untreated.

Dr. Sherry: The question that might be asked is, could you reproduce these results in a thrombocytopenic animal? Also, could you demonstrate whether there is an increased egress of thromboxane A_2, or one of its stable end-products, in the untreated group as compared to the treated group? That kind of information would help to determine whether platelets are involved in this, and also whether thromboxane is a mechanism regardless of its source of origin.

Dr. Moschos: As far as the first question is concerned, we have an application pending with the National Institutes of Health to determine the role of the platelet in a thrombocytopenic model. It's a very important question. We have to consider, of course, that this is an invasive method. The dog is intact, but we have to cut arteries and veins to pass catheters. We think that we will have to preinstrument the animal, then produce thrombocytopenia, and with remote control cause obstruction of the coronary artery. By so doing, it should be possible to reproduce the same type of experiment as presented here. As far as the second question is concerned, I don't think that I have the means and background to do such a study, but it would be very nice to collaborate with a biochemist and try to prove this possible effect of thromboxane, its egress in the environment, and its association with the arrhythmias and the counteracting effect, of course, of sulfinpyrazone in terms of protection and survival of the animals.

Dr. Cooper: In the group receiving a stat dose IV, how was that administered?

Dr. Moschos: A dose of 300 mg was dispersed in 150 ml of distilled water. The first 100 mg was given within the half hour which preceded the occlusion, and the rest was injected in the femoral vein for the following 2.5 to 3 h.

Dr. Cooper: It might not be germane, but in our laboratory some years ago several experiments failed to reproduce our effects when we gave sulfinpyrazone to the sheep. We suddenly had several experiments in which we did not have the protective effect. In tracking it down, we found that we had dispersed sulfinpyrazone into an IV solution and administered it over 30 to 45 min instead of injecting it into the circulation directly over 5 to 10 min as we usually did. Looking at the difference in blood level achieved with your intravenous and your oral dose, I would suggest that perhaps, in fact, the effect is related to the manner in which the drug is administered. When it was dispersed and run in over a drip of 30 to 45 min in our own laboratory, we did not achieve the effect that we obtained when it was given in bolus form.

Dr. Moschos: Our experience with acutely given antiplatelet agents has been very bad. In other words, the animals don't survive. I don't know what happens, but we have found that the 7-day model is essential if we are to obtain favorable results. We established this 8 or 9 years ago when we first started working with aspirin, not for any particular reason, but just because we arbitrarily set 7 days as a good time to be considered as "chronic treatment." Anything we gave just before the experiment didn't work, whether it was sulfinpyrazone, aspirin, or indomethacin.

Dr. McNicol: How do you identify the platelet-related radioactivity in these hearts?

Dr. Moschos: We cut out about 40 to 50 small samples of the left ventricle as high as possible from the obstructed and unobstructed vessels, and then we put these pieces in a counter scintillation well. We measure the radioactivity as a ratio of the circulating blood radioactivity. We combine the obstructed and unobstructed vessels, and express that as a ratio of the two.

Dr. McNicol: So that you're counting whole tissue samples, tissue blocks?

Dr. Moschos: Yes.

Dr. McNicol: The analogy I am going to talk about may seem remote, but we have been interested in looking at radiolabeled platelet accumulation in the uterus during menstruation. There is no doubt at all that in thrombocytopenia, or in von Willebrand's disease, there is major hemostatic failure in the uterus, and it is highly probable that platelets are involved in checking menstrual flow. We infused autologous ^{51}Cr-labeled platelets into women before menstruation, collected menstrual fluid, and then removed the uteri during menstruation. Astonishingly, there was negligible platelet-related radioactivity in the menstrual fluid, and in the uteri removed during menstruation there was less platelet-related radioactivity than could be anticipated from the blood content of the excised uterus (Aparicio, S.R. et al.: Effect of intrauterine contraceptive device on uterine haemostasis: A morphological study. Br. J. Obstet. Gynaecol. 86: 314-324, 1979). Thus I think that conclusions based on counting tissue blocks for platelet-related radioactivity have to be regarded with extreme caution. If one wants to identify a platelet contribution, I think that a label other than chromium — one which will permit detailed serial autoradiography — is essential before any firm statements can be made about the involvement of microplatelet accumulation.

Dr. McGregor: Is your own conclusion that treatment with sulfinpyrazone has substantially reduced the extent of cell death? Are you saying that there is not an electrical effect, an effect on electrical stability but that you simply preserved more live cells, as demonstrated by the fact that they retained a striking electrolyte gradient across the cellular border?

Dr. Moschos: Yes.

Dr. McGregor: Thus you have conserved tissue?

Dr. Moschos: One of the main factors is the swelling; I think that preservation of the cell by means of reduced swelling is the essential mechanism we've seen in this case.

Dr. McGregor: You took a sample of tissue right out of the middle of the most ischemic area. After treatment with sulfinpyrazone it had retained the high potassium levels that you expect in living tissue, as distinct from the control series in which the potassium had dropped, as you would expect in largely dead tissue. This seems to indicate to me the inescapable conclusion that you have preserved living cells by this treatment. I wondered if you concluded the same thing.

Dr. Moschos: Yes. Again, I have to refer to the swelling. We have to consider the possible mechanism which we postulate to be an effect upon the cellular membrane. In the untreated animal, at least, there is evidence of some degree of failure or complete failure of the sodium pump which pulls along chlorides and water, changing the intracellular electrical stability and pushing the potassium out. You have to consider the whole mechanism, what happens across the membrane, in order to explain the movements of cations and water, which seems to be minimized in the animals treated with sulfinpyrazone.

Effect of Sulfinpyrazone on Arrhythmia and Death Following Coronary Occlusion in Cats

G. J. Kelliher, Ph.D., R. K. Dix,
N. Jurkiewicz and T. L. Lawrence, M.D.

Introduction

We have reported previously that prostaglandins (PG) may exert an important arrhythmogenic effect on the ischemic heart during the first hour following left anterior descending (LAD) coronary artery occlusion. In this regard we have found that infusion of PGE_1 or prostacyclin (PGI_2) into the left atrium during LAD occlusion may increase the severity of arrhythmia [1, 2]. Moreover the arrhythmogenic effect of PGE_1 appears to be exerted by an action on the sympathetic nervous system [3].

It has been reported that sulfinpyrazone (Anturane ®) may reduce the incidence of sudden death in men who have had a previous myocardial infarction [4]. In addition to its uricosuric action sulfinpyrazone has been shown to inhibit PG synthesis [5]. Since sulfinpyrazone reduced the incidence of sudden death but not infarction, it is possible that it has an antiarrhythmic effect which may be dependent on its action to inhibit PG synthesis. The purpose of our study was to

G. J. Kelliher, Ph.D. and R. K. Dix, Department of Pharmacology, The Medical College of Pennsylvania; and N. Jurkiewicz and T. L. Lawrence, M.D., Veterans Administration Hospital, Philadelphia, Pa.

This work was supported in part by a grant (HL 23962) from the National Institutes of Health and by grants from the Veterans Administration and from the CIBA-GEIGY Corporation.

determine if sulfinpyrazone could reduce the incidence of ventricular fibrillation (VF), the amount of ventricular arrhythmia, or both, observed during the first hour following coronary artery occlusion in the anesthetized cat.

Methods

Cats of either sex, weighing between 2.5 and 3.8 kg, were anesthetized with α-chloralose (70 mg/kg IP). Body temperature was measured with a rectal probe and maintained between 36° and 38°C with a regulated hot-water pad. The electrocardiogram (ECG) lead II was monitored continuously for heart rate and rhythm. Arterial blood pressure was recorded from a femoral artery with a pressure transducer. A polyethylene catheter was placed in the right femoral vein for administration of sulfinpyrazone. The animals were ventilated with room air at a rate of 12 to 16 breaths per minute and a tidal volume of 20 to 25 cc/kg. Arterial pH was maintained between 7.40 and 7.50 by adjusting the respiratory rate.

In one group of animals the vagus nerves were left intact while in another they were isolated and sectioned. The latter group is referred to in the text as vagotomized animals.

In all cats a left thoracotomy was performed through the fifth intercostal space and the pericardium incised. The LAD was isolated from the left coronary artery and circumflex artery by dissection and a ligature placed around the vessel at its origin.

Fifteen minutes after completion of the surgery when the blood pressure and heart rate had stabilized, either sulfinpyrazone (100 mg/kg) or an appropriate volume of vehicle was administered intravenously during a 3-min period. Sulfinpyrazone, as the free acid, was dissolved in a sodium bicarbonate-carbonate buffer (0.1 M, pH 8.8) to achieve a final concentration of 20 mg/ml. After the addition of sulfinpyrazone the final pH of the solution was 7.7. One hour following the infusion of sulfinpyrazone the LAD was tied abruptly. The incidence of VF occurring during the first hour after occlusion was noted. In animals that did not develop VF, the total number of ventricular ectopic beats (premature ventricular contractions, PVC), the incidence of ventricular tachycardia (VT), and the duration of tachycardia were determined for the first 30 min following occlusion. The ECG and blood pressure were monitored for up to 5 h following coronary occlusion. When the animal died or was sacrificed, the heart was removed and the coronary ligation verified by dissection. Only animals in which complete occlusion of the LAD could be demonstrated at autopsy were included in the results.

Five hours after occlusion the animals were sacrificed, the hearts were removed, and the extent of infarction was determined using the method of Nachlas and Shnitka [6], which employs a tetrazolium salt, nitro-blue tetrazolium (NBT), to delineate infarcted from noninfarcted tissue. This method is based on the capacity of NBT to stain tissue with dehydrogenase enzyme activity linked to either NAD or NADP. Since infarcted tissue has been shown to be depleted of dehydrogenase activity [7], NBT will stain the noninfarcted tissue leaving the infarcted tissue without stain or only lightly stained. This procedure for determining infarct size has been reported previously and has been shown to be reproducible in quantifying infarct size [8-11].

Venous blood (5 ml) was collected in a heparinized syringe 5 min before and 1 h after sulfinpyrazone was administered so that the degree of PG synthesis inhibition, as reflected by inhibition of platelet aggregation, could be determined. Platelet-rich plasma was obtained by centrifuging the heparinized blood at 1000 rev/min for 20 min. Arachidonic acid (1.25 mM) was added to produce platelet aggregation. This procedure was carried out in a platelet aggregometer (Chronolog), which measures platelet aggregation as a function of light transmission, i.e., as aggregation increases, more light is transmitted through the cuvette and 100% transmission of light indicates complete aggregation of the sample.

The values presented in the text are expressed as mean ± SE. The incidence of VF was determined by chi square analysis. Changes in heart rate, blood pressure, and number of PVC were analyzed using Student's t test (paired and unpaired). Values less than 0.05 were considered significant.

Results

Effect of Sulfinpyrazone on Arrhythmia and Death

Administration of vehicle or sulfinpyrazone did not produce any alteration in cardiac rhythm during the hour before LAD occlusion. Abrupt ligation of the LAD in all groups of cats resulted in ECG signs of ischemia, such as T-wave inversion and ST segment changes in all of the cats within 1 min following occlusion. Occlusion of the LAD produced ventricular arrhythmias in all the cats. PVC started approximately 5 min after occlusion and persisted for about 30 min. The ventricular arrhythmias seen in these animals ranged from isolated to unifocal and multifocal ectopic ventricular complexes and VT (six or more consecutive PVC). Most of the arrhythmia occurred during the first 30 min after occlusion and there was very little beyond this time.

The time to the onset of ventricular arrhythmia was substantially abbreviated in cats with vagotomy when compared with cats with intact vagus nerves, i.e., 1 ± 1 versus 5 ± 2 sec, respectively. Although sulfinpyrazone did not alter the onset of arrhythmia when the vagus nerves were intact (7 ± 2 sec), it prevented the abbreviation in onset found in the vagotomy control group (4 ± 1 versus 1 ± 1 sec).

The number of PVC occurring in the first 30 min after occlusion ranged from 53 to 500 beats in the group with vagus nerves intact, while in the corresponding group with sulfinpyrazone, the range was 7 to 102 beats. Thus, sulfinpyrazone significantly reduced the mean number of PVC following LAD occlusion ($p < 0.02$; Fig. 1). In the control cats with vagotomy, the low survival rate did not permit this comparison to be made. Another indication of the antiarrhythmic action of sulfinpyrazone is evident in the incidence and duration of VT. In the control group with vagus nerves intact, VT occurred in 71% of the animals surviving LAD occlusion, while in the corresponding group treated with sulfinpyrazone VT occurred in only 17% ($p < 0.05$; Table 1). In addition, sulfinpyrazone reduced the duration of VT in both vagus-intact and vagotomy groups by 60 and 40%, respectively (Table 1).

Acute occlusion of the LAD in ten control animals with intact vagus nerves produced VF in 30% of these animals. Administration of sulfinpyrazone 1 h prior to occlusion reduced the incidence of VF to 14% (Fig. 1). Bilateral vagotomy increased the incidence of VF in control animals to 57%, while the incidence of VF in a corresponding group of animals treated with sulfinpyrazone was only 17% (Table 1).

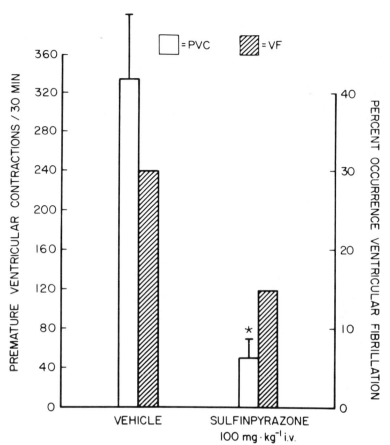

FIG. 1. Effect of sulfinpyrazone on PVC and VF. Vehicle or sulfinpyrazone (100 mg/kg IV) was administered to cats with vagus nerves intact 1 h
before LAD occlusion. Values represent the mean number of PVC and the
percent incidence of VF for the first 30 min after occlusion. Control
group, n = 10; sulfinpyrazone group, n = 7. *p< 0.02 vs. control.

Effect of Sulfinpyrazone on Heart Rate and Blood Pressure

Bilateral vagotomy produced a slight but significant increase
in heart rate in the control group (p<0.05), while in the group
subsequently treated with sulfinpyrazone there was no change
in initial heart rate (Table 2). Administration of vehicle to
either of the control groups did not produce any change in
heart rate (Table 2, Heart Rate Before Occlusion). Administra-

Table 1. Effect of Sulfinpyrazone on Ventricular Tachycardia and Death

Treatment Group	n	Incidence of VT*	Duration of VT* (sec)	Incidence of VF
Control	10	5/7	25 ± 5	3/10
Sulfinpyrazone	7	1/6†	10	1/7
Control and Vagotomy	7	2/3	25	4/7
Sulfinpyrazone and Vagotomy	6	2/5	15	1/6

*Determined in survivors.
†p < 0.05 vs. control.

tion of sulfinpyrazone in the vagus-intact and vagotomy groups increased heart rates by 11 and 12 beats/min; in the latter group this difference was statistically significant.

LAD occlusion produced a marked bradycardia prior to development of ventricular arrhythmia in both groups of animals with intact vagus nerves (Table 2). The heart rate prior to onset of arrhythmia was similar in the two groups (p>0.05). The heart rate returned toward preocclusion values in both groups during the 60 min following occlusion.

In the control group with vagotomy, LAD occlusion produced a significant increase in heart rate (p<0.02; Table 2), while no change occurred in the group treated with sulfinpyrazone. In the former group heart rate remained elevated during the hour following occlusion.

Infusion of either vehicle or sulfinpyrazone produced no change in blood pressure in cats with vagus nerves intact or with vagotomy (Table 3). In cats with vagus nerves intact, acute occlusion produced a marked hypotensive response (p<0.05; Table 3) which returned toward the preocclusion value during the following hour. Cats with vagotomy demonstrated a different response to occlusion. Blood pressure dropped after occlusion in the group treated with sulfinpyrazone, whereas this was not seen in the control vagotomy group. The increase in heart rate after occlusion in the latter group was probably responsible for the lack of a hypotensive response.

Effect of Sulfinpyrazone on Infarct Size

All animals that did not develop VF survived for 5 h following occlusion. At this time they were sacrificed and infarct size was determined by dehydrogenase (NBT) staining

Table 2. Effect of Sulfinpyrazone on Heart Rate (HR)

Treatment Group	Initial	After Vagotomy	Before Occlusion*	Heart Rate (beats/min) After Occlusion† 5 min	15 min	30 min	1 h
Control	230 ± 13	—	225 ± 14	168 ± 12[a]	205 ± 13[b]	209 ± 14	212 ± 13
Sulfinpyrazone	188 ± 10[c]	—	200 ± 14	163 ± 10[b]	191 ± 10	194 ± 13	186 ± 12
Control and Vagotomy	217 ± 9	227 ± 9[d]	233 ± 11	258 ± 10[b]	254 ± 9	252 ± 7	251 ± 1
Sulfinpyrazone and Vagotomy	224 ± 4	217 ± 6	228 ± 3[d]	230 ± 6	230 ± 4	230 ± 4	228 ± 11

*1 h after administration of vehicle or drug.

†Determined in survivors.

[a]p < 0.001 vs. preceding value; [b]p < 0.02 vs. preceding value; [c]p < 0.05 vs. control; [d]p < 0.05 vs. preceding value.

Table 3. Effect of Sulfinpyrazone on Blood Pressure

| | | | Blood Pressure (mm Hg) | | | | |
| | | | | After Occlusion† | | | |
Treatment Group	Initial	After Vagotomy	Before Occlusion*	5 min	15 min	30 min	1 h
Control	122 ± 9	—	124 ± 6	77 ± 5^a	97 ± 4^b	101 ± 5^c	101 ± 4^c
Sulfinpyrazone	116 ± 9	—	109 ± 8	79 ± 5^d	91 ± 6^c	96 ± 6^c	97 ± 8^c
Control and Vagotomy	146 ± 7	151 ± 7	146 ± 9	142 ± 14	142 ± 9	148 ± 15	137 ± 12
Sulfinpyrazone and Vagotomy	129 ± 8	124 ± 13	124 ± 10	107 ± 12^d	105 ± 13^c	99 ± 14^c	99 ± 15^c

*1 h after administration of vehicle or drug.
†Determined in survivors.
$^a p < 0.001$, $^b p < 0.005$, $^c p < 0.05$, $^d p < 0.02$, vs. pre-occlusion value.

(Fig. 2). In every cat LAD occlusion produced infarction of the left ventricle involving approximately 28% of the total ventricular mass. There was no difference between the control or sulfinpyrazone groups, i.e., those with or without vagotomy. There also was extensive involvement of the interventricular septum in each cat, resulting in infarction of approximately 70% of the septum. Again there was no difference between any of the groups. These data indicate that although sulfinpyrazone

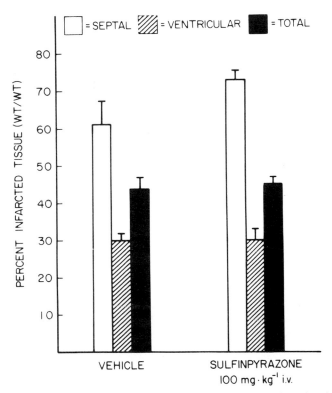

FIG. 2. Effect of sulfinpyrazone on infarct size in cats 5 h after LAD occlusion. On the ordinate the amount of infarcted tissue in each area examined is expressed as a percentage of the tissue. Vehicle or sulfinpyrazone was administered 1 h before LAD occlusion. At 5 h after LAD occlusion, control (vehicle) and treated (sulfinpyrazone) animals were sacrificed and infarct size in the septum, ventricular wall, and total tissue was determined by NBT staining. Control group, n = 7; sulfinpyrazone group, n = 5. There were no significant differences between the vehicle control and the sulfinpyrazone-treated group.

significantly reduced the amount of ventricular arrhythmia following occlusion, it did not reduce the extent of infarction as determined by NBT stain.

Effect of Sulfinpyrazone on Platelet Aggregation

The capacity of sulfinpyrazone to inhibit platelet aggregation was studied in two cats. Platelet-rich plasma was obtained from these animals prior to and 1 h after administration of sulfinpyrazone, just before occlusion of the LAD. Platelet aggregation was produced by addition of arachidonic acid (sodium salt; 1.25 mM). In the pretreatment plasma addition of arachidonic acid produced complete platelet aggregation, whereas this same concentration of arachidonic acid failed to produce aggregation in the plasma obtained 1 h after administration of sulfinpyrazone. Since arachidonic acid is thought to produce platelet aggregation by production of thromboxane, these data indicate that this dose of sulfinpyrazone completely inhibits the cyclooxygenase enzyme system responsible for thromboxane synthesis in platelets.

Discussion

We initiated the present study with sulfinpyrazone to determine if this compound had a beneficial effect on the ventricular arrhythmias and sudden death produced by abrupt ligation of the LAD in cats. Our initial findings are intriguing in that they indicate that sulfinpyrazone may possess an anti-arrhythmic action in the setting of myocardial ischemia. This action is apparent from the dramatic reduction in PVC after occlusion in the sulfinpyrazone-treated animals, as well as the absence of VT in five of six of these animals. It should be noted that in the animals in the control group that survived for 5 h after occlusion, not only was there more arrhythmia, but also five of seven animals had episodes of VT. Thus, sulfinpyrazone reduced both the total amount of arrhythmia, as well as its severity.

The results that we obtained with sulfinpyrazone on the incidence of VF suggest that use of this agent may lead to a reduction in the occurrence of this fatal rhythm disorder. The incidence of VF that we attain in our model in our control group is approximately 30%. In order to increase the severity of arrhythmia in our cat model, bilateral vagotomy was performed. Gillis and co-workers [12] have reported that vagotomy prior to occlusion in chloralose-anesthetized cats increases the incidence of VF to approximately 60% in the control group. Even though vagotomy nearly doubled the incidence of VF in our studies, i.e., from 30% to 57%, it is important to note that it still did not increase the incidence of VF in the sulfinpyrazone-treated group. In fact, the incidence of VF was similar in both groups treated with sulfinpyrazone, i.e., 14% and 17%.

The basis for the beneficial action of sulfinpyrazone on arrhythmia is not apparent from the results of our study; however, several possible explanations exist. In this regard, an action on (a) uric acid, (b) cardiac excitability, (c) infarct size, (d) platelet function, or (e) PG synthesis could contribute to an antiarrhythmic action.

It is unlikely that the uricosuric action of the drug contributed to the antiarrhythmic response due to the short onset of action which would not be consistent with an action of the drug on urate handling in the proximal tubule. However, we did not measure the effect of the drug on serum urate levels in our study.

The finding that this agent affects rhythm disorders much faster than previously thought is of considerable interest. It appears from our data that this action is manifest within 1 h of drug administration. This finding suggests that the delayed onset of effect observed in the clinical study may reflect the need to achieve a critical tissue level of the drug in the myocardium. Intravenous administration of the drug at the dose we employed most likely produced these high levels within 1 h.

The possibility that sulfinpyrazone has a direct action on cardiac excitability at the dose employed in our study cannot be dismissed since it was not evaluated in our study. However, Bandura et al. [13] have presented preliminary evidence of microelectrode studies with dog Purkinje fibers that sulfinpyrazone in concentrations of 2 to 100 μg/ml had no effect on six electrophysiologic parameters. They also reported that sulfinpyrazone (2 or 20 μg/ml) inhibited human platelet function and PG synthesis by 37% and 89%, respectively. Additional studies directed toward an examination of its effects directly on the heart are needed before an action on cardiac excitability can be discarded as a basis for the antiarrhythmic action of sulfinpyrazone.

In recent years there has been a great deal of interest in studying the relationship between infarct size and the severity of arrhythmia, but for the most part, the results have been inconclusive. For example, Roberts et al. [14] have shown a relationship between CPK-estimated infarct size and arrhythmia. They demonstrated that the larger the infarct, the more the ventricular ectopic complexes were recorded. On the other hand, Thomas et al. [15] have demonstrated no relationship between infarct size and arrhythmia. We examined the effect of sulfinpyrazone on infarct size in our study and were unable to detect any change from that found in the control animals with or without vagotomy. Bolli et al. [16] have recently reported a similar finding in the dog. They found that administration of sulfinpyrazone (30 mg/kg) 10 min before and at 3 and 6 h after LAD occlusion did not alter infarct size measured at 72 h after occlusion. It is interesting to note that the extent of infarction of the left ventricle after sulfinpyrazone was similar to our own results, i.e., 30 ± 5% versus 29 ± 3%, respectively. Thus, it is unlikely that the antiarrhythmic effect of sulfinpyrazone can be attributed to a reduction in infarct size.

Two likely explanations for the antiarrhythmic action of sulfinpyrazone are inhibition of platelet function and inhibition of prostaglandin synthesis. The dose of sulfinpyrazone employed (100 mg/kg) was sufficient to prevent platelet aggregation in the two animals tested and it is tempting to attribute the antiarrhythmic action of the drug to this effect. In fact, Bandura et al. [13] have suggested that since sulfinpyrazone did not produce any effects on isolated Purkinje fibers that were consistent with an antiarrhythmic action, it may produce its beneficial effects against sudden cardiac death through an action to inhibit PG synthesis and hence platelet function. However, Moschos et al. [17] reported recently that pretreatment of dogs with aspirin (600 mg/dog) for 7 days prior to LAD occlusion significantly reduced the incidence of VF without altering platelet accumulation in the myocardium. Studies with thrombocytopenic animals may help to resolve this question in the future. In any event the results of our study and that of Bolli et al. [16] clearly show that platelet inhibition produced by sulfinpyrazone does not produce a reduction in infarct size in the cat or dog following coronary artery occlusion.

Finally, the action of sulfinpyrazone to inhibit platelet aggregation probably is a reflection of its action to inhibit PG synthesis. It is felt that generation of thromboxane produces the clumping of platelets so that any agent which inihibits at the cyclooxygenase step should produce similar results. In this regard sulfinpyrazone has been reported to inhibit PG synthesis *in vitro* in platelets [5] and cultured endothelial cells [18], as well as the coronary vasodilator response induced with arachidonic acid *in vivo* in dogs [19].

Inhibition of platelet PG synthesis does not necessarily indicate inhibition of cardiac PG synthesis, and additional studies are needed to evaluate this possibility. If cardiac PG synthesis is inhibited, it indicates that these substances may play an important role in the severity of ventricular arrhythmia following coronary occlusion. This is of particular importance since we have shown previously [1] that PGs may enhance development of ventricular arrhythmia and VF after coronary occlusion in cats. We proposed that these substances may interact with cardiac sympathetic nerves to facilitate the development of VF [3]. The present study suggests that sulfinpyrazone may produce its beneficial effect by inhibiting the formation of PGs that facilitate arrhythmia.

Acknowledgments

The authors wish to express their appreciation to Ms. Beverly Burak and Mrs. Frances Dix for their help in the preparation of this manuscript.

References

1. Kelliher, G.J., Lawrence, L.T., Jurkiewicz, N. and Dix, R.K.: Comparison of the effects of prostaglandin E_1 and A_1 on coronary occlusion-induced arrhythmia. Prostaglandins 17: 163-177, 1979.
2. Dix, R.K., Kelliher, G.J., Jurkiewicz, N. and Lawrence, T.L.: Effect of prostacyclin on ventricular arrhythmia after coronary occlusion in the cat. *In* Ramwell, P., Samuelsson, B. and Paoletti, R. (eds.): Proceedings of International Conference on Prostaglandins, in press.

3. Kelliher, G.J., Lawrence, T., Jurkiewicz, N. and Dix, R.K.: Role of sympathetic nervous system in prostaglandin-induced ventricular arrhythmia (Abst.). Pharmacologist 20: 444, 1978.

4. Anturane Reinfarction Trial Research Group: Sulfinpyrazone in the prevention of cardiac death after myocardial infarction. N. Engl. J. Med. 298: 289-295, 1978.

5. Ali, M. and McDonald, J.W.D.: Effect of sulfinpyrazone on platelet prostaglandin synthesis and release of serotonin. J. Lab. Clin. Med. 89: 868-875, 1977.

6. Nachlas, M.M. and Shnitka, T.K.: Macroscopic identification of early myocardial infarcts by alterations in dehydrogenase activity. Am. J. Pathol. 42: 379-405, 1963.

7. Wachstein, M. and Meisel, E.: Succinic dehydrogenase activity in myocardial infarction and in induced myocardial necrosis. Am. J. Pathol. 31: 353-365, 1955.

8. Althaus, V., Janett, J., Scholl, E. and Riedwyl, H.: Effects of myocardial revascularization following acute coronary occlusion in pigs. Eur. J. Clin. Invest. 6: 7-15, 1976.

9. Shatney, C.H., MacCarter, D.J. and Lillehei, R.C.: Temporal factors in the reduction of myocardial infarction volume by methylprednisolone. Surgery 80: 61-69, 1976.

10. Vogel, W.M., Zannon, V.G., Abrams, G.D. and Lucchesi, B.R.: Inability of methylprednisolone sodium succinate to decrease infarct size or preserve enzyme activity measured 24 hours after coronary occlusion in the dog. Circulation 55: 588-595, 1977.

11. Ritchie, D.M., Kelliher, G.J., MacMillan, A., Fasolak, W., Roberts, J. and Mansukhani, S.: The cat as a model for myocardial infraction. Cardiovasc. Res., in press.

12. Corr, P.B. and Gillis, R.A.: Role of vagus nerves in the cardiovascular changes induced by coronary occlusion. Circulation 49: 86-97, 1974.

13. Bandura, J.P., Iansmith, D.H.S., Nash, C.B. and Sullivan, J.M.: Microelectrophysiologic and antiplatelet effects of sulfinpyrazone (Abst.). Clin. Res. 27: 150, 1979.

14. Roberts, R., Husain, A., Ambos, H.D., Oliver, G.C., Cos, J.R. and Sobel, B.E.: Relation between infarct size and ventricular arrhythmia. Br. Heart J. 37: 1169-1175, 1975.

15. Thomas, M., Shulman, G. and Opie, L.: Arteriovenous potassium changes and ventricular arrhythmias after coronary artery occlusion. Cardiovasc. Res. 4: 327-333, 1970.

16. Bolli, R., Goldstein, R.E., Davenport, N. and Epstein, S.E.: Effect of naproxen and sulfinpyrazone on myocardial infarction size (Abst.). Clin. Res. 27: 155, 1979.

17. Moschos, C.B., Haider, B., Cruze, D.C., Lyons, M. and Regan, T.: Antiarrhythmic effects of aspirin during nonthrombotic coronary occlusion. Circulation 57: 681-684, 1978.

18. Gordon, J.L. and Pearson, J.D.: Effects of sulfinpyrazone and aspirin on prostaglandin I_2 (prostacyclin) synthesis by endothelial cells. Br. J. Pharmacol. 64:481-483, 1978.

19. Lipson, L.C., Goldstein, R.E., Davenport, N., Bonow, R.O., Capurro, N.L., Shulman, N.R. and Epstein, S.F.: Ibuprofen and sulfinpyrazone inhibit coronary vasodilatation induced by arachidonic acid (Abst.). Clin. Res. 27: 184, 1979.

Discussion

Dr. McGregor: I was puzzled by the very substantial difference in initial heart rates of the control and test animals, far outside what you could get by chance. I wondered what accounted for the difference between the two series — was it anesthesia, temperature, or what? Have you any comment on the probability that these differences in initial heart rate might have some bearing on the incidence of tachycardias?

Dr. Kelliher: Because of the difference in initial heart rates prior to administration of sulfinpyrazone, we did experiments in more cats. When we used control animals with initial heart rates in the 215 or 220 range, we got the same type of effect, so that it does not appear to be a heart rate-mediated effect.

Dr. Minick: You said that you had data showing that infarct size didn't relate to ventricular arrhythmias, I believe. In the data you presented, it seemed to me that there was a very small variance in the amount of infarcted tissue between groups. I wondered how you could demonstrate whether there was or was not a correlation with infarcts that were essentially the same in size.

Dr. Kelliher: Are you referring to a correlation of severity of arrhythmia with the size of the infarct?

Dr. Minick: I think you made a statement concerning the correlation of VF with size of the infarct, did you not?

Dr. Kelliher: There is no correlation between the two in the cat model. In the cat model, when the LAD is tied off, there will be very slight variation in infarct size, about a 3% standard error. It is very reproducible, appears in the same location of the left ventricle every time, and is of the same size. Of course, these are the survivors, not the animals that fibrillated, and thus represent a somewhat selected population. The point I was making was that one of the possible mechanisms of action of sulfinpyrazone might have been a reduction in infarct size and in severity of arrhythmia, as suggested by Sobel's group but not corroborated by Thomas' group. We found no such results; in fact, sulfinpyrazone did not change the infarct size in survivors and my conclusion is that it's unlikely that sulfinpyrazone produces an antiarrhythmic or antifibrillatory effect by preserving the ischemic myocardium.

Dr. Sherry: Concerning your speculation that prostaglandins might be stimulating a release of norepinephrine, where do you think these prostaglandins are rising from, an ischemic myocardium or elsewhere?

Dr. Kelliher: Burger et al. at Yale University measured prostaglandins coming out of the great cardiac vein, compared them with those appearing in the coronary sinus, and reported that prostaglandins are released from all over the heart after acute coronary artery occlusion. However, there seems to be a differential release, in that the E-type prostaglandins are released on a general basis, whereas more of the F series of prostaglandins are released from the ischemic myocardium. With regard to norepinephrine release from sympathetic nerve endings, these two series of prostaglandins have just the opposite effects; the E series provides a feedback to reduce norepinephrine release, whereas the F series tends to facilitate norepinephrine release.

Dr. Sherry: If your speculation is correct, wouldn't one find a more striking effect with aspirin or indomethacin? Have you tested this?

Dr. Kelliher: Not yet, just with sulfinpyrazone so far. Concerning one of your earlier comments, Dr. Sherry, about the role of thromboxane, we have done a radioimmunoassay for thromboxane in blood collected from the great cardiac vein, which drains the ischemic area, and have been unable to find thromboxane being released after the occlusion.

Dr. Oliver: Have you studied the effect of sulfinpyrazone when you have pretreated the animal with a catechol such as isoproterenol.

Dr. Kelliher: You mean by a continuous infusion of isoproterenol to exacerbate the arrhythmia?

Dr. Oliver: Yes.

Dr. Kelliher: I'm doing it the other way around. I'm pretreating the animal with sulfinpyrazone and reinfusing the prostaglandin to see if I can come back to my high incidence of VF in that particular model.

Dr. Oliver: You should be able to set up a system where you can almost titrate the isoproterenol and the prostaglandin and sulfinpyrazone against each other.

Dr. Kelliher: An interesting comment I should make is that in this particular model if 6-hydroxy-dopamine, which destroys the nerve ending and releases norepinephrine, is administered during the occlusion so that norepinephrine is released, the animals fibrillate, every one of them. I think that there is a very high catecholamine involvement in this early arrhythmia in the cat.

Dr. Folts: When I was a student in 1970, Dr. Kramer and I demonstrated that prostaglandins are indeed released from ischemic myocardium; I believe we were the first to show that. Secondly, if one watches the anesthesia and the time of drawing the sample very carefully, it appears that sulfinpyrazone does indeed reduce circulating catecholamines to a statistically significant amount. We have data to show that sulfinpyrazone at a dose of 30 mg/kg does indeed lower circulating catechol-amines.

Inhibition of Platelet Plugging in Stenosed Dog Coronary Arteries with Sulfinpyrazone

J. D. Folts, Ph.D. and R. A. Beck

Introduction

In recent years there has been considerable interest generated with regard to the role of blood platelets in the genesis of atherosclerosis and in the mechanism of sudden death. While it is accepted that atherosclerotic narrowing of coronary arteries is the primary pathologic lesion, on postmortem examination those dying suddenly often fail to show evidence of recent sudden total occlusion of vessels or recent myocardial infarction [1]. Furthermore, those resuscitated after cardiac arrest commonly do not have myocardial infarction. Thus, the mechanisms leading to the fatal arrhythmia remain to be elucidated.

Platelet aggregation has been implicated, and it has been postulated that platelet plugs form in stenosed coronary and cerebral arteries and lead to sudden coronary death and stroke [2-4].

We have previously shown this in a dog model, where the animal was given a 60% to 80% fixed stenosis of a branch of the coronary artery [5]. Platelet plugs were shown to develop, producing cyclical reductions in coronary flow, which led to fatal arrhythmias when the coronary flow was low. These flow reductions caused by platelet plugging could be abolished with aspirin in a dose of 35 mg/kg [5]. However, these platelet plugs could be caused to return with infusions of epinephrine [6].

J. D. Folts, Ph.D. and R. A. Beck, Cardiovascular Section, Clinical Science Center, University of Wisconisn, Madison, Wis.

We present experimental evidence here that with a fixed stenosis in a narrowed coronary artery, platelet plugs form acutely, reducing the flow and that these flow reductions can be abolished with sulfinpyrazone.

Methods

Fifteen, healthy, adult, mongrel dogs of either sex were premedicated with morphine sulfate, 3 mg/kg, followed 30 min later with sodium pentobarbital, 30 mg/kg. Respiration was maintained with positive pressure from a Foregger anesthesia machine utilizing 75% nitrous oxide and 25% oxygen. The heart and coronary arteries were exposed through a left thoracotomy at the 5th intercostal space in the usual fashion.

Electromagnetic flowmeter probes were placed on the ascending aorta and the left circumflex coronary artery for measuring blood flow. A 2-0 silk ligature was placed loosely around the distal coronary artery to permit temporary complete occlusions so that the reactive hyperemic response could be measured and the baseline stability checked (Fig. 1). A cardiac catheter was passed down the carotid artery with its tip in the ascending aorta for arterial blood pressure measurement. An epicardial electrocardiograph (ECG) lead was placed in the area of the distal circumflex bed (Fig. 1). Two ultrasonic crystals were placed in the distal circumflex bed and used to measure regional myocardial cord length as a measure of "contractility." Control coronary and aortic flow was recorded along with ECG and contractility, as determined by rate of change in dimension measured with a Preyz Precision Instruments Sonomicrometer.

Stenosis was then produced with the plastic cylinder (3 mm in length) and the tapered fish line, as shown in Figure 1 (inset). These cylinders are made in a range of internal diameters, and one is chosen which just eliminates the reactive hyperemic response to a 20-sec complete occlusion [7, 8]. This has been called "critical stenosis" [9] and found to be approximately a 72% reduction in lumen diameter [8]. The plastic cylinder was then tied shut with a 2-0 Tevdek suture through the two small holes near the V, so that the stenosis would remain unchanged in size. (With this procedure, the reactive hyperemic response should remain abolished but coronary flow should approach normal levels. If necessary, fine adjustments of the amount of

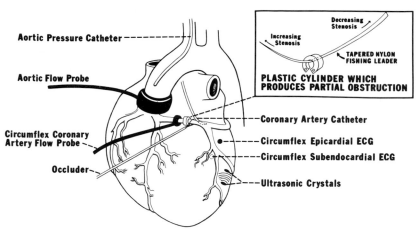

FIG. 1. Technique for producing fixed partial obstruction in the left circumflex coronary artery. The outside diameter of the artery is measured with a caliper, and an electromagnetic flowprobe of appropriate size is placed on the artery. Then a plastic cylinder, 3 mm in length (upper righthand corner) and with an internal diameter which will narrow the outside diameter by 60% to 80%, is placed on the vessel. The tapered monofilament fishline is placed in the lumen and the cylinder is tied shut with a 2-0 silk suture passed through the two small holes near the V. Small adjustments in the amount of stenosis can be made by pulling the fishline in either direction. Ultrasonic crystals are placed in the distal circumflex bed so that myocardial cord length can be determined as a measure of myocardial contractility.

fixed stenosis can be made by pulling the tapered fish line in either direction, thus slightly increasing or decreasing it.) The animal preparation was then studied as follows.

First the animal was monitored continuously for 45 min, during the time that cyclical flow reductions due to platelet accumulation were occurring. Several 20-sec complete occlusions were done so that lack of reactive hyperemic response could be confirmed, suggesting that with this level of fixed obstruction, the arterioles were maximally dilated. Control blood samples were taken for platelet aggregation studies (Sienco aggregometer), platelet counts, and plasma catecholamine determinations (Cat-O-Kit ®, Upjohn Co., Kalamazoo).

A reactive hyperemic response was determined and phasic coronary flow was recorded when the coronary flow was at its highest level, that is, not during a cyclical flow reduction. The phasic coronary flow record was divided into systolic and diastolic components, with the QRS complex used to denote the onset of systole and the dicrotic notch of the aortic pressure tracing used to depict the end of systole and the beginning of diastole. Ten consecutive cycles were planimetered and the ratio of diastolic to systolic flow was determined [10]. Heart rate, blood pressure, and ECG were also recorded.

During the next decline in coronary flow, sulfinpyrazone, 30 mg/kg, was administered IV over approximately 1 min. The animal was then continuously monitored for 1.5 h. Twenty minutes after the sulfinpyrazone was administered, blood samples were drawn again for platelet studies, and the plasma catecholamine and hemodynamic measurements were repeated. Phasic coronary flow was recorded and the diastolic:systolic flow ratio determined. The reactive hyperemic response was then repeated by total occlusion for 20 sec. In 7 of the 15 dogs, 30 min after the sulfinpyrazone had been given, 10 μg of epinephrine per minute was infused IV for 10 min.

Platelet Aggregation Studies

Twenty milliliters of venous blood was drawn into a plastic syringe and diluted with one part 3.8% trisodium citrate to nine parts blood in a polystyrene tube. Platelet-rich plasma (PRP) was obtained by centrifuging this mixture for 15 min at room temperature. If the platelet count in the PRP was greater than 300,000/cu mm, it was adjusted to that figure using autologous platelet-poor plasma (PPP).

Aggregation studies were done with a Sienco aggregometer by a modification of the method of Born [11]. PRP, 0.4 ml, was placed at 37°C in a siliconized cuvette in the aggregometer with a siliconized stirring bar. The aggregometer was adjusted to give 5 and 95 light transmission units (LTU) readings on the Sienco recorder with PRP and PPP, respectively. An addition of 0.1 ml of aggregating substance (ADP, 50 μg/ml) was made, and the change in light transmission was measured to the point where the tracing reached a plateau or began to decline. The aggregation tendency of each test sample was then reported in units ranging from 5 to 95 LTU, with the higher numbers indicating greater aggregation of platelets by ADP.

Although canine platelets do not aggregate in response to epinephrine alone, studies were done to determine the synergistic effects of low-dose ADP and low-dose epinephrine as a combined aggregating stimulus. Twenty microliters of 1:100,000 (55 μM) epinephrine was administered with 0.1 ml of ADP (10 μg/ml) so that the inhibitory effect of sulfinpyrazone on this synergistic aggregating effect could be determined.

Results

There were cyclical reductions in flow in all 15 dogs. Three of these flow reductions are shown in Figure 2. We feel that the rate at which flow declines is related directly to the rate of platelet accumulation in the narrowed lumen (slope m) and that the size of the flow jump (y) is a function of the size of the platelet plug which broke loose. A reactive hyperemic response to a 20-sec complete occlusion, done at a time when flow was not declining, is shown in Figure 3. During the occlusion, the ECG shows mild ST segment deviation and the ultrasonic

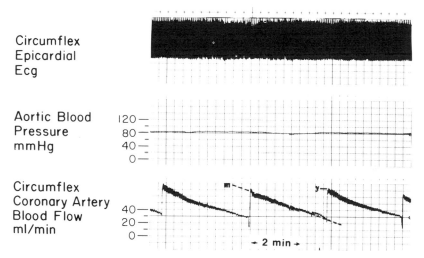

FIG. 2. Mean aortic pressure and mean coronary flow showing three cyclical reductions in coronary blood flow in an artery stenosed 70%. The flow reductions are caused by platelet plugs forming in the stenosed lumen and then breaking loose and being carried downstream. The rate of decline in flow indicated by the slope is related to the rate at which the platelets are accumulating in the lumen. The size of the flow jump (y) is related to the size of the platelet mass which breaks loose and is carried downstream.

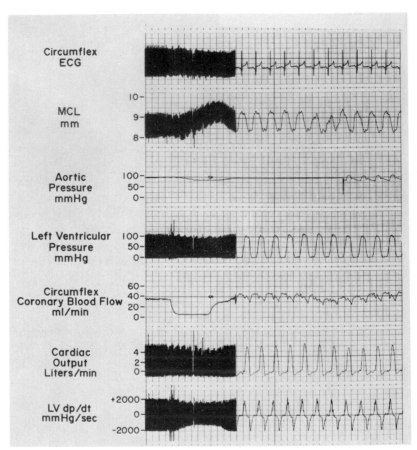

FIG. 3. The epicardial ECG in the distal circumflex bed is shown at the top, followed by myocardial cord length (MCL) or "contractility," as measured with the ultrasonic crystals. Note the increased MCL that occurs with a 20-sec complete occlusion of the circumflex coronary artery. The sudden increase in MCL cord length or decrease in "contractility" shows the sensitivity of the crystals in detecting impaired contractility during the temporary complete occlusion of the circumflex coronary artery. The aortic pressure falls, and left ventricular dp/dt decreases from the ischemic insult. It should be noted that with this level of fixed mechanical stenosis there is no reactive hyperemic response to the 20-sec complete occlusion. A similar phenomenon occurs when the flow declines as a result of platelet plug formation. On the right, at fast paper speed the phasic coronary flow shows a diastolic:systolic flow ratio of 1.4, which suggests severe stenosis of the circumflex coronary artery.

crystals show impaired "contractility" as indicated by the increased myocardial cord length. Figure 4 shows the effect of giving the sulfinpyrazone during a decline in flow. The arrow indicates the beginning of the infusion. There is an abrupt reversal of the decline and coronary flow increases although arterial blood pressure remains unchanged. The phasic flow pattern (Fig. 4, left) shows a low diastolic:systolic flow ratio, indicating severe stenosis.

Figure 5 (right) shows the increased diastolic:systolic flow ratio and a hyperemic response to the 20-sec complete occlusion now occurring even though the obstructing cylinder is still tied closed and the tapered fish line has not been moved, i.e., the mechanical external cause of the fixed stenoses applied earlier has not been changed.

Table 1 shows hemodynamic measurements before and after administration of sulfinpyrazone. The heart rate declined from 127 ± 30 beats/min to 97 ± 23 beats/min (p<0.001), and the blood pressure did not change. The mean coronary flow increased from 38 ± 9 ml/min to 40 ± 6 ml/min but the increase was not statistically significant. There was a reactive hyperemic response of 23 ± 8 ml/min after administration of sulfin-pyrazone. The average diastolic:systolic flow ratio was 1.7 ± 0.4 before and 2.4 ± 0.3 after administration of sulfinpyrazone (p<0.01).

The results of the platelet aggregation studies are shown in Figure 6. Sulfinpyrazone at this dose significantly decreased the aggregation response to all three concentrations of ADP. The synergistic effect of low-dose ADP and epinephrine was reduced more than the effect of ADP alone. In the seven dogs that received epinephrine infusions there were no cyclical flow reductions after administration of sulfinpyrazone in response to epinephrine. The only other agent we know of which protects against epinephrine-induced platelet plugging is phentolamine (J. D. Folts, unpublished data).

The epinephrine and norepinephrine levels did not change to a statistically significant degree after administration of sulfinpyrazone. The cyclical reductions in flow were abolished for an average of 85 ± 14 min, after which they gradually returned.

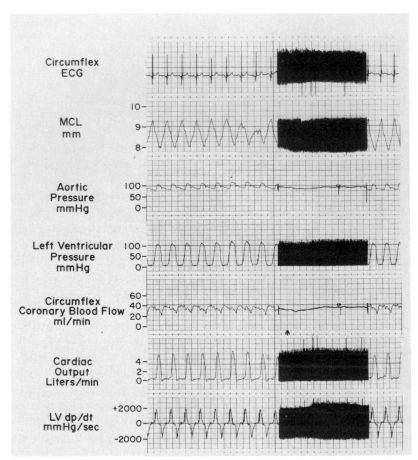

FIG. 4. On the left, at fast paper speed, the circumflex coronary blood flow has begun to decline, representing the accumulation of another platelet plug in the stenosed lumen. At the arrow in the center, while the coronary flow is falling, the IV infusion of sulfinpyrazone is begun. Within 2 min the flow stops declining and begins to rise again, suggesting that the sulfinpyrazone has already begun to clear the lumen of residual platelet masses. The myocardial cord length begins to decrease, suggesting improved regional contractility, and the left ventricular LV dp/dt increases, suggesting an improvement in global function.

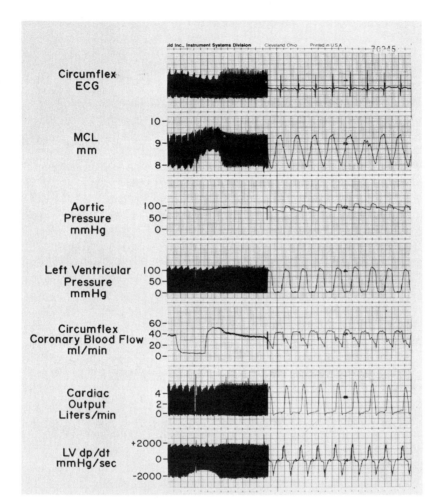

FIG. 5. Record taken 20 min after sulfinpyrazone has been given. On the left there is now a reactive hyperemic response to the temporary 20-sec complete occlusion (compared to Fig. 3 where there was none), even though the externally applied mechanical stenosis has not changed. On the right the myocardial cord length has decreased, suggesting improved regional contractility, and the circumflex phasic flow pattern has improved, with a greater diastolic:systolic flow ratio of 2.5 indicating that there is now less stenosis in the lumen of the circumflex coronary artery in the area of the fixed obstruction.

Table 1. Hemodynamic Effects of Sulfinpyrazone in Anesthetized Dogs

	Before Sulfinpyrazone	After Sulfinpyrazone	p
Coronary Blood Flow (ml/min)	38 ± 9	40 ± 11	NS
Reactive Hyperemia (ml/min)	0	23 ± 8	p<0.001
Arterial Blood Pressure (mm Hg)	96 ± 11	96 ± 12	NS
Heart Rate (beats/min)	127 ± 30	97 ± 23	p<0.001
Plasma Epinephrine Levels (pg/ml)	531 ± 767	331 ± 286	p<0.4
Diastolic:Systolic Flow Ratio	1.7 ± .4	2.4 ± 3	p<0.01

Dogs (n = 15) were given sulfinpyrazone 30 mg/kg IV. NS = Not significant.

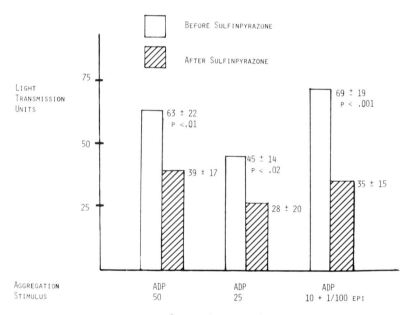

FIG. 6. Bar graphs showing the decrease in *in vitro* aggregation before and 20 min after sulfinpyrazone, 30 mg/kg IV, in response to three standard aggregating stimuli: ADP 50: 0.1 ml of ADP, 50 μg/ml; ADP 25: 0.1 ml of ADP, 25 μg/ml; and ADP 10 + 1/100 EPI: 0.1 ml of ADP, 10 μg/ml and a 1:100 dilution of epinephrine (55 μM, total epinephrine). The greatest change after administration of sulfinpyrazone occurred in the synergistic effect of low-dose ADP and epinephrine.

Discussion

The concept of pharmacologic inhibition of platelet activity as an approach to antithrombotic therapy has gained considerable support in recent years. Platelet microemboli have been demonstrated in the epicardial arteries of man [12] and in the intramyocardial vessels of patients dying suddenly of coronary artery disease [13]. Platelet aggregates in human coronary arteries producing ischemia and sudden death have been postulated by many investigators [14-16]. Experimental models using brief intracoronary infusions of ADP, a potent platelet aggregator, have demonstrated focal ischemic myocardial necrosis, myocardial infarction, and sudden death in the pig [17].

Studies on platelet microthrombi and platelet plugs in sudden cardiac death are faced with one important methodological problem — the lability and apparent reversibility of the aggregates. This reversibility was a significant factor when the frequency of intramyocardial platelet microemboli arising from a pump oxygenator was related to the length of postoperative survival [18]. Platelet fibrin microemboli were five to ten times more common in patients surviving less than 24 h than in comparable patients who survived 24 to 48 h. If platelet aggregates formed, thereby reducing coronary flow, and then broke loose, the sudden restoration of flow could produce a fatal arrhythmia. The lethal platelet aggregate would no longer be in the narrowed segment of the lumen and could be difficult to find distally.

We have previously shown in a dog model that platelets do aggregate in coronary arteries given a 60% to 80% fixed mechanical stenosis [5]. These platelet plugs occur within 5 to 10 min and can lead to a fatal arrhythmia if not prevented with aspirin [5] or other means. We have also shown that by IV infusions of epinephrine [6] or nicotine [19], or by ventilating the dog with cigarette smoke [19], periodic platelet plugging can be caused to recur in spite of treatment with aspirin.

Our studies with sulfinpyrazone appear promising for several reasons. As a platelet inhibitor, sulfinpyrazone inhibits the platelet release reaction [20, 21], increases platelet survival time in patients with previously decreased platelet survival [22, 23], and decreases platelet adhesiveness [24]. It does not have an effect on bleeding time [25]. Most of sulfinpyrazone's antiplatelet properties have been attributed to the fact that it competitively inhibits cyclooxygenase in the platelet prostaglandin synthetic pathway [26]. Sulfinpyrazone has a half-life of approximately 2 h, and since it is a competitive inhibitor, it can be effective only as long as it circulates in the plasma. However, metabolic derivatives may be active for a longer period of time.

In our animal model, sulfinpyrazone does three things which appear to be beneficial. First, it is the only agent that we have studied which can reverse a progressive reduction in coronary flow due to platelet accumulation in the narrowed lumen, with return of flow to normal (Fig. 4). The other agents we have studied, including aspirin [6], indomethacin, and propranolol (J. D. Folts, unpublished observations), did not show this capacity to reverse platelet aggregation in the narrowed lumen after its onset, although they would prevent any repeated onset of the process. This may be due to sulfinpyrazone's ability to decrease platelet adhesiveness or possibly to a direct effect on the vessel wall [27]. At any rate, the sulfinpyrazone appears to clear the lumen, restoring to it the amount of fixed stenosis present before platelets and any other material began to accumulate there, and to allow maximal flow for the given amount of stenosis.

Secondly, although the fixed mechanical stenosis applied initially is unchanged, administration of sulfinpyrazone increases the diastolic:systolic flow ratio. We have previously shown that an increase in stenosis produces a decrease in the diastolic:systolic flow ratio and a progressive loss in the reactive hyperemic response [28]. We have used this decrease in the flow ratio diagnostically to detect areas of stenosis in, or distal to, aortocoronary saphenous vein bypass grafts [10]. Conversely, any mechanism which decreases the stenosis increases the diastolic:systolic flow ratio and restores some reactive hyperemic response to a 20-sec complete occlusion. Sulfinpyrazone does this, possibly by clearing residual platelets from the stenosed lumen and thus reducing the total stenosis.

Thirdly, sulfinpyrazone appears to protect against epinephrine exacerbation of cyclical flow reductions due to platelet plugging. With the three other agents we studied, epinephrine infusions caused platelet plugging and cyclical flow reductions to recur, producing ischemia and sudden death. This did not occur when epinephrine infusions were given in the 1.5-h period after sulfinpyrazone administration.

The reduction in heart rate was unexpected and, at present, cannot be accounted for, although it occurred in every case. The return of the reactive hyperemic response may be due in part to the reduced heart rate. However, the improvement in phasic flow pattern would suggest a decrease in total obstruction at the stenosis.

If these mechanisms occur in man with stenosed coronary or other arteries, sulfinpyrazone could be beneficial in several ways. It might clear the stenosed lumen of adhering platelets and reduce the rate at which platelets reaccumulate there, thus preventing interaction between platelets and the damaged vessel wall. Mustard has postulated that platelets adhering to the atherosclerotic plaque are involved in several ways in exacerbating its development [29].

Secondly, sulfinpyrazone by its various antiplatelet actions may reduce the incidence of vessel obstruction from platelet plug formation, thereby reducing the incidence of sudden death. Since sulfinpyrazone appears to protect against epinephrine-exacerbated platelet plugging, this may account for another part of the apparent success in the Anturane Reinfarction Trial, which reported a 48% reduction in cardiac deaths as a result of sulfinpyrazone treatment compared to placebo [21]. The Type A patients and smokers in the studies of antiplatelet agents very likely have at least transient elevations of catecholamines, and if so, sulfinpyrazone might be more beneficial than other antiplatelet agents that do not negate catecholamine effects.

Thirdly, if sulfinpyrazone could clear the lumen of agglutinated platelets, thus increasing lumen diameter, restoring some coronary flow, and permitting reactive hyperemia, and reduce the heart rate as well, thus decreasing myocardial demand, it could retrieve a patient from preinfarction angina and prevent acute myocardial infarction. Since it does not alter bleeding time, it should not interfere with needed surgical or catheterization procedures.

In summary, it appears that sulfinpyrazone abolishes platelet plugging in stenosed dog coronary arteries, reduces heart rate, improves phasic coronary flow pattern, restores some arteriolar reserve, and protects against the epinephrine-exacerbated platelet plugging (as aspirin does not). Sulfinpyrazone is the only agent we have studied which at this dose protects against epinephrine-exacerbated cyclical coronary flow reductions due to platelet plugs.

References

1. Grace, W.J.: Sudden death and acute myocardial infarction — what are we talking about? Am. Heart J. 92: 1-2, 1976.
2. Schwartz, C.J. and Gerrity, R.G.: Anatomical pathology of sudden unexpected cardiac death. Circulation 51-52: III18-III26, 1975.
3. Blakely, J.A. and Gent, M.: Platelets, drugs and longevity in a geriatric population. In Hirsh, J., Cade, J.F., Gallus, A.S. and Schönbaum, E. (eds.): Platelets, Drugs, and Thrombosis. Basel: S. Karger, 1975, pp. 284-291.
4. Acheson, J. and Hutchinson, E.C.: Controlled trial of clofibrate in cerebral vascular disease. Atherosclerosis 15: 177-183, 1972.
5. Folts, J.D., Crowell, E.B. and Rowe, G.G.: Platelet aggregation in partially obstructed vessels and its elimination with aspirin. Circulation 54: 365-370, 1976.
6. Folts, J.D. and Rowe, G.G.: Platelet aggregation in stenosed coronary arteries: Mechanism of sudden death? (Abst.). Am. J. Cardiol. 41: 425, 1978.
7. Folts, J.D., Gallagher, K. and Rowe, G.G.: Hemodynamic effects of controlled amounts of coronary artery stenosis in short term and long term studies in dogs. J. Thorac. Cardiovasc. Surg. 73: 722-727, 1977.
8. Gallagher, K.P., Folts, J.D. and Rowe, G.G.: Comparison of coronary arteriograms with direct measurements of stenosed coronary arteries in dogs. Am. Heart J. 95: 338-347, 1978.
9. May, A.G., Van de Berg, L., DeWeese, J.A. and Rob, C.J.: Critical arterial stenosis. Surgery 54: 250-259, 1963.
10. Folts, J.D., Kahn, D.R., Bittar, N. and Rowe, G.G.: Effects of partial obstruction on phasic flow in aortocoronary grafts. Circulation 51-52: I48-I54, 1975.
11. Born, G.V.R.: Aggregation of blood platelets by adenosine diphosphate and its reversal. Nature 194: 927, 1962.
12. Haerem, J.W.: The occurrence of platelet aggregates in the epicardial arteries of man. Atherosclerosis 14: 417-423, 1971.
13. Haerem, J.W.: Platelet aggregates in intramyocardial vessels of patients dying suddenly and unexpectedly of coronary artery disease. Atherosclerosis 19: 529-541, 1974.
14. Genton, E., Gent, M., Hirsh, J. and Harker, L.A.: Platelet-inhibiting drugs in the prevention of clinical thrombotic disease. N. Engl. J. Med. 293: 1236-1240, 1975.

15. Weiss, H.J.: Antiplatelet drugs — A new pharmacologic approach to the prevention of thrombosis. Am. Heart J. 92: 86-102, 1976.
16. Mustard, J.F. and Packham, M.A.: Platelet function in myocardial infarction. Circulation 39: 20-25, 1969.
17. Jorgensen, L., Rowsell, H.C., Hovig, T., Glynn, M.F. and Mustard, J.F.: Adenosine diphosphate-induced platelet aggregation and myocardial infarction in swine. Lab. Invest. 17: 617-644, 1967.
18. Schwartz, C.J., Korns, M.E., Edwards, J.F. et al.: Pathologic sequelae and complications of ventriculotomy with particular reference to platelet thromboemboli in the small intramyocardial vessels. Arch. Pathol. 89: 56-64, 1970.
19. Folts, J.D., Bonebrake, F.C., Anderson, J.M. and Rowe, G.G.: Exacerbation of platelet aggregation in stenosed coronary arteries with cigarette smoke after aspirin (Abst.). Clin. Res. 26: 645, 1978.
20. Hirsh, J.: Clinical effects of platelet function suppressing drugs. In Mills, D.C.B. (ed.): Platelets and Thrombosis. New York: Academic Press, 1977, pp. 175-183.
21. The Anturane Reinfarction Trial Research Group: Sulfinpyrazone in the prevention of cardiac death after myocardial infarction. N. Engl. J. Med. 298: 289-295, 1978.
22. Smythe, H., Ogryzlo, M.A., Murphy, E.A. et al.: The effect of sulfinpyrazone (Anturan) on platelet economy and blood coagulation in man. Canad. Med. Assoc. J. 92: 818-821, 1965.
23. Weily, H. and Genton, E.: Altered platelet function in patients with prosthetic mitral valves. Effects of sulfinpyrazone therapy. Circulation 42: 967-972, 1970.
24. Cazenave, J.P.: Inhibition of platelet adherence to a collagen-coated surface by nonsteroidal anti-inflammatory drugs, pyrimido-pyrmidine, and tricyclic compounds and lidocaine. J. Lab. Clin. Med. 83: 797-806, 1974.
25. Winchester, J.: Effect of sulfinpyrazone and aspirin on platelet adhesion to activated charcoal and dialysis membranes in vitro. Thromb. Res. 11: 443-451, 1977.
26. Ali, M. and McDonald, J.W.D.: Effects of sulfinpyrazone on platelet prostaglandin synthesis and platelet release of serotonin. J. Lab. Clin. Med. 89: 868-875, 1977.
27. Verstraete, M.: Are agents affecting platelet functions clinically useful? Am. J. Med. 61: 897-913, 1976.
28. Folts, J.D., Gallagher, K.P. and Rowe, G.G.: Phasic coronary blood flow changes with partial coronary artery obstruction (Abst.). Physiologist 17: 233, 1974.
29. Mustard, J.F.: Platelets and thrombosis in acute myocardial infarction. Hosp. Pract., January 1972, pp. 115-128.

Discussion

Dr. White: I was surprised to see qualitative differences in your model with respect to effects on cyclical blood flow between papaverine, dipyridamole, and caffeine, because these are all inhbitors of phosphodiesterase. In the case of papaverine, the dose was very low, 1 mg/kg, and that could be the explanation.

Dr. Folts: We have not used higher doses of papaverine, because at the 1 mg/kg dose you can spread it topically on an artery in spasm; it makes it balloon right out, and surgeons commonly use it for spasm. One would have to use a higher dose, I think, to inhibit phosphodiesterase.

Dr. White: The effects of sulfinpyrazone on ADP-induced platelet aggregation are not readily understandable.

Dr. Folts: I don't understand them either, except that it may be a species-specific matter, and we do use a fairly high dose of ADP as the stimulus for aggregation.

Dr. Gordon: As was noted earlier, it's well established that in the dog platelets do not normally respond to thromboxane A_2, although they do make thromboxanes when they're stimulated. As far as I know, no one apart from yourself has looked at a dog platelet aggregation model *in vivo* in quite this way. This may be a useful comparative model for studying the effects of sulfinpyrazone, inasmuch as the actions of sulfinpyrazone that are independent of any effect on prostaglandin synthesis might be more evident in the dog than in another species. Have you had the opportunity to perform similar studies in other species?

Dr. Folts: Yes, we have studied one monkey and two pigs, but we have not given them sulfinpyrazone yet. In those animals aspirin does inhibit the spontaneous platelet plugs, but they can be brought back with epinephrine. We have used prostacyclin, and prostacyclin does abolish them very nicely.

Dr. Gordon: Aspirin, of course, is a cyclooxygenase inhibitor and therefore will prevent formation of all products distal to the cyclooxygenase enzyme; imidazole and some substituted imidazoles are specific inhibitors of thromboxane production. Have you looked at those compounds in the dog model?

Dr. Folts: Not yet; we are going to test some agents that are supposed to do that.

Dr. Gordon: In regard to Dr. White's comment, the question of sulfinpyrazone inhibiting ADP-induced aggregation *in vitro* is curious. When citrate is used as an anticoagulant, if there is any change in the hematocrit during the experiment, then the citrate concentration in the plasma will alter and thus affect the platelet aggregation response *in vitro*. Could a change in hematocrit have occurred in your experiments?

Dr. Folts: Hematocrits did not change. In the sulfinpyrazone experiments, we performed aggregation studies just before and after addition of sulfinpyrazone. When we gave epinephrine challenges to see if we could provoke platelet plugging again, we did not do any platelet aggregation studies, partly because the epinephrine causes emptying of the spleen and hematocrit does change rather dramatically in the dog. In the studies I reported here there was no change in hematocrit.

Dr. Minick: In man it is suggested that in coronary artery stenosis there must be alterations in the endothelium and fractures of plaques to promote thrombosis at the site of stenosis. Your studies would suggest that the stenosis alone might be enough to cause platelet aggregation and perhaps occlusion of the artery. Have you examined the arterial wall at these sites? What is the status of the endothelium in the remainder of the wall at the sites of narrowing that you produce with your clamp?

Dr. Folts: We have done histologic sections. Even if one puts on the plastic clyinder and manipulates the monofilament leader very carefully, there is some cracking and damage to the intima. If one then exacerbates it by pinching, poking, and beating the vessel, one gets greatly exacerbated platelet aggregation here. In some that were treated very, very carefully, within 5 min after placing a plastic cylinder, we still saw the cyclical flow reductions. Turbulence, damaging red cells and platelets which release ADP, might start the process, but that is combined with the fact that the endothelium is surely somewhat damaged, as well.

Dr. Mustard: Did you say that when aggregates form in the vessels, you can give sulfinpyrazone IV and reverse them, but if you give aspirin IV, they do not reverse?

Dr. Folts: That's correct.

Dr. Mustard: Have you measured PGI_2 production in your stenosed vessel, since stimulation of the vessel wall probably promotes PGI_2 production?

Dr. Folts: No, we haven't. I'm planning some experiments in which we can place fine catheters above and below the obstruction, and I'm trying to find a suitable assay for PGI_2. We hope to draw simultaneous samples and see if there is PGI_2.

Dr. Mustard: If you are studying thrombus formation at a site where there is strong stimulation for PGI_2 production, then PGI_2 will tend to decrease the amount of thrombus formation. If you then use too much aspirin and inhibit the PGI_2 production, you will potentiate the thrombus formation. In your aspirin experiments where you fail to get an effect, I wonder what would happen if you went to a lower dose of aspirin.

Dr. Folts: We have tried lower doses of aspirin and with doses of less than 15 mg/kg of aspirin we were unable to abolish even spontaneous platelet plugs.

Dr. Oliver: Dr. Harker has asked to present some data.

Dr. Harker: When we had a significant population of survivors from acute coronary events in Seattle, we sought evidence in these patients of platelet activation *in vivo*. The most sensitive indicator that we have available is a radioimmunoassay of platelet factor 4 (the platelet-specific protein released from the alpha granule).

When values are measured in a large number of individuals, it can be seen that in normal subjects the plasma levels are at a mean of <1 ng. Patients with idiopathic thrombocytopenic purpura have values similar to normal subjects; patients with coronary artery disease and peripheral vascular disease have significantly increased levels, with less than 10% of overlap with the normal subjects. Patients with aortic aneurysms undergoing resection and patients on oxygenator bypass can be shown to have markedly elevated levels. In patients that have survived ventricular fibrillation ("sudden death"), the levels are also significantly different. Although this is a small number of patients, the differences are quite striking.

When you look at platelet survival time in the same patients, there are no measurable differences beween the age- and sex-matched patients with coronary artery disease (without ventricular fibrillation). Therefore platelet factor 4 may serve as a useful indicator of platelet activation *in vitro* in patients with cardiovascular events.

Platelets, Sulfinpyrazone and Organ Graft Rejection

Stuart W. Jamieson, M.B., F.R.C.S., Nelson A. Burton, M.D. and Bruce A. Reitz, M.D.

Introduction

At the turn of the century, adrenal glands, thyroids, parathyroids, ovaries, legs, arms, loops of intestine, the lower half of the body, the head and neck, as well as kidneys and hearts, were all being transplanted experimentally. Failure occurred in every case, largely because of technical reasons. Then, in 1933, it was first documented that late failure might be due to "biological incompatibility," which, of course, we now call rejection. Thus organ transplantation did not become a clinical reality until the early 1960s, when chemical immunosuppression was first used. However, in the last 20 years there have been no real advances in the use of immunosuppressive agents available for clinical use, and in both renal and cardiac transplantation rejection remains the primary barrier to success.

In simple terms rejection takes place by two almost distinct mechanisms. The first is infiltration of the graft by lymphocytes, which cause rejection of the organ in the untreated host between one and two weeks, and the second is the production of antibodies by the host. The early, progressive, and cellular phase of rejection can be treated with drugs such as antithymocyte globulin, azathioprine, and steroids. The second, more insidious, form of transplant rejection is manifested by the development of arteriosclerosis, related to antibody. No

Stuart W. Jamieson, M.B., F.R.C.S., Nelson A. Burton, M.D. and Bruce A. Reitz, M.D., Department of Cardiovascular Surgery, Stanford University Hospital, Stanford, Calif.

effective treatment is currently available for this. This arteriosclerosis is seen in all organ transplants in all species and, after early rejection crises have been surmounted, is the major impediment to long-term organ graft survival.

The development of this atheroma is the result of the interaction of the antibody circulating within the vessel, the endothelial lining of the vessel wall, and platelets. We designed a study to determine the effect of platelet-active agents on the survival of heart transplants in rats. Rats were chosen because inbred strains were available. This made the experiments reproducible and the assessment of treatment possible. Hearts are a particularly suitable model because they are highly vascular. Their function is easily assessed and an advantage over renal transplants is that uremia, itself an immunosuppressant, is not encountered.

Methods

Heart Transplantation

Heterotopic cardiac transplantation was performed after modification of the method described by Ono and Lindsey [1]. After heparinization, the donor heart is removed by ligation of both venae cavae and all pulmonary veins and division of aorta and pulmonary artery. Anastomosis of donor aorta to recipient abdominal aorta and of donor pulmonary artery to recipient inferior vena cava is then made end-to-side. In this way recipient blood, via the aorta, perfuses the coronary circulation of the donor heart. Blood returns through the coronary sinus to the right atrium, then to the right ventricle, and to the recipient inferior vena cava via the pulmonary artery. The abdomen is closed and subsequent assessment of graft function is easily made by simple palpation of the heart through the abdominal wall or by placing ECG electrodes upon the surface of the abdomen.

Rats

Inbred ACI rats were used as donors and inbred Lewis-Brown Norway rats as recipients. These strains, mismatched at two Ag-B loci [2], represent a model of severe rejection [3].

Treatment

The following drugs were used:

azathioprine	30 mg/kg
methylprednisolone	20 mg/kg
dipyridamole	60 mg/kg
promethazine hydrochloride	20 mg/kg
sulfinpyrazone	150 mg/kg
sodium salicylate	200 mg/kg
aspirin	200 mg/kg
ibuprofen	80 mg/kg
indomethacin	4 mg/kg

Promethazine hydrochloride was given intraperitoneally; all other drugs were administered subcutaneously once daily.

Results and Further Experiments

Eighty transplants were performed and the animals divided into ten treatment groups (Table 1). Animals with no treatment

Table 1. Survival Times for Treatment Groups

Treatment	No. of Rats	Survival (days)	Mean ± SD			p
None	8	5,5,6,6,6,6,6,7	6	±	0.6	—
Azathioprine	8	6,6,6,6,6,6,7,7	6	±	0.5	NS
Azathioprine and prednisolone	8	6,6,7,7,7,7,8,50	12	±	15.3	NS
Azathioprine and dipyridamole	8	3,6,6,7,7,7,8,8	6.5	±	1.6	NS
Azathioprine and promethazine	8	7,7,9,15,17,22,39,42	20	±	4.9	<0.03
Azathioprine and sulfinpyrazone	8	6,7,12,16,31,32,>50,>50	26	±	18.0	<0.02
Azathioprine and sodium salicylate	8	all >50	50	±	0.0	<0.01
Azathioprine and aspirin	8	all >50	50	±	0.0	<0.01
Azathioprine and ibuprofen	8	6,6,6,6,6,6,7,7,	6	±	0.5	NS
Azathioprine and indomethacin	8	5,5,6,6,6,6,6,7	6	±	0.6	NS

NS = Not significant.

rejected their grafts with a mean survival time (MST) of 6 ± 0.6 (SD) days. Neither azathioprine nor azathioprine plus methylprednisolone, both in toxic doses, significantly delayed rejection, although one heart in the group receiving the latter treatment continued to beat weakly for 50 days.

Azathioprine was then combined with five antiplatelet agents: dipyridamole, promethazine hydrochloride, sulfinpyrazone, sodium salicylate, and aspirin. Azathioprine and dipyridamole did not produce a significant difference in survival as compared to the animals receiving no treatment or azathioprine alone, but rejection was modified in each of the other four groups. The MST with azathioprine and sulfinpyrazone was 26 days, a fourfold increase over that of the controls. When either sodium salicylate or aspirin was used, all hearts were beating normally at 50 days. In an earlier series of experiments, all animals died when azathioprine was given continuously with sodium salicylate or aspirin. In these groups, therefore, drugs were given in combination for the first week only, and thereafter sodium salicylate or aspirin was given alone.

The latter two combinations were obviously the best. They were studied intensively in rats and then used in dogs and monkeys. Unfortunately, it soon became apparent that the action of azathioprine with salicylates was not only an antiplatelet one, as profound leukopenia developed through bone marrow suppression. Despite varying the dosage and the time of administration of the drugs, a regimen could not be found that prevented rejection but did not kill the animals. These combinations were therefore abandoned in this study.

To determine whether similar results as those obtained with azathioprine and sulfinpyrazone could be obtained with prostaglandin inhibitors, we treated 16 rats with a combination of azathioprine and either ibuprofen or indomethacin. There was no increase in survival in either of these two groups. This indicated that the prolongation of survival seen with promethazine and sulfinpyrazone was independent of prostaglandin inhibition.

The next question was whether sulfinpyrazone was depressing circulating antibody levels. Cytotoxic antibody was determined by the method of Floersheim and Ruskiewicz [4]. Figure 1 shows the antibody levels in recipient rats that were

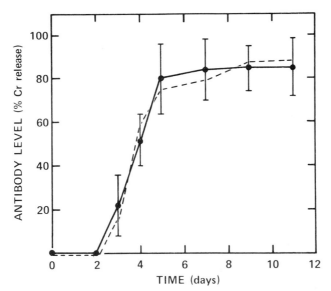

FIG. 1. Antibody levels in recipient animals. (——) no treatment; (- - - -) treated with azathioprine and sulfinpyrazone.

either untreated or treated with azathioprine and sulfinpyra-zone. Circulating antibody was detected after two days and rose to high levels by five days. There was no inhibition of cytotoxic antibody formation by azathioprine and sulfinpyrazone.

For determination of the effect of circulating antibody in a cardiac transplant, guinea pig hearts were transplanted into Lewis-Brown Norway rats. Rats possess preexisting antibody against guinea pigs, and rejection of guinea pig hearts is immediate or hyperacute [5]. This model has the advantage that inbred strains can be used, and the rejection process is very finely reproducible. Biopsies of 40 such transplants were taken at minute intervals for 10 minutes, when rejection was complete.

Figures 2 to 6 show representative appearances of such biopsies. They demonstrate the sequence of events that occurs in a transplant when antibody begins to circulate.

Figure 2 shows a large capillary 2 min after revascularization of the graft and its exposure to antibody. Red blood cells (rbc) are shown within the lumen. An endothelial cell nucleus (n) and the endothelial cytoplasm (end) are seen. Two platelets (pl) are present.

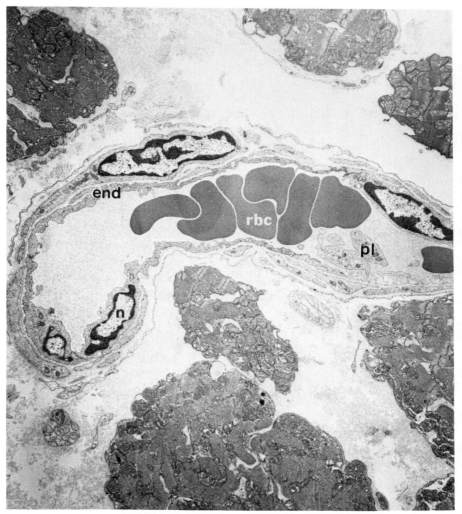

FIG. 2. Guinea pig heart 2 min after revascularization (original magnification: × 5,500). *rbc*, red blood cells; *end*, endothelial cell cytoplasm; *pl*, platelets; *n*, endothelial cell nucleus.

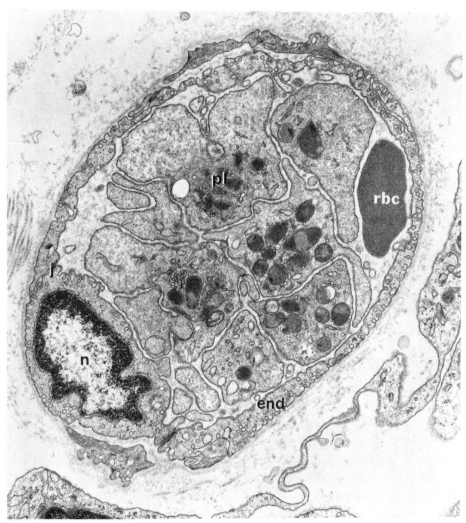

FIG. 3. Capillary at 4 min (original magnification: ×33,500). *j*, tight junction of endothelial cell (*end*).

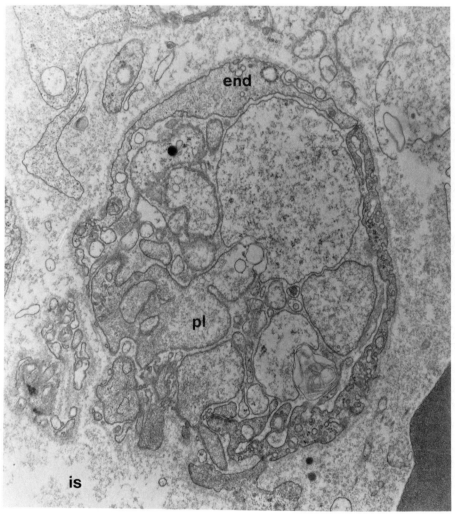

FIG. 4. Capillary at 6 min (original magnification: × 23,300). *end*, endothelium; *pl*, platelet (degranulated); *is*, interstitium.

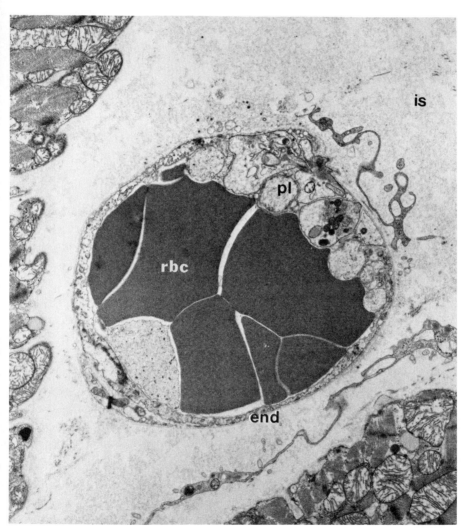

FIG. 5. Capillary at 6 min (original magnification: ×23,300). *rbc*, red blood cell; *pl*, platelets; *is*, interstitium.

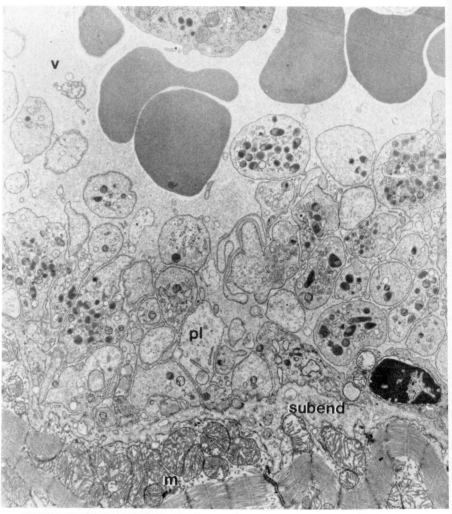

FIG. 6. Vein at 8 min (original magnification: × 23,300). *v*, lumen of vein; *pl*, platelet; *subend*, subendothelium; *m*, cardiac muscle.

A capillary at 4 min is seen in Figure 3. This is a smaller capillary, but platelets (*pl*) are seen almost occluding the lumen. Part of a red cell (*rbc*) is shown. This was a constant appearance at 4 min. We found to our surprise that platelets were aggregating when the endothelium was morphologically normal. We had assumed that the endothelium would first be damaged by antibody and platelet aggregation would then occur on damaged endothelium. This was clearly not the case, even when platelets had begun to degranulate.

At 4 and 5 min all the platelets at the periphery of the vessels began to degranulate, although the endothelium remained normal. At 6 min (Fig. 4) endothelial cell damage was seen. Next to degranulated platelets the endothelium became edematous and was finally destroyed. This appearance was seen only in those vessels containing platelets, and then only next to degranulated platelets.

This is exemplified in Figure 5, which shows a capillary at 6 min containing both erythrocytes and platelets. The endothelium is normal next to the erythrocytes but has been damaged and removed next to the platelets, which are now leaking out into the interstitium (*is*).

The final process is seen in Figure 6, a large vein at 10 min. The endothelium has been removed, and the platelets are now adhering to the naked subendothelium (*subend*), next to a pyknotic and damaged endothelial cell nucleus. This is the process previously recognized to occur — that platelets would adhere to the subendothelium. However, because the process is so rapid, and because a reproducible model was not previously available, it was not appreciated that platelet aggregation and degranulation always took place before morphological damage occurred to the endothelium.

Discussion

The possibility that platelets play a role in the pathogenesis of arteriosclerotic lesions was first proposed by Duguid in 1946 [6]. When transplantation of organs became a clinical reality and vascular lesions were encountered, it was proposed that these lesions were the result of either an antigen-antibody reaction in the vessel wall or the deposition of immune complexes at this site [7]. Supporting this, a very close association was noted between the appearance of humoral antibodies in patients with renal allografts and the appearance of vascular lesions in the transplants [8]. Mowbray [9] found that there was an accumulation of platelets in rejection episodes and it was realized that prompt treatment with steroids during rejection episodes could be successful in inducing a diuresis from a renal allograft shortly before it ceased to function. This was correlated with the fact that *in vitro* platelet aggregation, induced by soluble collagen, could be prevented by both hydrocortisone and 6-mercaptopurine, which block the release of adenosine diphosphate.

Platelet aggregation was thought to be induced by the exposed basement membrane, which was the result of endothelial cell damage after an antibody insult, and it was postulated that platelet aggregation was followed by platelet lysis and the appearance of fibrin, and that then the process became irreversible [10]. A mixture of antigen-antibody complexes, complement, platelets, and fibrin now became covered with a new layer of endothelium and incorporated into the vessel wall. In this way repair would lead to narrowing of the arteriolar, arterial, and capillary lumina, and repeated episodes of immunological injury and repair would eventually result in obliteration of vessels in renal grafts [7].

However, from the studies reported here, it seems likely that platelets play a role in the arteriosclerosis of transplantation not only by adhering to the exposed basement membrane, but also by taking an active part in removing the endothelium. The sequence of events is hypothesized as follows. The donor endothelium acts as a source of antigen to which the recipient circulation is exposed. After a period of time (and in the rat allograft model described here, after two days) host antiendothelial antibody is made. Host antibody, together with complement, combines with donor antigen and provides the stimulus for platelet aggregation. Platelet aggregation is a critical event in the history of graft rejection. If platelet degranulation occurs, the endothelium is stripped and successive platelet aggregation occurs on the subendothelium, leading to the accelerated atheroma encountered in graft rejection.

The experiments described here have also demonstrated that certain platelet-active agents can be more effective than conventional immunosuppression in preventing the early form of graft rejection, which is infiltration by lymphocytes. Lymphocytes can only enter a graft via the circulation. A lymphocyte within a blood vessel may enter the graft in two ways: it can insinuate itself between two endothelial cells or actually traverse the endothelial cytoplasm itself. Both these mechanisms are known to occur [11]. It seems reasonable to suppose, however, that it is more difficult for cells to achieve passage through a vessel wall if the endothelium is intact than if it has been removed. It is therefore suggested that the maintenance of endothelial cell integrity not only prevents late intimal proliferation and vessel thickening subsequent to a repair process but also serves to inhibit lymphocytic invasion of the graft by maintaining a physical barrier. Endothelial cell integrity is vital, to inhibit both cellular rejection and the later long-term intimal thickening of the vessels. It is therefore proposed that the addition of sulfinpyrazone to the immuno-suppressive regimen was interrupting, at some point, the chain of events that led to endothelial damage (Fig. 7).

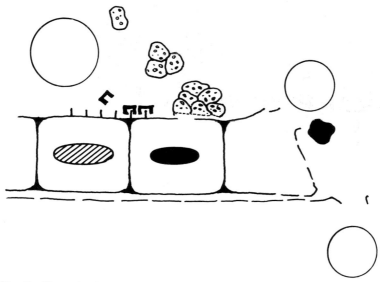

FIG. 7. Hypothesis of interaction of platelets (⊘⊜), antigen (ᴜᴜᴜ), antibody (⊓), and lymphocytes (◯).

To confirm this hypothesis, we tested the combination of sulfinpyrazone and azathioprine on skin grafts between inbred ACI and Lewis-Brown Norway rats. If the mechanism of action of sulfinpyrazone was through preservation of the integrity of the endothelium, then the survival of a nonvascularized organ graft, such as skin, should not be prolonged. Ten skin grafts were performed and treated with azathioprine only. Another ten were treated with azathioprine and sulfinpyrazone, in the same doses as were used for the cardiac grafts. The results are shown in Figure 8. Although there was a fourfold increase in survival when sulfinpyrazone was used in cardiac grafts, there was no increase in survival with skin grafts.

Conclusions

The combination of azathioprine and sulfinpyrazone is more effective than azathioprine and steroids in preventing cardiac allograft rejection between severely mismatched rats.

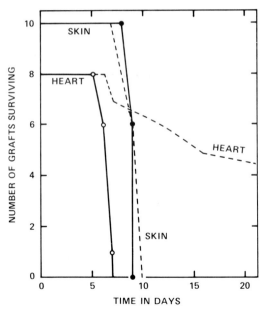

FIG. 8. Results of heart and skin transplantation. (——) azathioprine; (----) azathioprine and sulfinpyrazone.

Circulating antibody in a cardiac graft leads to platelet aggregation and platelets then appear to directly damage the endothelium. Removal of the endothelium gives rise to both enhanced cellular infiltration of the graft and progressive atherosclerosis by the repeated deposition of platelets. The mechanism of action of sulfinpyrazone in prolonging organ graft survival appears to be the protection of endothelial cells against damage.

Acknowledgments

Dr. Charles Bieber and Randi Shorthouse performed the antibody assays. The electron micrographs were performed by Dr. Margaret Billingham and Marilyn Masek.

References

1. Ono, K. and Lindsey, E.S.: Improved technique of heart transplantation in rats. J. Thorac. Cardiovasc. Surg. 57: 225-229, 1969.
2. Palm, J.: Classification of inbred rat strains for Ag-B list of compatibility antigens. Transplant Proc. 3:169-171, 1971.
3. Guttman, R.D.: Genetics of acute rejection of rat cardiac allografts and a model of hyperacute rejection. Transplantation 17: 383-386, 1974.
4. Floersheim, G.L. and Ruszkiewicz, M.: Bone marrow transplantation after antilymphocytic serum and lethal chemotherapy. Nature 222: 854-857, 1969.
5. Jamieson, S.W.: Xenograft hyperacute rejection. Transplantation 17: 533-534, 1974.
6. Duguid, J.B.: Thrombosis as a factor in pathogenesis of coronary atherosclerosis. J. Pathol. Bacteriol. 58: 207-212, 1946.
7. Porter, K.A.: Clinical renal transplantation. Int. Rev. Exp. Pathol. 11: 73-176, 1972.
8. Jeannet, M., Pinn, V.W., Flax, M.H., Winn, H.J. and Russel, P.S.: Humoral antibodies in renal transplantation in man. New Engl. J. Med. 282: 111-117, 1970.
9. Mowbray, J.F.: Methods of suppression of immune responses. Integration Intern. Med., Proc. Int. Congr. 9th, 1966. Excerpta Med. Found. Int. Congr. Ser. No. 137, pp. 106-110.
10. Porter, K.A.: Rejection in treated renal allografts. J. Clin. Pathol. 20: 518-534, 1967.
11. Schoefl, G.I.: The migration of lymphocytes across the vascular endothelium in lymphoid tissue. A reexamination. J. Exp. Med. 136: 568-588, 1972.

Discussion

Dr. Minick: Have you examined the arteries in detail in the allografts in the controls and drug-treated animals? If so, what did you find?

Dr. Jamieson: Unfortunately, because the rejection takes place over 6 days or so, it's not possible to pinpoint the sequence of events exactly. I can't state with certainty that endothelial cells are damaged by platelets, although I believe it to be so.

Dr. Minick: Concerning the type of lesion in the human heart, which has probably developed over several days, will sulfinpyrazone and various types of immunosuppressives have an effect on the development of that kind of lesion in allografts?

Dr. Jamieson: We haven't yet started to use sulfinpyrazone in our human hearts. We do biopsy them quite regularly; we hope not to pick up many vessels in biopsy, of course. We do see capillaries, and during rejection crises we do see platelet aggregates within the vessels and endothelial damage. They seem to represent what we see in hyperacute rejection. At present, at Stanford, we treat our patients with dipyridamole, and during a rejection crisis we treat them with heparin. That will shortly be changed, largely as a result of these studies.

Dr. Minick: It should be very interesting to use some of these regimens and look during the later stages at the large arteries, namely, the arteries that show atherosclerosis, to see if the development of atherosclerosis can actually be prevented in these animals. The best way to do that might be with some morphometric studies on perfused animals at autopsy.

Dr. Jamieson: Yes. One of the problems of using this particular model is that we chose a too aggressive match, so that at 5 days in the controls, we don't really have any atherosclerosis. Of course, even if the animals are treated with azathioprine and steroids in lethal doses, they still reject before they develop large-vessel atherosclerosis, so that with this model you would have nothing to compare other regimens to. You would have to go to an intermediate model.

Dr. Minick: You might consider using rabbits. In our experience with rabbits we could extend the survival of the grafts up to 100 days with azathioprine at moderate doses, but we did not prevent development of atherosclerosis. It would be very interesting in this type of model system to see if platelet inhibitory drugs would prevent development of atherosclerosis.

Dr. Jamieson: When we removed the hearts from rats that had been treated with azathioprine and sulfinpyrazone and survived for 50 days, they had developed atherosclerosis. We had found in previous studies with a less aggressive model that although atherosclerosis still developed in these animals, it was to a very considerably less degree than in those treated with azathioprine alone. Of course, in this model we have nothing to compare it to.

Dr. McDonald: I am a little confused about what happened with aspirin treatment, ibuprofen treatment, and indomethacin treatment. Did you abandon the aspirin treatment because of some problem with the deaths?

Dr. Jamieson: I am also a little confused about what happened with the aspirin-treated animals. Certainly an entirely different mechanism was involved. The animals became leukopenic, and there was a marked suppressor cell activity on mixed lymphocyte culture; it was quite plainly not an antiplatelet action. The animals survived but it was through a different mechanism.

Dr. McDonald: What was the manner of death of the ibuprofen- and indomethacin-treated animals? Was it rejection?

Dr. Jamieson: No, they died of gastric perforation and peritonitis.

Dr. Sherry: I noted in your interesting observations that there was no interference with antibody production. Do you have any data on whether sulfinpyrazone is able to combine with, or inactivate, activated components of complement?

Dr. Jamieson: No. We tried sulfinpyrazone in the hyperacute model, transplanting guinea pig hearts into rats, and we measured platelets and complement in the venous circulation of the heart from the coronary sinus. Sulfinpyrazone didn't change the amount of complement, but it prevented massive retention of platelets in the transplanted heart, so that rejection, instead of occurring within 2 or 3 min, was prolonged about 20-fold. Eventually, it still occurred. We have performed some more studies in dogs, in which we're examining complement levels in the coronary sinus, and we should have data at some future date.

Dr. Sherry: Are these total complement levels, and not specific ones, like C1-esterase or C3?

Dr. Jamieson: Yes.

Dr. Folts: Why did you give such a large dose of ibuprofen as 80 mg/kg?

Dr. Jamieson: Quite simply, I just thought that if we used a small dose and it didn't work, we would then have to increase the dose to be sure of getting the maximal effect of the drug.

Dr. Folts: In the studies we've done with ibuprofen, it appears that with a dose of more than 30 or 40 mg/kg, there is a reversal and it becomes less effective.

Dr. Jamieson: I didn't know that.

Dr. White: These results are extremely gratifying to us, since in the Forssman reaction the results with sulfinpyrazone were also qualitatively different from those with indomethacin. We now seem to have two examples of heterophile antibody-induced endothelial damage in which this pharmacologic distinction can be seen. In fact, all your electron micrographs were highly reminiscent of what we see in the Forssman reaction. In the Forssman reaction the endothelial edema is platelet-dependent, so that again we see this subtle interaction between damage to the endothelium and the requirement of platelets, which I think you have also seen.

Dr. Jamieson: In regard to a previous discussion as to whether sulfinpyrazone might be encouraging PGI_2 production in preference to thromboxane, we not only tried to use azathioprine and indomethacin together, but also a combination of azathioprine, indomethacin, and sulfinpyrazone, reasoning that if sulfinpyrazone was working through the PGI_2 mechanism, that would be inhibited by the indomethacin. The effect of azathioprine, indomethacin, and sulfinpyrazone was no different from that of just azathioprine and sulfinpyrazone.

Dr. Mustard: There is a pattern of data presented here which may mean that an important mechanism of sulfinpyrazone's action involves endothelial injury. The work of Harry Jacob's group indicates that activation of complement leads to leukocyte adherence to the endothelium and superoxide formation. In Dr. Cooper's experiments, he can apparently block the

leukocyte-mediated changes in pulmonary vessels with sulfinpyrazone. If you consider the experiments Dr. White presented,
and those presented by Dr. Clopath, about the protection
provided by sulfinpyrazone in antigen-antibody induced atherosclerosis, it is possible the action of sulfinpyrazone is on the
mechanisms causing endothelial injury, such as superoxide
production, rather than platelet aggregation.

Experimental Animal Studies: Chairman's Summary

Michael F. Oliver, M.D.

Before my summation I am going to make a very brief presentation concerning some preliminary studies into the possibility that sulfinpyrazone might have an antiarrhythmic action in the presence of acute myocardial ischemia.

We have had many years' experience using an open-chest dog preparation to induce regional myocardial ischemia by placing a light spring clip around different branches of the left anterior descending coronary artery. This provides a model with which it is possible to induce ischemia in various parts of the myocardium for periods of 5 or 10 min, and with a recovery period of about 30 min it is possible to use this dog heart as its own control for the testing of the effectiveness of various forms of metabolic intervention or of antiarrhythmic drugs. A pacing electrode is sewn into the right atrium. The left atrium is cannulated for the introduction of radioisotope-labeled microspheres for assessment of endocardial and epicardial blood flow. The local vein serving the area of myocardial ischemia is cannulated for estimation of various metabolites, and the coronary sinus is also cannulated for this purpose. Thus, it is possible to calculate the arterial-local vein differences in various concentrates.

This preparation also permits electrophysiological measurements. We have been particularly interested in action potential, and epicardial and endocardial conduction delay. These are measured by floating microelectrodes inserted into the exposed myocardium [1]. It is also possible to measure the refractory

Michael F. Oliver, M.D., The Duke of Edinburgh Professor of Cardiology, University of Edinburgh, Edinburgh, Scotland.

period in various parts of the ischemic and normal myocardium and to assess the degree of divergence of refractoriness in a given preparation and the extent to which this is affected by drug manipulation [2]. Furthermore, this preparation permits assessment of a ventricular premature beat (VPB) threshold [3]. This is an arbitrary threshold which permits definition of the current in milliamps required to produce a particular sequence of VPB, and it has the advantage over a ventricular fibrillation threshold of not requiring a defibrillation current for restitution to normal. At present, we have only studied five dogs, but we have been interested to find that sulfinpyrazone given at a dose concentration of 30 mg/kg reduced the conduction delay between 30 and 60 min after its administration in leads taken from the center of the ischemic area. We were also interested to find that there was an increase in VPB threshold and a decrease in the actual number of VPB when sulfinpyrazone was given. This suggests that it reduced the vulnerability of the ischemic myocardium to VPB production. All that can be said at present is that sulfinpyrazone might have, in our preparation, an anti-arrhythmic effect; more studies are clearly indicated.

In comment about this session, the most important aspect is to emphasize that we really have been talking about sudden cardiac death, although not always actually saying so. The reason why we are interested in sudden cardiac death is because of the very striking findings in the published Anturane trial, where sudden cardiac death was significantly reduced but non-fatal myocardial infarction was not. These were surprising findings. The only other drug which has been shown to reduce sudden cardiac death in a similar way is practolol, one of the beta-adrenergic blockers (but not all beta-blocking drugs have had the same effect). More often, trials of drugs after myocardial infarction, such as the Coronary Drug Project, have shown a reduction in nonfatal myocardial infarction but no effect on sudden cardiac death. One distinctive aspect of the Anturane trial, is, therefore, that it focuses our attention on sudden cardiac death, which is effectively ventricular fibrillation. In constructing a clinical trial, it is important to differentiate between the end-point of sudden cardiac death and that of nonfatal myocardial infarction, and trials should be constructed from the outset to discriminate between these. Any future

Anturane trial should certainly have sufficient numbers to allow this discrimination.

We have in this session been considering what can be learned from experimental preparations in relation to lethal ventricular arrhythmias. Most people here have experience of animal investigations and most are probably aware of the inadequacy of any given animal model to represent the situation which one supposes takes place in man. We should be under no illusion about the difficulty, for example, of controlling and reproducing the extent of ischemia, the depth of anesthesia, the extent of the catecholamine response during induction of anesthesia, and the differences in species response to the procedures. One of the most serious problems in cardiac experimentation in animals is to know how deeply anesthetized the animal is. We know, for example, that the deeper the animal is anesthetized, the less the response so far as arrhythmias are concerned and also the less the metabolic response. For example, we have made many studies of the effects of raising free fatty acids in the ischemic myocardium in dogs, and under certain circumstances we have produced arrhythmias, while in others we have not; to a considerable extent, this depends on the depth of anesthesia induced. The same applies to potassium concentrations. The method of producing the ischemia is also important; a clip occlusion (such as we use) is quite different in effect from a ligature which interferes with the small sympathetic nerves running down the arterioles. These are both different from methods of producing occlusion internally, such as a balloon or a wire helix producing platelet emboli. It is exceedingly important to define precisely the model which is used when any drug is being examined.

One of the speakers, in examining possible mechanisms of action of sulfinpyrazone, dismissed — rightly in my opinion — the possibility that its putative antiarrhythmic effect might be due to an effect on the size of the myocardial infarct. The size of an infarct has little to do with the initial reentry arrhythmia. It takes several hours for an infarct to develop and the majority of sudden deaths in man occur within 1 h and are associated with potentially reversible acute myocardial ischemia, not infarction. Furthermore, I do not think that it would be useful to examine the effect of sulfinpyrazone on ST segment changes or creatine kinase MB isoenzymes, because neither of these would necessarily give useful information concerning the sensitivity of the preparation to the development of arrhythmias.

It has been suggested that sulfinpyrazone may have a direct antiarrhythmic action. This is certainly a viable hypothesis, although I do not understand the mechanism of action. It might, of course, have some immediate effect on platelet aggregates. This would presumably be through the prostacyclin or thromboxane-A_2 pathway but it could also have an effect on PGE_1 series, which are produced by the myocardium and which have a profound vasodilating effect. I put forward another hypothesis a year ago — for which I have no evidence at all — that sulfinpyrazone might have a secondary inhibitory effect on production of arrhythmias by blocking xanthine oxidase activity. This could cause accumulation of vasodilating adenine nucleotides, such as inosine and adenosine. We know that these can be recycled back into the higher adenine nucleotides and that an increase in the concentration of adenosine causes reduction in cyclic-AMP production. It has been shown that there is a relationship between increased concentrations of cyclic-AMP in the ischemic myocardium and its susceptibility to develop ventricular fibrillation. If sulfinpyrazone is truly shown to be antiarrhythmic, these speculations will go on for years.

Finally, there are many causes of sudden cardiac death:

> Coronary vasospasm
> Rupture of atheromatous plaque
> Thrombosis in a large vessel
> Platelet emboli
> Increased myocardial O_2 demand
> Myocardial metabolic disequilibrium
> Myocytosis.

Unfortunately none of us will ever know which operates in a given individual. Sudden death is sudden and autopsies, regrettably, are slow. Many changes take place in the intervening time and it is highly unlikely, for example, that coronary vasospasm could be identified 24 h later. Nor will it necessarily follow that platelet emboli will be identifiable. I do not think that we should look for a single explanation of sudden cardiac death; by so doing we run the risk of narrowing our outlook. For example, sulfinpyrazone might be effective on two or three of the above mechanisms but ineffective in the others. It is going to be very difficult to explain or examine further the effects of a given treatment on sudden cardiac death. This is a negative statement and negative statements are not popular, but the fact is that we have to explain the cause of lethal ventricular arrhythmias first before we can explain the effectiveness, if it is effective, of sulfinpyrazone as an antiarrhythmic drug.

It is an exciting possibility that sulfinpyrazone might have an antiarrhythmic action, but much more work is required. This should be undertaken in electrophysiological laboratories experienced with the difficulties of controlling and providing reproducible experiments of acute myocardial ischemia.

References

1. Russell, D.C., Oliver, M.F. and Wocjtak, J.: Combined electrophysiological technique for assessment of the cellular basis of early ventricular arrhythmias. Lancet 2: 686-688, 1977.
2. Russell, D.C. and Oliver, M.F.: Refractoriness during acute myocardial ischaemia and its relationship to ventricular fibrillation. Cardiovasc. Res. 12: 221-227, 1978.
3. Russell, D.C. and Oliver, M.F.: The effect of intravenous glucose on ventricular vulnerability following acute coronary artery occlusion in the dog. J. Molec. Cell. Cardiol. 11: 31-44, 1979.

Clinical Studies

Effects of Sulfinpyrazone on Platelet Coagulant Activities in Patients with Thromboembolic Disorders

Peter N. Walsh, M.D., Ph.D. and Paul D. Mintz, M.D.

Investigations of the contributions of human platelets to the interaction and activation of intrinsic coagulation proteins have demonstrated catalytic and protective functions of platelets at various stages of intrinsic coagulation [1]. Although platelets have long been thought to participate in coagulation as passive providers of phospholipids which can accelerate the rate of prothrombin activation [2], a contrasting view, arising from recent experiments on platelet-coagulant protein interactions holds that the events of primary hemostasis and blood coagulation are intimately linked and that platelets are specifically and actively involved in promoting a variety of zymogen-to-enzyme conversions at every stage of intrinsic coagulation [1].

Evidence from studies carried out in our laboratory on the reactions of platelets isolated by albumin density gradient centrifugation [3] with plasma samples obtained from patients with coagulation protein deficiencies suggested that human platelets can participate in the initiation of intrinsic coagulation by two alternative mechanisms, one requiring coagulation factor XII [4] and the other independent of it [5]. Recent experi-

Peter N. Walsh, M.D., Ph.D., Specialized Center for Thrombosis Research, and Paul D. Mintz, M.D., Department of Medicine, Temple University School of Medicine, Philadelphia, Pa.

This work was supported in part by a research grant (HL14217) from the National Institutes of Health and a grant from the CIBA-GEIGY Corporation.

257

ments with highly purified radiolabeled contact factors, including factor XII, factor XI, high-molecular-weight kininogen, and prekallikrein, confirm these hypotheses and indicate that ADP- or collagen-treated platelets can promote the proteolytic activation of factor XII and that collagen-treated platelets can greatly enhance the proteolytic activation of factor XI in the presence of kallikrein, even in the absence of high-molecular-weight kininogen and factor XII [6]. Subsequently platelets protect factor XI_a from inactivation by its natural inhibitor in plasma, antithrombin III [7]. Furthermore, platelets have a factor-XI-like activity [3, 8] which is specifically localized in the plasma membrane, which can participate in "contact phase" reactions, which is protected from inactivation by anti-factor-XI antibody [9], and which appears to be similar to purified plasma factor XI, since immunofluorescent studies have recently demonstrated that it is recognized by an antibody to plasma factor XI [10]. It has been shown that phospholipids [11] and platelets [7] can form a complex with factor IX_a, factor VIII, and calcium, which comprises the factor-X activator. Factor X_a thus formed is protected by platelets [7] and by phospholipids [12] from inactivation by its natural inhibitor in plasma, antithrombin III. Furthermore factor X_a has been shown to bind to a highly specific receptor in platelet membranes which has been identified as factor V [13]. Thereby a complex is formed of factor X_a, factor V, calcium, and platelets [14], which comprises a potent prothrombin activator with greatly enhanced activity compared with a similar complex in which phospholipids replace platelets [13].

Assays for platelet coagulant activities at various stages of intrinsic coagulation have been developed [15] and applied to the study of patients with various thromboembolic disorders affecting the venous and arterial circulations. For example, to determine whether platelets play a part in the pathogenesis of transient cerebrovascular ischemia, we studied 22 patients with transient cerebral ischemic attacks (TIAs), 18 control patients, and 38 normal subjects [16]. Platelet aggregation and ^{14}C-serotonin release by ADP, epinephrine, and collagen were normal in all patients, as were plasma coagulation assays, except for shortened partial thromboplastin times in the patients with TIAs. In contrast, platelet coagulant activities concerned with the initiation and early stages of intrinsic coagulation were increased two to three times in 12 patients with TIAs and normal serum lipids but normal in ten other patients with TIAs associated with Type IV hyperlipoproteinemia. These results indicate an association which could be important in pathogenesis between platelet coagulant hyperactivity and TIA in a group of patients with normal serum lipids.

Similar abnormalities of platelet coagulant activities were found in two additional separate studies, one of patients with acute primary retinal vein occlusion [17] and the other in patients with acute primary retinal arterial occlusion [18] without traditional risk factors. In contrast, those patients with either retinal vein occlusion or retinal artery occlusion secondary to other conditions, such as hypertension, diabetes mellitus, type IV hyperlipoproteinemia, or generalized atherosclerosis, had platelets which gave normal results in assays for platelet coagulant activities. These results are consistent with a platelet contribution to retinal arterial and venous occlusive disease in patients without other known contributing factors, such as hypertension, serum lipid abnormalities, diabetes mellitus, and generalized atherosclerosis, and may have important implications for prophylaxis. We were therefore motivated to determine whether abnormalities of platelet coagulant activities observed in patients with cerebral and retinal vascular disease were normalized by treatment with a variety of platelet inhibitor medications.

The mechanism of action of aspirin as a platelet inhibitor medication has been intensively studied and is well understood, and yet the results of clinical trials of aspirin in the prophylaxis of venous and arterial thrombotic diseases have been disappointing [19]. In contrast, although the mechanism of action of sulfinpyrazone as a platelet inhibitor drug is poorly understood, it has been shown to be effective in preventing arteriovenous shunt thromboembolism occurring in patients on chronic hemodialysis, in correcting the shortened platelet survival observed in a variety of thromboembolic disorders [19], and in significantly reducing the frequency of sudden death in patients with myocardial infarction [20]. Therefore we have examined the effects of sulfinpyrazone therapy on platelet coagulant activities, aggregation, and secretion in normal donors and also in patients with various thromboembolic disorders found to have platelet coagulant hyperactivity.

Clinical Material

Normal Donors

Sixteen normal subjects (nine males, seven females) ranging in age from 20 to 30 were identified for study in our laboratory. All subjects denied a history of hemorrhagic or thrombotic events and were instructed to refrain from taking any medications known to affect platelet function (e.g., nonsteroidal anti-inflammatory agents, oral anovulatory agents, tranquilizers) during the 2 weeks prior to the study and during the time interval between portions of the study. All participants had been previously studied in our laboratory and found to have normal results for platelet count, platelet coagulant activity, aggregation and secretion, and coagulation studies, including partial thromboplastin time, prothrombin time, and plasma fibrinogen. Normal subjects were studied in pairs. Initially baseline determinations were performed as follows: platelet aggregation and secretion of ^{14}C-5-hydroxytryptamine; platelet coagulant activities; peripheral whole blood platelet counts; and bleeding times. One of the subjects then received sulfinpyrazone, 200 mg four times daily for 2 days, and all the determinations were repeated, the other donor serving as a control. After an additional 8 days of administration of sulfinpyrazone, 200 mg four times daily (total, 10 days), the studies were again repeated, and both donors were instructed to refrain from receiving any medications, including sulfinpyrazone, for a period of at least 1 month. Thereafter, baseline determinations were repeated in both individuals of the pair, after which the trial was repeated with the previous normal donor now receiving sulfinpyrazone and the previous recipient of sulfinpyrazone now designated the normal control.

Patient Studies

Twenty patients were selected for study on the basis of baseline studies, repeated on two to eight separate occasions, demonstrating reproducible and significant increases in the results of assays for platelet coagulant activities. Six patients with juvenile diabetes mellitus and either background or proliferative retinopathy (three male, three female) ranging in age from 20 to 40 (mean age, 29) were included as participants in the study. Significant elevations of platelet coagulant activities occurred in patients with background or proliferative retinopathy and normal results in diabetic patients without retinopathy. Eight patients with retinal vein occlusion were studied, none of whom had hypertension, diabetes mellitus, serum lipid abnormalities, or other conditions known to predispose to retinal vascular disease. They ranged in age from 25 to 58 (mean age, 44). Six patients were male, and two female. Five patients with cerebral vascular disease (one male, four female) ranged in age from 24 to 58 (mean age, 37 years), none of whom had serum lipid abnormalities, hypertension, diabetes mellitus, or other conditions known to predispose to cerebral vascular occlusive disease.

After baseline determinations of platelet coagulant activities, platelet aggregation and secretion, platelet counts, coagulation screening tests, and serum lipid determinations after a 14-h period of fasting, patients were treated with sulfinpyrazone, 200 mg four times daily, for periods ranging between 1 and 3 months, following which the studies were repeated. Usually sulfinpyrazone therapy was then stopped and studies were repeated after a period of approximately 1 month after therapy. Thereafter treatment with sulfinpyrazone, 200 mg four times daily, was reinstituted, and studies were repeated.

Materials and Methods

Preparative Procedures

Nine volumes of blood were collected by clean venipuncture directly into 1 vol of 3.8% trisodium citrate with plastic containers and equipment. Platelet-rich plasma (PRP) and platelet-poor plasma (PPP) were prepared [15], and platelets were washed and suspensions stored as previously described [21]. Platelets were counted by phase-contrast microscopy [22] and electronically with a model ZBI particle counter (Coulter Electronicis, Hialeah, Fla.).

Platelet Aggregation and Serotonin Release

Platelet aggregation and ^{14}C-5-hydroxytryptamine release studies were done with ADP, epinephrine and collagen as previously described [16]. Threshold concentrations of each agent resulting in secondary aggregation and release of more than 20% of ^{14}C-5HT were determined. The method for quantitative detection of platelet aggregates [23] was carried out by comparing platelet counts in PRP obtained from blood collected either in EDTA/formalin or EDTA alone. The result was expressed as a platelet aggregate ratio obtained by dividing the platelet count in EDTA PRP into the platelet count in EDTA/formalin PRP. A decrease in the ratio denoted an increase in platelet aggregates.

Platelet Coagulant Activities

The platelet coagulant activities assayed included: (1) contact-product-forming activity, the capacity of normal platelets to respond to ADP and participate in the activation of factor XII [4]; (2) collagen-induced coagulant activity, the capacity of collagen-stimulated platelets to participate in the initiation of intrinsic coagulation by an alternative mechanism in the apparent absence of factor XII [5]; (3) intrinsic factor X_a-forming activity, by which platelet membrane components become available and promote the interactions of factors XI_a, VIII, and IX to activate factor X in the presence of calcium [7]; and (4) platelet factor 3 activity, by which platelet membrane phospholipoproteins become available to promote the interactions of factors X_a and V to activate prothrombin in the presence of calcium [14]. These platelet coagulant activities were assayed by modifications [16] of previously described methods [15] and were expressed as percentages of normal platelets by reference to a double logarithmic plot of clotting time and platelet concentration. Results obtained in normal donors were normally distributed when the logarithms of these percentages were examined.

Bleeding Times

Bleeding times were carried out by a template modification [24] of the method of Ivy.

Statistical Methods

Results are expressed as mean and standard deviation (SD) or standard error of the mean (SEM), and groups were compared by Student's *t* test or by Chi square analysis.

Table 1. Effects of Sulfinpyrazone on Platelet Count, Bleeding Time,
and Circulating Platelet Aggregate Ratio in Normal Donors

Time of Measurement	Whole Blood Platelet Count (n = 16)	Bleeding Time (min) (n = 10)	Circulating Platelet Aggregate Ratio (n = 16)
Before therapy	257,000 ± 16,000	4.0 ± 0.37	0.89 ± 0.04
After 2 days	247,000 ± 10,000	4.5 ± 0.38	0.95 ± 0.02
After 10 days	252,000 ± 14,000	5.25 ± 0.66	0.89 ± 0.04

Sulfinpyrazone was given at a dose of 200 mg PO four times daily. Results are mean ± SEM.

Results

Studies in Normal Donors

When normal donors were examined before and during short-term (2-day) and sustained (10-day) treatment with sulfinpyrazone, 200 mg four times daily, no significant effects on platelet counts, bleeding time, or circulating platelet aggregate ratios were observed (Table 1). Data satisfactory for adequate analysis of platelet aggregation and ^{14}C-5HT release were available in eleven normal donors before and after 2 days and 10 days therapy with sulfinpyrazone, 200 mg four times daily (Table 2). Ten normal donors had platelets which released more than 20% of prelabeled ^{14}C-5HT prior to therapy with sulfinpyrazone. Only five of these demonstrated adequate release in response to the higher concentration of ADP tested (usually 8 μM) after 2 days or 10 days of therapy with sulfinpyrazone, 200 mg four times daily. In contrast, of those donors whose platelets released serotonin in response to epinephrine or collagen before therapy, a majority underwent

Table 2. Effect of Sulfinpyrazone on Serotonin Release ($\geq 20\%$) in Normal Donors

Aggregating Agent	Proportion of Positive Release Results		
	Before Therapy	After 2 Days	After 10 Days
ADP	10/10	5/10	5/10
Epinephrine	11/11	9/11	10/11
Collagen	11/11	11/11	11/11

Sulfinpyrazone was given at a dose of 200 mg PO four times daily for 2 or 10 days.

Table 3. Effect of Short-Term Sulfinpyrazone Therapy on
Serontonin Release in Normal Donors

Aggregating Agent	n	Threshold Concentration		Serotonin Release (%)	
		Before Therapy	After 2 Days	Before Therapy	After 2 Days
ADP	5	3.6 μM	3.6 μM	40	24*
Epinephrine	9	1.2 μM	2.0 μM*	52	39
Collagen	11	0.9 μg/ml	1.0 μg/ml	40	28*

Sulfinpyrazone was given at a dose of 200 mg PO four times daily for 2 days.
*p < 0.05.

release after either 2 days or 10 days of therapy with
sulfinpyrazone (Table 2).

The threshold concentrations of aggregating agents effecting
^{14}C-5HT release and the percentage of ^{14}C-5HT released at
those threshold concentrations for normal donors whose platelets released serotonin in response to the agents tested are
shown in Tables 3 (2 days' therapy) and 4 (10 days' therapy).
After 2 days of treatment with sulfinpyrazone, 200 mg four
times daily, although the threshold concentration of ADP
effecting ^{14}C-5HT release remained the same (3.6 μM), the
percentage of ^{14}C-5HT released at this concentration was
significantly reduced. Similar findings were observed for collagen-induced release, whereas the threshold concentration of
epinephrine increased from 1.2 μM to 2.0 μM, a significant
increase (Table 3). Similar findings were observed after 10 days
of treatment with sulfinpyrazone (Table 4).

Effects on platelet coagulant activities of sulfinpyrazone
therapy, 200 mg four times daily, given to normal donors for

Table 4. Effect of Sustained Sulfinpyrazone Therapy on
Serotonin Release in Normal Donors

Aggregating Agent	n	Threshold Concentration		Serotonin Release (%)	
		Before Therapy	After 10 Days	Before Therapy	After 10 Days
ADP	5	2.4 μM	3.8 μM	46	35
Epinephrine	10	1.1 μM	3.0 μM*	54	39*
Collagen	11	0.9 μg/ml	1.4 μg/ml	40	27*

Sulfinpyrazone was given at a dose of 20 mg PO four times daily for 10 days.
*p < 0.05.

either 2 days or 10 days are shown in Table 5. The results are expressed as ratios of platelet coagulant activities during therapy divided by the baseline results. Thus the baseline result is defined as a ratio of 1 and the effects of short-term (2-day) and sustained (10-day) therapy are related to the baseline results and expressed as ratios. No significant effect of short-term therapy with sulfinpyrazone on any of the platelet coagulant activities was observed. However, after treatment for 10 days, collagen-induced coagulant activity and intrinsic factor X_a-forming activity were significantly decreased compared with baseline values. Contact-product-forming activity and platelet factor 3 activity in response to collagen and kaolin were unaffected by sustained therapy.

Results in Patients

Patients with juvenile diabetes mellitus and background or proliferative retinopathy (six patients), retinal venous occlusion (eight patients) and cerebrovascular occlusive disease (five patients) were studied without administration of drugs on two to eight separate occasions and thereafter on two to four separate occasions while receiving sulfinpyrazone, 200 mg four

Table 5. Effects of Sulfinpyrazone on Platelet
Coagulant Activities in Normal Donors

Type of Activity	Before Therapy	After 2 Days	After 10 Days
Contact-Product-Forming Activity	1.0	1.46 ± 0.22	1.14 ± 0.08
Collagen-Induced Coagulant Activity	1.0	1.19 ± 0.15	0.74 ± 0.10 (p < 0.005)
Intrinsic Factor X_a-Forming Activity	1.0	0.96 ± 0.17	0.82 ± 0.10 (p < 0.025)
Platelet Factor 3 with Kaolin	1.0	1.35 ± 0.18	1.23 ± 0.15
Platelet Factor 3 with Collagen	1.0	1.30 ± 0.37	1.03 ± 0.11

Sulfinpyrazone was given at a dose of 200 mg four times daily for 2 or 10 days. Results are mean ± SEM for measurements in 16 normal donors and expressed as the ratio to the baseline measurements taken before therapy.

Table 6. Effect of Sulfinpyrazone on Serotonin Release
in Six Patients with Diabetic Retinopathy

Aggregating	Threshold Concentration		Serotonin Release (%)	
Agent	Baseline	Treated	Baseline	Treated
ADP	2.8 μM	4.3 μM*	25	11*
Epinephrine	1.4 μM	3.7 μM*	31	12*
Collagen	0.6 μg/ml	1.2 μg/ml*	30	17

Patients were given sulfinpyrazone at a dose of 200 mg PO four times daily for 1 to 3 months. *$p < 0.05$.

times daily. Baseline values and treatment values were then expressed as the means of the following data: threshold concentrations of ADP, epinephrine, and collagen resulting in $\geq 20\%$ [14]C-5HT release; percent release of [14]C-5HT at the threshold concentration of the aggregating agent; and platelet coagulant activities including contact-product-forming activity, collagen-induced coagulant activity, intrinsic factor X_a-forming activity and platelet factor 3 activity in response to collagen or kaolin.

The effects of sulfinpyrazone therapy, 200 mg four times daily, for 1 to 3 months on release of [14]C-5HT are shown for six patients with diabetic retinopathy (Table 6), eight patients with retinal vein occlusion (Table 7) and five patients with cerebral vascular disease (Table 8). Threshold concentrations of ADP, epinephrine, and collagen leading to release of $\geq 20\%$ of [14]C-5HT were significantly increased during treatment with sulfinpyrazone in six patients with diabetic retinopathy, whereas the percentage release of [14]C-5HT in response to ADP and epinephrine at threshold concentrations was significantly reduced during the treatment phase (Table 6). Similar trends were

Table 7. Effect of Sulfinpyrazone on Serotonin Release
in Eight Patients with Retinal Vein Occlusion

Aggregating	Threshold Concentration		Serotonin Release (%)	
Agent	Baseline	Treated	Baseline	Treated
ADP	4.1 μM	4.7 μM	22	13*
Epinephrine	2.8 μM	4.3 μM	30	22
Collagen	1.6 μg/ml	1.9 μg/ml	23	15*

Patients were given sulfinpyrazone at a dose of 200 mg PO four times daily for 1 to 3 months. *$p < 0.05$.

Table 8. Effect of Sulfinpyrazone on Serotonin Release
in Five Patients with Cerebrovascular Disease

Aggregating Agent	Threshold Concentration		Serotonin Release (%)	
	Baseline	Treated	Baseline	Treated
ADP	3.9 μM	4.4 μM	41	22*
Epinephrine	3.0 μM	5.5 μM	33	19
Collagen	0.8 μg/ml	0.9 μg/ml	27	31

Patients were given sulfinpyrazone at a dose of 200 mg PO four times daily for 1 to 3 months. *$p < 0.05$.

observed in patients with retinal vein occlusion and cerebral vascular disease, but the results were not generally significant except for percent release at the threshold concentrations of ADP (Tables 7 and 8).

The results of baseline platelet coagulant activities in these patients with diabetic retinopathy, retinal vein occlusion, and cerebral vascular disease are shown in Table 9. Previously we have shown two- to threefold elevations of platelet coagulant activities concerned with the initiation (contact-product-forming activity and collagen-induced coagulant activity) and early stages (intrinsic factor X_a-forming activity) of coagulation in patients with retinal vein occlusion [17] and cerebral vascular disease [16] without other risk factors when these

Table 9. Platelet Coagulant Activities Before Sulfinpyrazone Therapy
in Patients with Diabetes Mellitus, Retinal Vein Occlusion,
or Cerebral Vascular Disease

	Diabetic Retinopathy ($n = 6$)	Retinal Vein Occlusion ($n = 8$)	Cerebral Vascular Disease ($n = 5$)
Contact-Product-Forming Activity	130 ± 24	116 ± 16	159 ± 38
Collagen-Induced Coagulant Activity	171 ± 19	141 ± 14	164 ± 38
Intrinsic Factor X_a-Forming Activity	202 ± 11	157 ± 26	176 ± 28
Platelet Factor 3 with Collagen	108 ± 8	129 ± 21	144 ± 14
Platelet Factor 3 with Kaolin	132 ± 21	107 ± 12	102 ± 20

Results are mean ± SEM.

results were compared with similar studies in control patients or normal donors. The results shown in Table 9 are consistent with these previous findings. The effects of sulfinpyrazone therapy, 200 mg four times daily for periods ranging between 1 and 3 months, on platelet coagulant activities in these three groups of patients are shown in Figure 1 (diabetic retinopathy), Figure 2 (retinal vein occlusion), and Figure 3 (cerebral vascular disease). No significant effects on any of the platelet coagulant activities were observed during treatment with sulfinpyrazone.

Discussion

Previous studies from our laboratory have suggested that platelet coagulant activities concerned with the initiation and early stages of intrinsic coagulation may be important determinants of normal hemostasis, since deficiencies of the platelet contribution to contact activation in patients with thrombasthenia [15] and the hereditary giant platelet (Bernard-

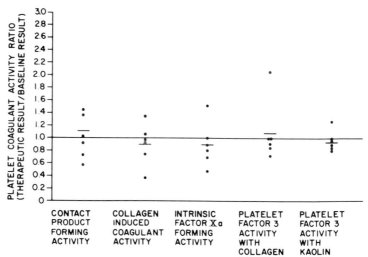

FIG. 1. The effects of sulfinpyrazone on platelet coagulant activities in patients with diabetic retinopathy. Each point represents a platelet coagulant activity ratio expressed as the mean of assay results obtained during therapy with sulfinpyrazone divided by the mean of assay results obtained when patients were receiving no platelet inhibitor medication. The short horizontal bars represent the means of platelet coagulant activity ratios. (See text for further details.)

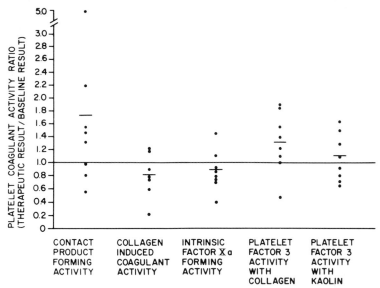

FIG. 2. The effects of sulfinpyrazone on platelet coagulant activities in patients with retinal vein occlusion. (See text and the legend to Fig. 1 for details.)

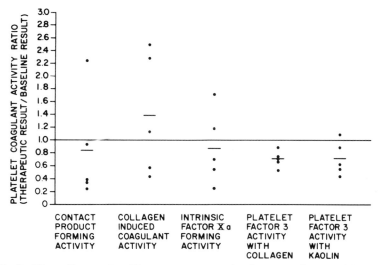

FIG. 3. The effects of sulfinpyrazone on platelet coagulant activities in patients with cerebral vascular disease. (See text and the legend to Fig. 1 for details.)

Soulier) syndrome [25] are associated with defective hemo-stasis. Complementary studies in patients with thromboembolic disorders have demonstrated two- to threefold elevations of platelet coagulant activities concerned with the initiation and early stages of coagulation in patients with postoperative deep venous thrombosis [26], TIAs [16], retinal artery throm-bosis [18], and retinal vein thrombosis [17], without tradi-tional risk factors for these disorders. Thus the contribution of platelets to coagulation reactions occurring prior to the activa-tion of factor X may play an important part in the pathogenesis of various venous and arterial thromboembolic disorders. It seems reasonable to suggest that hemodynamic, vascular, or other factors may determine the type and location of throm-bosis and that hyperactive platelets may provide a trigger mechanism under certain clinical conditions.

Although the mechanism by which platelet coagulant hyperactivity develops is unknown, our studies provide a rational basis for patient management. In patients with vascular occlusive disease and platelet coagulant hyperactivity without associated hypertension, hyperlipidemia, or evidence of other potentially controllable risk factors, it would seem rational to evaluate drugs that inhibit platelet function in preventing recurrences. On the other hand, attempts should be made with diet, drugs, and other measures to control associated diseases, such as hypertension, hyperlipidemia and diabetes mellitus, in patients with vascular occlusive diseases in whom platelet abnormalities cannot be demonstrated. Obviously our findings do not preclude a possible therapeutic role of platelet-inhibiting drugs in patients with normal platelets in whom other risk factors are present. However, the results of therapeutic trials might well be influenced if antiplatelet agents were ineffective in this subset.

These considerations motivated us to study the effects of sulfinpyrazone on platelet aggregation, serotonin secretion, and platelet coagulant activities in normal donors and in patients with venous and arterial thrombotic diseases. Our results indicate variable inhibition of serotonin secretion in response to ADP, epinephrine, and collagen both in normal donors and in patients with diabetic retinopathy, retinal vein occlusion, or cerebral vascular occlusive disease. In normal donors we observed significant decreases in collagen-induced coagulant activity and intrinsic factor X_a-forming activity after 10 days of treatment with sulfinpyrazone, but no effects were observed on platelet coagulant activities after 2 days of therapy with sulfinpyrazone at a similar dosage level. No effects of sulfinpyrazone therapy were seen on elevated platelet coagulant activities in patients with diabetic retinopathy or retinal or cerebral vascular occlusive disease. However, preliminary observations in small numbers of patients suggest that combinations of sulfinpyrazone and aspirin may have a greater effect in these patients than either sulfinpyrazone or aspirin alone. If confirmed, this observation would be consistent with the synergistic effect of combined aspirin and sulfinpyrazone therapy on collagen-induced platelet aggregation in guinea pigs previously observed by Wong, Zawidzka, and Thomas [27].

Acknowledgments

We thank Cheryl Beckett, Sarah Caspar, and Beverly White for excellent technical assistance; Mary Kate Cunningham for invaluable assistance in data retrieval and analysis; and Anne Arker for typing the manuscript.

References

1. Walsh, P.N.: Platelet coagulant activities and hemostasis: an hypothesis. Blood 43: 597-605, 1974.
2. Aggeler, P.M., Sahud, M.A. and Robinson, A.J.: The role of platelets in blood coagulation. *In* Brinkhous, K.M., Shermer, R.W. and Mostof, F.K. (eds.): The Platelet. Baltimore:Williams and Wilkins, 1971, pp. 172-182.
3. Walsh, P.N.: Albumin density gradient separation and washing of platelets and the study of platelet coagulant activities. Br. J. Haematol. 22: 205-217, 1972.
4. Walsh, P.N.: The role of platelets in the contact phase of blood coagulation. Br. J. Haematol. 22: 237-254, 1972.
5. Walsh, P.N.: The effects of collagen and kaolin on the intrinsic coagulant activity of platelets. Evidence for an alternative pathway in intrinsic coagulation not requiring factor XII. Br. J. Haematol. 22: 393-405, 1972.
6. Walsh, P.N. and Griffin, J.H.: The role of human platelets in the contact phase of blood coagulation (Abst.). Clin. Res. 26: 509A, 1978.

7. Walsh, P.N. and Biggs, R.: The role of platelets in intrinsic factor-X_a formation. Br. J. Haematol. 22: 743-760, 1972.

8. Schiffman, S., Rapaport, S.I. and Chong, M.M.Y.: Platelets and initiation of intrinsic clotting. Br. J. Haematol. 24: 633-642, 1973.

9. Lipscomb, M.S. and Walsh, P.N.: Human platelets and factor XI. Localization in platelet membranes of factor-XI-like activity and its functional distinction from plasma factor XI. J. Clin. Invest. 63: 1006-1014, 1979.

10. Tuszynski, G.P., Camp, E., Bevacqua, S. et al.: Factor XI antigen in human platelets (Abst.). Fed. Proc. 38: 1307, 1979.

11. Lundblad, R.L. and Davie, E.W.: The activation of antihemophilic factor (Factor VIII) by activated Christmas factor (activated factor IX). Biochemistry 3: 1720-1725, 1964.

12. Marciniak, E.: Factor-X_a inactivation by antithrombin III: evidence for biological stabilization of factor X_a by factor V-phospholipid complex. Br. J. Haematol. 24: 391-400, 1973.

13. Miletich, J.P., Jackson, C.M. and Majerus, P.W.: Properties of the factor X_a binding site on human platelets. J. Biol. Chem. 253: 6903-6916, 1978.

14. Milstone, J.H.: Thrombokinase as prime activator of prothrombin: Historical perspectives and present status. Fed. Proc. 23: 742-748, 1964.

15. Walsh, P.N.: Platelet coagulant activities in thrombasthenia. Br. J. Hamatol. 23: 553-569, 1972.

16. Walsh, P.N., Pareti, F.I. and Crobett, J.J.: Platelet coagulant activities and serum lipids in transient cerebral ischemia. N. Engl. J. Med. 295: 854-858, 1976.

17. Walsh, P.N., Goldberg, R.E., Tax, R.L. et al.: Platelet coagulant activities and retinal vein thrombosis. Thromb. Haemostas. 38: 399-405, 1977.

18. Walsh, P.N., Kansu, T.A., Savino, P.J. et al.: Platelet coagulant activities in arterial occlusive disease of the eye. Stroke, in press.

19. Genton, E., Gent, M., Hirsh, J. et al.: Platelet-inhibiting drugs in the prevention of clinical thrombotic disease. N. Engl. J. Med. 293: 1174-1178, 1236-1240, 1296-1300, 1975.

20. Anturane Reinfarction Trial Research Group: Sulfinpyrazone in the prevention of cardiac death after myocardial infarction. N. Engl. J. Med. 298: 289-295, 1978.

21. Walsh, P.N., Mills, D.C.B. and White, J.G.: Metabolism and function of human platelets washed by albumin density gradient separation. Br. J. Haematol. 36: 285-300, 1971.

22. Brecher, G. and Cronkite, E.P.: Morphology and enumeration of human blood platelets. J. Appl. Physiol. 3: 365-377, 1950.

23. Wu, K.K. and Hoak, J.C.: A new method for the quantitative detection of platelet aggregates in patients with arterial insuffiency. Lancet 2: 294-296, 1974.

24. Mielke, C.H., Kaneshiro, M.M., Maher, I.A. et al.: The standardized normal Ivy bleeding time and its prolongation by aspirin. Blood 34: 204-215, 1969.

25. Walsh, P.N., Mills, D.C.B., Pareti, F.I. et al.: Hereditary giant platelet syndrome. Absence of collagen-induced coagulant activity and deficiency of factor-XI binding to platelets. Br. J. Haematol. 29: 639-655, 1975.
26. Walsh, P.N., Rogers, P.H., Marder, V.J. et al.: The relationship of platelet coagulant activities to venous thrombosis following hip surgery. Br. J. Haematol. 32: 423-439, 1976.
27. Wong, L.T., Zawidzka, Z. and Thomas, B.H.: Effect of acetylsalicylic acid, sulfinpyrazone and their combination on collagen-induced platelet aggregation in guinea pigs. Pharm. Res. Comm. 10: 939-949, 1978.

Discussion

Dr. Sherry: If sulfinpyrazone has reversible effects on the platelet membrane, would you detect this in a test system where sulfinpyrazone was no longer present?

Dr. Walsh: We have detected the effects of sulfinpyrazone in washed platelet suspensions obtained from sulfinpyrazone-treated individuals, which implies that the platelets have somehow been altered and that the effect does not require the presence of sulfinpyrazone.

Dr. Sherry: If sulfinpyrazone is added to the medium, do you get different effects from those in the absence of sulfinpyrazone?

Dr. Walsh: We haven't done *in vitro* studies on these platelet coagulant activities.

Dr. Sherry: Am I to conclude then that although we've heard that sulfinpyrazone may have important effects in terms of the vessel wall—platelet interaction, in terms of those aspects related to more extensive thrombus formation, it is much more difficult to demonstrate that there is any interaction between platelets and the coagulation mechanism?

Dr. Walsh: That's probably true.

Controlled Clinical Trial
of Aspirin and Sulfinpyrazone
in Threatened Stroke

David L. Sackett, M.D. for the Canadian
Cooperative Study Group

Introduction

It may be useful to distinguish between two sorts of randomized clinical trial. In the first sort of trial, the intent is one of *explanation*: does this drug cause a specific biologic effect? The recruitment of an unusual subset of highly compliant patients can be justified, as can the idealized application of the experimental maneuver (even though it violates contemporaneous practice). Similarly, the exclusion of certain events (such as those that occur between randomization and the beginning of treatment, or before treatment can "take hold," or after treatment ends) can be justified as long as assessment is "blind" and their removal does not bias the comparisons between different treatment groups. Finally, the events selected for answering the explanatory question will often be "hard" end-points, such as survival time, tumor size, or discrete clinical catastrophes.

The second sort of randomized trial asks a therapeutic rather than an explanatory question: Does this drug do more good than harm to patients with illness X? The intent is management and the question concerns evaluation of the intention to embark down a specific therapeutic pathway.

David L. Sackett, M.D., Professor of Medicine, Departments of Clinical Epidemiology and Biostatistics, McMaster University, Hamilton, Ont., Canada.

This research was supported by a grant (MA-4535) from the Medical Research Council of Canada.

275

Accordingly, it is sensible to include all eligible patients (rather than just those who are highly compliant) and to apply and monitor the experimental therapy in a fashion that replicates contemporaneous clinical practice. Furthermore, the inclusion of all outcomes (rather than just those explained by known mechanisms of the experimental therapy) can be justified, as can the inclusion of "softer" outcomes, such as social function, emotional function, and peace of mind.

In this report of the Canadian Cooperative Study, the findings of which have already been reported elsewhere [1], analyses of the trial from the viewpoints of both explanation and management are presented.

Patients and Methods

The study was a multicenter, double-blind, factorial, randomized clinical trial, conducted by the Canadian Cooperative Study Group (see Appendix).

Eligibility

Patients were eligible if they had experienced at least one cerebral or retinal ischemic attack in the 3 months before entry. (During the first year of the trial only patients with multiple attacks were admitted, and the protocol was then revised to include patients with single attacks.) Definitions for symptoms of transient ischemic attacks (TIAs) were developed and agreed upon by all participants. Certain symptoms were sufficient for entry when they constituted the only manifestation of an attack, whereas others had to occur in predefined combinations. Patients with residual symptoms beyond the 24-h limit were eligible only if the symptoms were both stable and capable of subsequent observable further deterioration.

Exclusions

Neurologically stable patients were nonetheless excluded if they had coexisting morbid conditions that could explain their symptoms, if they were likely to die from other illness within 12 months, or if they were unable to take the test drugs. Participating centers were asked to submit information on all patients excluded from the trial.

Baseline Studies

Neurologic assessment at entry included an extensive documentation of TIAs (number of attacks in the prior 1, 3, 6, and 12 months; dates of first and most recent ischemic episodes; occurrence of residua; and presence or absence of appropriate symptoms) and a detailed neurologic examination. Cerebral angiography (followed by another neurologic assessment) was encouraged but optional. This evaluation at entry also included determination of smoking habits, drug use within the prior month, and any past history of diabetes mellitus, cardiomegaly, heart failure, angina pectoris, myocardial infarction, intermittent claudication, hypertension, or cardiovascular surgical procedures. A detailed cardiovascular examination was carried out, as was an electrocardiography, a chest x-ray study, and a series of hematologic determinations and blood chemical tests. Mandatory tests of platelet function consisted of template bleeding times, platelet aggregation, and glass-bead retention. Optional studies included ^{51}Cr-labeled platelet survival and tests for circulating platelet aggregates.

Allocation

When baseline studies had been completed, contact was made with the Methods Center at McMaster University, which was staffed 24 h per day. Patients were stratified according to the presumed site of ischemia and the presence or absence of a residual deficit and were entered into a previously established randomization schedule. (A separate randomization schedule, balanced every four patients, had been constructed for each stratum within each participating center.) The trial medications were started immediately.

Regimens

Patients were randomized to one of four regimens throughout the study. Each regimen was taken four times daily and consisted of: a 200-mg tablet of sulfinpyrazone plus a placebo capsule; a 325-mg capsule of aspirin plus a placebo tablet; both active drugs; or both placebos. Each active drug and its corresponding placebo were identical in size, shape, weight, and color, and they were shipped to the participating centers in identical bottles of 130, labeled with four-digit random numbers. Neither the patients nor their physicians were told which regimen had been assigned, but both were given a 24-h telephone number for emergency code-breaking. So that participating neurologists would not inadvertently break the code by discovering the hypouricemia that sulfinpyrazone produces, uric acid values were not included in local laboratory reports but were sent directly to the Methods Center. At the end of the trial (but before the code was broken), the neurologists were asked to predict both the overall study results and the regimens for each of their patients.

Compliance and Contamination

Patients were asked to return unused medication at each follow-up visit, and pills were counted as an estimate of medication compliance. Additional compliance information was obtained from changes in serum uric acid and determinations of sulfinpyrazone blood levels and of platelet aggregation in the presence of epinephrine (the latter measure was also used to assess contamination with aspirin). The results of all these tests remained unavailable to the treating neurologist during the course of the study. Because of the ubiquity of aspirin-containing compounds, all patients were urged to avoid cold remedies and other over-the-counter nostrums, and acetaminophen was recommended when an analgesic was needed. Finally, because many psychoactive drugs also affect platelet function, clinicians were advised to restrict their choice of tranquilizers to diazepam or chlordiazepoxide.

Follow-up Data

Patients were reevaluated at 1 and 3 months and every 3 months therafter. At each follow-up visit, the interim neurologic history was obtained, and the detailed neurologic and cardiovascular examinations were repeated. Smoking status, compliance, and contamination were reassessed, and a brief, standardized search was made for side effects and toxicity. Hematologic, blood chemical, and selected platelet-function studies were repeated at each follow-up visit, and electrocardiograms and chest x-ray films were obtained annually (or more frequently, if clinically indicated). Finally, the Methods Center was approached by telephone, and a new supply of study drugs was identified.

Withdrawals

It was recognized at the outset that many patients might be withdrawn from the trial because of discontinuation of study drugs, initiation of contaminating medications, submission to surgery, or change of residence. Furthermore, both study drugs were thought capable of producing side effects that would demand their discontinuation. Accordingly, it was decided that such patients would constitute withdrawals but that their follow-up observation would continue despite cessation of the study drugs.

Events

Follow-up data were examined for the three events of TIAs, stroke, and death. This report will focus on the events of stroke and death.

Stroke. Two groups of possible strokes were identified from follow-up data and submitted for adjudication. The first group consisted of patients in whom neurologists reported a stroke in a follow-up narrative summary; the second group had complained of one or more ischemic events with a residual neurologic deficit lasting for more than 24 h at a follow-up visit. The records of both groups (purged of any information about their study drugs) were reviewed independently by two senior neurologists, and disagreements were resolved by discussion in the presence of one of the directors of the Methods Center, who was also blind to the patient's therapy. These judges also ruled whether the stroke was minor (no impairment in activities of daily living), moderate (impairment in activities of daily living but residing at home and out of bed for all or part of the day), or severe (bedfast or institutionalized for reasons of disability). Since dead patients cannot proceed to stroke, death was included in these analyses.

Death. Each death was documented. Cause-specific deaths (e.g., death due to stroke or heart attack) could not be ascertained with certainty because most deaths occurred outside of hospital, few autopsies of the dead patients were performed, and almost none were attended by study physicians. Accordingly, they were considered in the aggregate in these analyses.

Eligibility of Events

For analyses of the explanatory question, certain events were excluded from the calculations. First, because it was believed that sulfinpyrazone takes 1 week to produce a biologically appreciable effect [2], any event occurring in the first week of any of the four treatment regimens was excluded. Second, all events following withdrawal of study drugs were also excluded from one set of explanatory analyses. However, since the withdrawal of patients from the trial might be precipitated by a deterioration in their neurologic status (and thus their exclusion from subsequent analyses might bias the results in favor of their study regimen), any events occurring within the first 6 months after withdrawal were charged against the corresponding study regimen (even if the patient stopped taking the study medication at the time of withdrawal) in a second set of explanatory analyses.

For analyses of the management or intervention question, all events occurring from the instant of randomization to the end of the study (regardless of whether the patient remained in the study regimen) were included in the calculations.

Statistical Analysis

Appropriate parametric and nonparametric tests were used to analyze baseline differences among study groups, associated hematologic investigations, and compliance. Outcome analyses were carried out with the log-rank, life-table method suggested by Peto et al. [3].

The primary analysis was related to the overall assessment of benefit of aspirin and sulfinpyrazone. However, it was also judged important to examine the relative efficacy of these drugs among clinically sensible subgroups. The findings from these secondary analyses must be interpreted with some caution since the true significance levels are affected by the repeated challenging of the data.

The number of patients required was estimated on the assumption that the annual incidence of stroke was 7% and the annual death rate 4%, and that one or other of the two drugs would reduce these rates by 50%. The Type 1 error, α, was chosen to be 0.05, and the Type 2 error, β, 0.20. Allowing for withdrawals, we estimated that some 600 patients would be required if they were entered uniformly over a 5-year period and followed for at least 1 year, and possibly up to 6 years.

Withdrawals were monitored for possible drug toxicity. The data were first examined for efficacy in April 1976, when 569 patients had been entered into the study. At that time there was a trend favoring aspirin that was not statistically significant. It was decided to continue admitting patients until June 30, 1976 (by which time it was expected that the target of 600 patients would be reached) and to follow them for a further 12 months; the data were then to be analyzed and reported.

Results

Enrollment

Twenty-four centers entered patients into the trial between November 1, 1971, and June 30, 1976, and follow-up observation on the study drugs was concluded on June 30, 1977. During this time 649 patients were entered, of whom 64 were later found to be ineligible according to protocol entry requirements, resulting in a study population of 585. There was some imbalance among the ineligible subjects across the four treatment groups in that 25 were on placebo, 17 on sulfinpyrazone, 12 on aspirin and 10 on the combination therapy.

Six hundred ninety-two patients were reported as exclusions; these subjects, plus the 64 ineligible patients, made the total number of 756 known exclusions. Of these patients, 174 had coexisting morbid conditions that might account for their symptoms, 43 were considered likely to die from other illness within 12 months, 160 were unable to take the test drugs, and 72 underwent surgery. Of the remaining 307 exclusions, 141 refused randomization, 53 had single attacks (excluded in the first year of the trial), 30 were misdiagnosed, 73 had a completed stroke before entry, and 7 had a stroke and 3 had continuing ischemic episodes within the first 7 days of therapy.

Characteristics at Entry

Definitions of TIA symptoms were developed and applied consistently throughout this trial. The four treatment groups were found to be comparable in regard to the distribution of various ischemic events before entry, neurologic signs at entry, coexisting cardiovascular morbidity, and risk factors at entry [1].

Stratification and randomization produced reasonably comparable treatment groups. Single-attack cases (admitted from the second year onward) constituted one fifth of entrants, and the number of attacks occurring in the 3 months before entry was evenly distributed among the four treatment groups. Roughly 65% of entrants had ischemic-event symptoms referable to the carotid circulation, 25% to the vertebrobasilar, and 10% to both. For each site, more than half the patients were free of residua. Again, the distribution of sites and residua was well balanced among the four treatments, as were neurologic symptoms and signs, coexisting cardiovascular morbidity and risk factors, and other laboratory results. Four hundred thirty-four patients (74%) underwent cerebral angiography before admission to the trial; when symptoms in the carotid territory had led to admission, the angiography rate was 77%.

Maintenance of Blindness

The treatment code was broken for only one patient during the course of the trial, and blindness appeared to have been well maintained. Neurologists were incorrect in their written predictions of the relative efficacy of the trial drugs, and they correctly predicted which of the four regimens individual patients had been assigned in only 18% of cases (as compared with a chance value of 25%).

Compliance

Pill counts were performed at each follow-up visit. For the final follow-up visit the compliance rate was 92% across all treatment groups. Compliance appeared to be remarkably high, clearly exceeding that observed for most other long-term medications.

Follow-up Observation, Side Effects, and Withdrawals

Follow-up from the seventh day in the study to death, June 30, 1977, or 6 months after withdrawal (events during this period were included in one of the "explanatory" analyses) was achieved for 99% of study patients. The duration of follow-up observation averaged 26 months and did not differ among the four treatment groups; 92% of this period involved treatment with the study drugs.

Among side effects reported at the 3-month follow-up visit, pain in the upper abdomen ($p < 0.001$) and heartburn ($p < 0.05$) were more common among patients allocated to aspirin-containing regimens. A total of 12 patients experienced sufficient gastrointestinal bleeding to produce hematemesis or melena during the trial: 6 were in the combination-therapy group; 4 were receiving sulfinpyrazone, 2 placebo, and none aspirin alone.

Forty-one per cent of study subjects stopped taking the trial medication before the close of the study. Of these 15% had suffered strokes, 42% had experienced further TIAs only, and 43% were free of either of these events. Although total withdrawals were evenly distributed across treatment groups, there were some interesting differences. Among withdrawals due to drug side effects (24% of all withdrawals), 72% of patients were receiving aspirin ($p < 0.005$). There were also statistically significant differences ($p < 0.01$) across treatment groups among patients whose trial drugs were stopped by their physician (28% of all withdrawals), placebo (41%), sulfinpyrazone (26%), aspirin (20%) and the combination threatment (14%). No differences among treatment groups were observed for the other reasons for withdrawal, including trial drugs stopped by patient (28%), anticoagulants added (14%), patient referred for operation (4%), and patient moved away (3%).

Events

The primary analyses of the trial have already been published [1]. The explanatory analyses are summarized for men and women in the trial (Table 1). Table 1*A* summarizes the risk reductions (and attendant p-values) associated with the experimental therapy in men and women, excluding events in the first 7 days of therapy and after withdrawal of study drugs, thus addressing the question: *Can* the study drugs reduce the risk of stroke and death? Table 1*B* recognizes that withdrawal of patients from the study may have been precipitated by a deterioration in their neurological status and includes events

Table 1. Change in Risk of Stroke or Death Associated
with Aspirin or Sulfinpyrazone Treatment,
Excluding Events in the First 7 Days of Therapy

| | Change in Risk | | | | Drug |
| | Aspirin | | Sulfinpyrazone | | Interaction |
	(%)	(p)	(%)	(p)	(χ^2)
A. Excluding Events after Withdrawal of Drugs					
Men	−51	0.003	− 5	0.84	1.91
Women	+ 44	0.35	−25	0.44	0.05
B. Including Events in First 6 Months after Withdrawal of Drugs					
Men	−48	0.003	− 3	0.91	1.93
Women	+ 42	0.36	−28	0.38	0.17

occurring up to 6 months following withdrawal. These same events are depicted for men in Figure 1. These data illustrate a substantial biologic effect of aspirin, but not sulfinpyrazone, in men and no significant effect of either drug in women.

Table 2 addresses the management or intervention question: Does the initiation of one or both study drugs do more good than harm? Accordingly, all events, from the instant of randomization to the termination of the study, are included in the analysis. The analysis indicates that treating men with aspirin, but not sulfinpyrazone, is of significant value and that neither drug significantly benefits women.

Formal analysis showed that the benefit of aspirin was consistent from center to center. Of 24 centers, 14 (contributing 75% of the study patients) exhibited trends in the occurrence of stroke or death that favored aspirin, 5 (contributing 10% of study patients) exhibited no trend, and the remaining 5 (contributing 15% of study patients) exhibited a reverse trend.

The original design called for an examination of potential interactions between clinically cogent subgroups of patients and the trial drugs. No statistically significant differences were observed in therapeutic responses to either drug for the different vascular sites of the TIAs, for the presence or absence of residua, or for single or multiple attacks before entry. In addition, there was no statistically significant difference in drug response with age at entry or with the presence or absence of amaurosis fugax, demonstrated hypertension, hypercholesterolemia, cigarette smoking, or obesity.

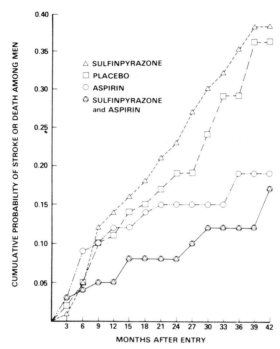

FIG. 1. Cumulative probability of stroke or death among men in the trial. (Reprinted, with permission, from [1].)

Statistically significant differences were found in the response to aspirin with the presence or absence of diabetes ($p < 0.02$) and prior myocardial infarction ($p < 0.04$) at entry; the benefit of aspirin was restricted to patients with negative histories for these conditions. When the life-table analyses were repeated, with simultaneous adjustment for sex, diabetes, and prior myocardial infarction, the risk reduction for stroke and

Table 2. Change in Risk of Stroke or Death Associated
with Aspirin or Sulfinpyrazone Treatment,
Including All Events from Randomization to the End of the Trial

| | Change in Risk | | | | Drug Interaction (x^2) |
| | Aspirin | | Sulfinpyrazone | | |
	(%)	(p)	(%)	(p)	
Men	−47	0.002	−6	0.76	3.66
Women	+22	0.55	−8	0.79	.046

death was 35% for aspirin (χ^2 = 5.11; p<0.03) and 15% for sulfinpyrazone (χ^2 = 0.77; p<0.38).

The adjusted life-table analysis also revealed that the lack of benefit with aspirin for diabetic patients was restricted to women. For men, the risk reduction with aspirin was 51% for those with diabetes and 47% for those without diabetes. Thus, the greatest response was found among the 331 men who entered the trial without a prior myocardial infarction. Within this subgroup the observed benefit of aspirin was a risk reduction of 62% for stroke or death (χ^2 = 12.38; p<0.001).

Discussion

Whether analyzed as an explanatory or management trial, this experiment demonstrated the efficacy of aspirin in men with threatened stroke. This conclusion receives additional support from other experiments in both man and rabbit. The point-estimate of the risk reduction for stroke and death among men in the U.S. aspirin trial was identical to that observed in the Canadian trial, and the U.S. trial also failed to demonstrate any benefit of aspirin among women (W.S. Fields, unpublished data). Furthermore, Kelton et al. have demonstrated that aspirin protects male, but not female, rabbits in an experimental thrombosis model [4].

In the original publication of the results of the Canadian trial [1], it was noted that there was a trend (although not statistically significant) toward an interaction between aspirin and sulfinpyrazone in the prevention of stroke or death among men in the trial (Fig. 1). In subsequent discussions of the trial it has been noted that the interaction trend derives from two sources of roughly equal magnitude: men treated with the combination fared better than those treated with aspirin alone and men treated with sulfinpyrazone fared worse than those treated with placebo. Indeed, the estimated sample sizes required to confirm these two contributions (should they persist) at conventional levels of statistical significance are within 10% of one another [5].

In conclusion, both explanatory and intervention analyses of the Canadian trial support the conclusion that aspirin, but not sulfinpyrazone, is efficacious in reducing the risk of stroke or death in men and that neither drug is useful in women with threatened stroke.

References

1. The Canadian Cooperative Study Group: A randomized trial of aspirin and sulfinpyrazone in threatened stroke. New Engl. J. Med. 299: 53-59, 1978.
2. Kaegi, A., Pineo, G.F., Shimizu, A. et al.: The role of sulfinpyrazone in the prevention of arterio-venous shunt thrombosis. Circulation 52: 497-499, 1975.
3. Peto, R., Pike, M.C., Armitage, P. et al.: Design and analysis of randomized clinical trials requiring prolonged observation of each patient. II. Analysis and examples. Br. J. Cancer 35: 1-39, 1977.
4. Kelton, J.E., Hirsh, J., Carter, C.J. and Buchanan, M.R.: Sex differences in the antithrombotic effects of aspirin. Blood 52: 1073-1076, 1978.
5. Sackett, D.L.: Response to the summary. In Price, T.R. and Nelson, E. (eds.): Cerebrovascular Diseases. New York: Raven Press, 1979, pp. 265-266.

Appendix:
The Canadian Cooperative Study Group

Neurologic Center

University of Western Ontario:
  H. J. M. Barnett, Principal Investigator*

Methods Center

McMaster University:
  M. Gent, Co-Principal Investigator*
  D. L. Sackett, Co-Principal Investigator*
  D. W. Taylor, Chief Statistician*

Hematology

Toronto:
  J. A. Blakely*
McMaster University:
  J. Hirsh*
  J. F. Mustard*
Western Ontario:
  R. K. Stuart*

Participating Centers

St. John's:
  W. Pryse-Phillips
Halifax:
  T. J. Murray
Montreal:
  D. W. Baxter
  J. Meloche
Quebec:
  M. Drolet
  D. Simard
Ottawa:
  E. Atack
  F. Nelson
  D. Preston
Kingston:
  H. B. Dinsdale*
Toronto:
  R. D. G. Blair
  J. Edmeads
  R. Gladstone

*Members of Executive Committee and Editorial Committee.

Participating Centers

M. Hill
O. Kofman
B. Steward
R. Wilson
London:
 H. J. M. Barnett
 C. Bolton
 J. Brown
 N. Jaatoul
 A. Kertesz
 J. D. Spence
 S. Stewart
Calgary:
 F. Leblanc*
 R. Lee
 F. W. Ramsay
 T. Seland

Vancouver:
 V. Sweeney
 M. J. Wong
Victoria:
 C. A. Simpson
New Westminster:
 R. D. Grosch
 M. Knazan

Research Staff

University of Western Ontario:
 P. Doucett
 F. Geoghegan
 S. Mann
McMaster University:
 J. Sicurella
 G. Smith

Discussion

Dr. Fontanilles: This trial offers a peculiarity in that the patients admitted to the trial not only had experienced classic transient ischemic attacks (TIAs), in the sense of Millikan's definition, but about 40% of them also had neurologic residua. Of the 166 patients with neurologic residiua at entry (patients who possibly had experienced strokes, mild or complete), 52, or 31%, were in the sulfinpyrazone group, and 36, or 21%, were in the placebo group. Admittedly, this difference is not statistically significant, but I am wondering whether there is another possible imbalance. This concerns the severity of the neurologic residua at entry. This is something that is not evident from the publication or from the data presented here. Could the severity of these neurologic residua at entry have differed among the different treatment groups?

Dr. Sackett: One of the interesting things we discovered at the beginning of the trial was that there is no such thing as a classic TIA. Diagnosis of TIA is extraordinarily variable, both between clinicians and within a clinician examining the same patient on two occasions. That was the reason we developed the rather explicit criteria. Our biologist collaborators in the trial felt that from the point of view of the pathogenesis of the disorder, it would be appropriate, and indeed important, to include that quite substantial subset of individuals who were called TIA cases by most physicians, but who, upon careful neurologic examination, were, in fact, demonstrated to have minor neurologic residua. It was therefore decided to admit to the trial individuals who had neurologic residua, as long as it was possible with the progression of their disease to have a worsening of the specific neurologic sign that was currently present. For example, a patient with minor weakness in a limb, which could proceed to more severe weakness or plegia, could be admitted.

With regard to the balance between groups in general, in conducting an experiment this can be handled in five different ways. One can carry out stratified sampling, one can do individual pair-wise matching, one can randomize, one can carry out a stratified analysis, and one can develop multivariate risk-factor scores. In this trial we used three such procedures. There was a stratification which preceded randomization, and we carried out a stratified analysis as well. Thus there was a stratification prior to randomization with respect to whether or not individuals had residual neurologic deficits. This produced groups which were not statistically significantly different with respect to balance. In addition, we carried out a stratified analysis, which would eliminate any trend toward differential severity or differential distribution of those individuals with or without residua. That stratified analysis indicated the same conclusions with respect to both the explanatory and the intervention types of analysis.

In summary, when a thorough neurologic examination was done, about 40% of these patients could be demonstrated to have quite minor, but discrete, neurologic residua, as would 40% of patients with so-called TIA anywhere. However, neither the distribution nor the course of those patients with residua affected the outcome of the investigation.

Dr. Sherry: If those with minor strokes were analyzed separately from those with major strokes, would the results have been any different?

Dr. Sackett: In terms of the hierarchies, of course, one wouldn't separate minor strokes, since if you have a major stroke or die, you can't have a minor stroke.

Dr. Sherry: You've already admitted that TIA episodes could be followed by neurologic residua; therefore, a minor stroke might be simply a residuum of a TIA episode, rather than a true stroke.

Dr. Sackett: Yes, but the appropriate analysis would be restricted to major strokes and death. This has been done and produces the same conclusions as we've shown.

Dr. Margulies: Dr. Sackett, I very much appreciated your explanation of the difference between an explanatory trial and an intervention trial. I've received many lectures that there are particular cardinal rules involved in doing studies like this, which must never be violated. Is it safe to assume from your explanation and the format in which you presented the results of this trial that you do not agree with those cardinal rules, particularly those in displaying results in the intervention trial format? Do you feel that it's most appropriate for trials such as this one, and particularly the Anturane Reinfarction Trial, for the results to be published in a format similar to the way in which you presented them today, that is, describing both the explanatory and the intervention results?

Dr. Sackett: To a certain extent, the investigator faces a dilemma. One may want to consider a staging, or a stepwise approach, to clinical trials, in which the first trial might well be an explanatory trial. One would severely restrict admission to the trial to compliant patients. One would want to focus on a very high-risk, but presumably highly responsive, subset of patients at entry, because indeed the chi-square value actually falls (even though sample size goes up) when low-risk or low-response patients are included in a trial. One might want to begin with an explanatory trial, such as the VA trials in hypertension, and then move to a more open intervention trial.

If one carries out the appropriate methodology, particularly with respect to explicit criteria and blinding (for the prevention of cointervention and diagnostic suspicion bias) and establishes rules beforehand for handling individuals who don't follow the protocol, one can justify, both in a scientific and a clinically credible fashion, the exclusion of specific end-points, with respect to either time or regimen. From that point of view, the 7-day rule in the Anturane Reinfarction Trial, for example, is quite appropriate.

The dilemma one faces under those circumstances relates to how far one then wants to extend the interpretation of the subsequent analysis. It would seem to me, for example, that the interpretation of the Anturane Reinfarction Trial in explanatory terms, as has been done, is quite appropriate. I am not sure that I would agree with the appropriateness of the interpretation and the generalization of the overall treatment results, however, because in this latter case the issue becomes one of intervention rather than explanation.

Dr. Walsh: Your analysis showed that patients without diabetes or hypertension responded to therapy, whereas those with these risk factors did not. This is consistent with our findings in patients with TIAs, showing that platelet abnormalities are present in patients without associated risk factors. Have you analyzed fasting plasma triglyceride results in the same way? In our studies we found platelet abnormalities in patients without lipid abnormalities, whereas patients with type IV hyperlipoproteinemia and elevated triglyceride levels had normal platelets. Do patients with hypertriglyceridemia fail to respond to platelet inhibitor drugs?

Dr. Sackett: The triglyceride measurements of our patients at entry suggested that there had been a lack of adherence to fasting before the specimens were drawn. Furthermore, the laboratory determinations in the 26 centers were sometimes quite spotty. Consequently we could not draw any valid conclusions about those entry characteristics. One of the other features that has come out of this particular trial, and of similar trials, is that one can no longer carry out randomized trials of cardiovascular disease, particularly in regard to factors affecting atherosclerosis, platelet function, and coagulation generally, without recognizing at the outset the need for doing analyses with respect to sex and other cardiovascular risk factors, such as glucose tolerance, hypertension, and (judging from your work) hyperlipidemia.

Dr. Sherry: It's well recognized that the rate of strokes and death in patients who have TIAs is very much higher during the first year as compared to subsequent years. The Canadian Cooperative Study evaluated patients who had been experiencing TIAs on an average of 11 months before entry into the trial. Do your data reflect at all on the possibility that these agents might have had a different effect during a high-risk period as compared to the risk period which you studied?

Dr. Sackett: For entry into the trial a patient had to have had at least one TIA during the previous 3 months. The prior histories of TIAs for our patients varied quite substantially; there were some who, in fact, had had their first TIA in the 3 months prior to entry and, of course, that was particularly so as the trial progressed. At the start of the trial, however, there were some so-called prevalent cases, patients who had been having TIAs for quite some time. It is intriguing that we really didn't see much difference between the response of those with long-standing prior histories and those of so-called incident histories of TIAs. Nor did we see, as we expected, much difference within duration in the trial. The average duration in the trial was about one thousand days, but, of course, there were individuals entered for 4 or 5 years. We didn't see much variation in the accumulation rate of these other events. This has suggested to us that we may have to rethink the natural history of TIAs. There are certainly periods during which individuals with TIAs appear to be at extreme risk. It also appears that patients with TIAs may have wide fluctuations in their risks, so that they may have a flurry of TIAs and be at exceptional risk at that period of time. We need to consider issues related to the point in the natural history of the disorder at which intervention occurs. It may well be that we'll be able to demonstrate different effects of different interventions at different stages in the natural history of these conditions.

Dr. McGregor: It's important to make this distinction between those who were entered shortly after their episode and those who weren't. Could you give me a qualitative idea of what you mean by shortly — a week, a month, 3 months?

Dr. Sackett: Thirty-six percent of the patients had their first TIA within 1 month of entry and 57% had their first TIA within 3 months of entry. In looking at the data, it appears that there are bursts of transient ischemic events, much as you described in the natural history of angina pectoris, I suppose. There are episodes during which the risk of some of these more devastating events appears to be substantially altered in individuals. The stage of the cycle the patient is in may be of more importance than the total duration since the first cycle began.

Dr. Fontanilles: In the course of this trial, you also conducted platelet function studies. It is generally accepted that sulfinpyrazone modifies platelet survival time, it lengthens or normalizes it, whereas aspirin does not. Can you tell us anything about the behavior of platelet survival time in the different treatment groups?

Dr. Sackett: We have an agreement with the investigators in the trial that before we publish or present various analyses, they will be informed of results first. Since we have not given them those results yet, I cannot say much about them here. I can say that, in general, there was no dramatic breakthrough in terms of the hematologic studies that were done in this trial.

Dr. White: Are there any hypotheses with respect to the sex difference that is occurring in these various trials? Here we have a situation where both premenopausal and postmenopausal women don't seem to benefit, whereas men do. If you wanted to be the Devil's advocate, you could say that that really eliminates the platelet hypothesis in favor of one for sex, because platelet inhibition is the same in men and women.

Dr. Sackett: As I stated in Utah last year, although some suggest that good clinical trials can only be conducted on the basis of sound basic biomedical research, sound basic biomedical research, of course, relies on good clinical trials for the generation of hypotheses. John Kelton has taken the results of this trial back into some animal models and has demonstrated that in an experimental thrombosis situation, he can protect male, but not female, rabbits with low doses of aspirin. I'm not enough of a biomedical research worker to be able to offer an interpretation of that work. At least those sorts of results have been replicated in an animal model, and some clues as to the explanation may come out of that.

Dr. McDonald: I think you summarized the findings of Dr. Kelton's work quite well. It is an animal model in which there is a platelet contribution, as well as thrombin generation and fibrin formation. When stroke occurs in patients with TIAs probably a number of factors come into play, including platelets and the vessel wall, and perhaps coagulation factors. These may not all contribute to the same extent in various patients. Vascular factors, for example, may be more important in female than in male subjects.

Dr. Clopath: Regarding the question of a sex difference in the mode of action, we measured prostacyclin-generating capacities in various arteries in swine and found that in males prostacyclin generation was lower than in females. If this were true in man, it might be an explanation for your observation that aspirin is effective in males and not in females.

Dr. Ellis: One of the factors in the Anturane trial was the extent to which patients had used beta blockers; I would be interested to know if in the Canadian Study you analyzed confounding concomitant medications. Some of the differences might be due to such confounding and I wonder if you had looked at that?

Dr. Sackett: Yes, we have. Of course, the ones of particular interest to us were the beta blockers. Over the course of the trial, only a very few individuals had received beta blockers and they were distributed evenly among the groups. Of course, in a trial using aspirin, one had to be terribly concerned about contamination, that is, the inadvertent administration of aspirin to individuals who were assigned to either sulfinpyrazone alone or placebo. For that reason, we distributed acetaminophen to everyone in the trial for use if they were ill. We did not find very much of concomitant medication and only about seven patients were taking beta blockers.

Sulfinpyrazone Treatment of Patients with Prosthetic Cardiac Valves

Peter P. Steele, M.D. and R. A. Vogel, M.D.

Systemic embolism continues to be a frequent and serious problem for patients with prosthetic cardiac valves. In recent years improvements in design and materials have been associated with a decreasing frequency of thromboembolic risk in these patients, but in consideration of the large numbers of patients who have prosthetic valves and the number of years these valves are expected to function, the thromboembolic risk is substantial.

Anticoagulant therapy with warfarin has not been shown to decrease the risk of embolism in patients with prosthetic mitral valves [1], although anticoagulation may have favorable effects in patients with both older prosthetic aortic valves [1] and more recently introduced aortic valves [2, 3]. Platelet-suppressant therapy has been considered for valve replacement patients. A controlled trial of one potential platelet-suppressant drug, dipyridamole, suggested that less thromboembolism occurred in patients receiving dipyridamole and warfarin than in patients receiving warfarin alone [4]. Platelet survival time is usually shortened in patients with prosthetic aortic and mitral valves, particularly in patients with prior embolism, and plate-

P. P. Steele, M.D., Associate Professor of Medicine, University of Colorado Medical Center; Chief, Cardiology, Veterans Administration Hospital; and R. A. Vogel, M.D., Assistant Professor of Medicine, University of Colorado Medical Center, Denver, Colo.

Supported by research funds of the Veterans Administration, a grant from the Colorado Heart Association, and a grant from the CIBA-GEIGY Corporation.

let-suppressant treatment with dipyridamole or sulfinpyrazone increases platelet survival [5-8].

In the present study the results of measurement of platelet survival time in patients with various prosthetic cardiac valves and in patients with valvular heart disease are presented. A prospective study of the effect of sulfinpyrazone on platelet survival and systemic embolism in these patients has been undertaken. In addition, the effect of sulfinpyrazone on platelet survival in relation to its effect on thromboembolism is defined.

Patients and Methods

Platelet Survival Studies

Platelet survival time was measured in a number of patient groups with valvular heart disease. One group included 96 patients with rheumatic heart disease who had undergone replacement of the mitral valve. Platelet survival was measured in 7 patients before and after mitral replacement with a new prosthetic valve, the Bjork-Shiley, and in 8 patients with rheumatic heart disease before and after mitral replacement with the porcine aortic heterograft. Platelet survival was also measured in another group of 76 patients with aortic valve disease, aortic stenosis and regurgitation judged to be caused by a process other than rheumatic disease, who had undergone aortic valve replacement and in 22 patients with aortic valve disease prior to cardiac surgery. Platelet survival was measured before and after valve replacement in 19 patients. Studies in patients with aortic valve replacement were undertaken, as preoperative and postoperative thromboembolism occurs less frequently than in patients with rheumatic mitral valve disease.

Sulfinpyrazone Study

Most of the patients with aortic and mitral replacement who had shortened platelet survival time were treated with sulfinpyrazone (800 mg PO daily). Episodes of thromboembolism had occurred in 11 sulfinpyrazone-treated patients (Table 1), and these 11 were matched to patients who had shortened platelet survival time, but had not had thromboembolism, who had the same cardiac valvular disease and the same prosthetic cardiac valve, and who had been treated with sulfinpyrazone for

Table 1. Patients with Prosthetic Cardiac Valves and Shortened Platelet
Survival Treated with Sulfinpyrazone

Type of Prosthetic Valve	Patients with Thromboembolism	Patients without Thromboembolism
Mitral Replacement		
CAD, Beall valve	2 (2)	7 (5)
RHD, Beall valve	2 (2)	21 (17)
RHD, Starr-Edwards valve, Model 6300	1 (1)	9 (9)
Aortic Replacement		
Starr-Edwards, Model 1200-1260	2 (1)	16 (6)
Starr-Edwards, Model 2300-2320	3 (3)	17 (10)
Bjork-Shiley	1 (1)	13 (10)
Total	11 (10)	83 (57)

All patients were treated with sulfinpyrazone; numbers in parentheses represent those who also received warfarin. CAD = coronary artery disease; RHD = rheumatic heart disease. (Reprinted from [13] with permission of the American Heart Association, Inc.)

at least 12 months. In addition, 32 patients with the same cardiac disease and the same prosthetic valve as the patients with embolism, but who had normal postoperative platelet survival, were followed (Table 2). These 32 patients were not treated with sulfinpyrazone. The effectiveness of sulfinpyrazone in altering the occurrence of thromboembolism and in altering platelet survival was studied in these patients.

Platelet survival time was measured between 2 and 6 months following cardiac surgery and between 3 and 6 months of treatment with sulfinpyrazone in treated patients. Platelet survival was measured by labeling the platelets from approximately 400 ml of the patient's venous blood with 100 to 150 μCi of ^{51}Cr [9]. A single exponent was fitted to 6 or 7 days of platelet count-rate data and half-time was computed. Normal platelet survival half-time averaged 3.7 ± 0.03 days (mean ± SEM; n = 26), with a normal range of 3.3 to 4.2 days.

Results

Platelet Survival Studies

Rheumatic Heart Disease. Platelet survival time was usually abnormal after mitral valve replacement in patients with rheu-

Table 2. Patients with Prosthetic Cardiac Valves
and Normal Postoperative Platelet Survival Time

Type of Prosthetic Valve	No. of Patients
Mitral Replacement	
CAD, Beall valve	4 (2)
RHD, Beall valve	5 (5)
RHD, Starr-Edwards valve, Model 6300	2 (2)
Aortic Replacement	
Starr-Edwards, Model 1200-1260	6 (3)
Starr-Edwards, Model 2300-2320	7 (4)
Bjork-Shiley	8 (4)
Total	32 (20)

These patients generally received warfarin (numbers in parentheses) but were not treated with sulfinpyrazone. CAD = coronary artery disease; RHD = rheumatic heart disease. (Reprinted from [13] with permission of the American Heart Association, Inc.)

matic heart disease (Fig. 1). Statistically significant (unpaired t test) differences were observed between average platelet survival for patients with a history of thromboembolism, either after valve replacement or before cardiac surgery, and those without embolism for each of the substitute valves (except Kay-Shiley and Bjork-Shiley, where an insufficient number of patients were studied) (Fig. 1). For patients with mitral replacement there were significant differences between those without an embolic episode and those with thromboembolism, but no differences between patients with embolism preoperatively, as a complication of rheumatic heart disease, or postoperatively (Fig. 2). Thus, for patients with rheumatic heart disease and mitral replacement, the occurrence of thromboembolism is associated with shortened platelet survival time.

The relationship of shortened platelet survival after mitral valve replacement in patients with a history of embolism before surgery suggested that platelet survival would be shortened in patients with rheumatic heart disease. Measurement of platelet survival was undertaken in 170 patients with rheumatic heart disease (mitral stenosis with or without mitral regurgitation or aortic valve disease). Almost all patients with a history of thromboembolism had shortened platelet survival time (Fig. 3). With increasing patient age the specificity of platelet survival for

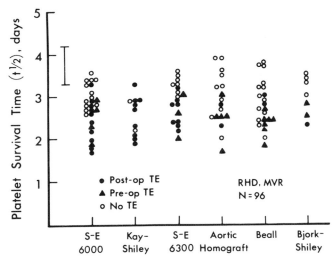

FIG. 1. Measurements of platelet survival time in 96 patients with rheumatic heart disease (RHD) who have undergone mitral valve replacement (MVR). The normal range is illustrated on the left. Open circles designate patients without a history of thromboembolism (TE); closed circles designate patients with postoperative embolism; and closed triangles designate patients with embolism before mitral replacement. S-E, 6000 = Starr-Edwards, series 6000 valve; S-E, 6300 = Starr-Edwards, model 6300 mitral valve.

thromboembolism increased. In young patients, aged less than 25 years or 26 to 35 years, platelet survival was shortened in about 75% of those who had not had embolism. In older patients, aged 56 to 65 years, the occurrence of shortened platelet survival in patients without a history of embolism was about 30%. Thus, a role for platelets in the pathogenesis of thromboembolism in patients with rheumatic heart disease is suggested.

Sulfinpyrazone increased platelet survival in patients with substitute mitral valves from 2.6 ± 0.13 to 3.1 ± 0.26 days (n = 35; $p < 0.001$, paired t test) and about 80% of patients had an increase in platelet survival of at least 0.2 days. Sulfinpyrazone also increased platelet survival in patients with rheumatic heart disease, from 2.5 ± 0.04 to 2.8 ± 0.04 days (n = 76; $p < 0.001$).

Replacement of the mitral valve with a newer prosthetic valve, the Bjork-Shiley, resulted in a small, but significant de-

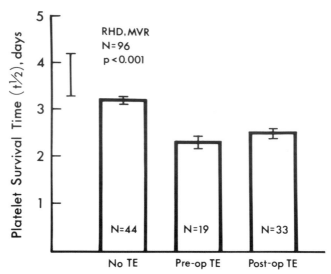

FIG. 2. Average platelet survival time (± SEM) for 96 patients with rheumatic heart disease (RHD) who have had mitral valve replacement (MVR). Average values are illustrated for patients without a history of thromboembolism (no TE); for patients with a history of thrombo-embolism before mitral replacement (pre-op TE); and for patients with a history of embolism following valve replacement surgery (post-op TE).

crease in platelet survival time from 3.1 ± 0.16 to 2.9 ± 0.15 days; $p < 0.05$). Replacement of the mitral valve with the stent-mounted porcine heterograft resulted in no significant altera-tion of platelet survival time (2.8 ± 0.11 to 2.7 ± 0.11).

Shortened platelet survival time in rheumatic heart disease is probably due to the combined effect of altered atrial endo-cardial surface [10] and turbulent blood flow induced by the stenotic mitral valve. After valve replacement with newer mitral substitute valves there may be only small alteration in the extent of surface abnormality and turbulence. These newer valves are associated with lower rates of thromboembolism than are older prosthetic valves.

Aortic Valve Disease. In patients with substitute aortic valves for nonrheumatic aortic valve disease, differences in average platelet survival time between patients with and without postoperative thromboembolism were observed (Fig. 4). In patients with less severe aortic valve disease who had not had valve replacement, platelet survival was normal in about half the

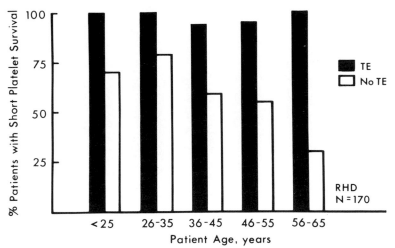

FIG. 3. Percentage of patients with shortened platelet survival who have a history of thromboembolism (TE) and who have not had thromboembolism in respect to patient age. All patients have rheumatic heart disease (RHD).

patients (Fig. 4). Platelet survival was not altered by valve replacement in patients who received the prosthetic Bjork-Shiley aortic valve (3.2 ± 0.10 to 3.2 ± 0.11 days; n = 9) or the porcine aortic valve (3.4 ± 0.10 to 3.3 ± 0.11 days; n = 10). Thus, a role for platelets in the thrombotic complications of aortic substitute valves is suggested as it is for mitral valves. Aortic valve disease is associated with less frequent occurrence of systemic embolism, and platelet survival is less often shortened than in patients with rheumatic heart disease. Replacement of the aortic valve with a current prosthetic valve, the Bjork-Shiley valve, does not appear to result in increased platelet consumption, which is consistent with the infrequent occurrence of thromboembolism with this valve.

Sulfinpyrazone Study

Platelet survival was shortened 2.4 ± 0.08 days in all 11 patients with prosthetic valves who subsequently had thrombosis and in none of these 11 patients was platelet survival increased with sulfinpyrazone treatment (2.3 ± 0.09 days; NS). Systemic embolism occurred between 10 and 47 months (avg. 25 months) after sulfinpyrazone treatment was started.

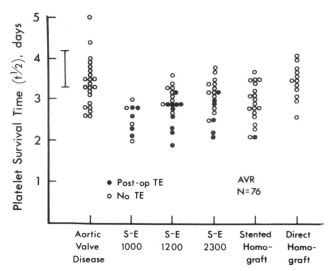

FIG. 4. Platelet survival time for 22 patients with aortic valve disease and for 76 patients who had undergone aortic valve replacement (AVR). The normal range for platelet survival is illustrated on the left. Patients with a history of postoperative thromboembolism (post-op TE) are designated as closed circles. Open circles are results from patients who have not had thromboembolism (no TE). S-E, 1000 = Starr-Edwards, model 1000; S-E, 1200 = Starr-Edwards, models 1200-1260; and S-E, 2300 = Starr-Edwards, model 2300 aortic valves.

Eighty-three patients have been treated with sulfinpyrazone and not had thromboembolism (Table 1). Platelet survival time was increased in 59 (71%) of these patients by at least 0.2 days (2.6 ± 0.05 to 2.9 ± 0.06 days; n = 83; $p < 0.001$). Embolism has not occurred in the group of 32 patients with normal postoperative platelet survival (Table 2) and in these patients platelet survival was not altered with time.

These patients frequently received anticoagulation therapy with warfarin. Sixty-seven of the 94 patients with shortened platelet survival treated with sulfinpyrazone also received warfarin, including 10 of the 11 who had embolism (Table 1), and 20 of the 32 patients with normal platelet survival received warfarin (Table 2).

This study suggests that patients with prosthetic aortic and mitral valves and shortened platelet survival in whom platelet survival does not increase with sulfinpyrazone treatment have a higher risk of thrombosis than patients in whom platelet survival increases (Fig. 5). Of 35 patients in whom platelet survival did not increase, 11 (31%) had embolism. Embolism did not occur in 59 patients in whom platelet survival increased. The antithrombotic effect of sulfinpyrazone by alteration of platelet survival time appears to be predictable in individual patients.

Discussion

Platelets appear to play a role in the thromboembolic complications of patients with prosthetic cardiac valves and in patients with rheumatic heart disease. A history of systemic embolism in these patients correlates with shortened platelet

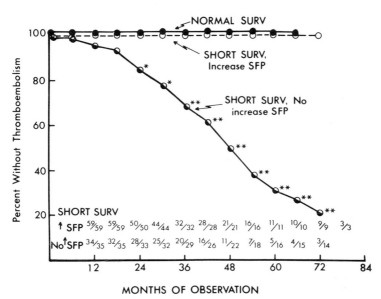

FIG. 5. Occurrence of thromboembolism with time plotted for patients with normal postoperative platelet survival time (normal SURV), shortened platelet survival with an increase in platelet survival with sulfinpyrazone treatment (short SURV, increase with SFP), and those with shortened platelet survival who did not respond to sulfinpyrazone (short SURV, no increase SFP). Chi square analysis yields significant differences at 24 through 72 months (*p< 0.05; **p< 0.01). Fractions are the number of patients without thromboembolism at each 6-month interval divided by the number followed and at risk. Standard errors at 24 months, 48 months, and 72 months for shortened platelet survival without an increase of sulfinpyrazone are 5%, 5%, and 7%, respectively. (Reprinted from [13] with permission of the American Heart Association, Inc.)

survival and shortened platelet survival appears to predict embolism in prosthetic valve patients and in rheumatic heart disease [11].

Sulfinpyrazone increases platelet survival in these patients and appears to decrease the frequency of embolism. In a recently completed prospective trial of sulfinpyrazone in patients with rheumatic heart disease, the reduction in new thromboembolism was demonstrated to be 30% in patients treated with sulfinpyrazone compared to 21% in patients receiving placebo.

Sulfinpyrazone appears to effectively decrease thromboembolism in patients with valvular heart disease and there appears to be a relationship between the favorable effect of the drug on platelet survival and on thromboembolism. Similar results were observed in patients with cerebral vascular disease and carotid transient ischemic episodes [12]. Platelet survival was shortened in 25 patients and in 10 patients sulfinpyrazone was remarkably effective in decreasing ischemic episodes. In 7 of these 10 sulfinpyrazone increased platelet survival as well. In 3 patients sulfinpyrazone treatment resulted in no improvement in ischemic episodes and platelet survival was not altered in any patient.

Acknowledgment

The authors acknowledge the expert technical assistance of Mrs. Jan Lacher, Carla Gilbert, Carol Vandello, Margie Anderson, and Mr. Michael Adams.

References

1. Duvoisin, G.E., Brandenburg, R.O. and McGoon, D.C.: Factors affecting thromboembolism associated with prosthetic heart valves. Circulation 35-36 (suppl. I): I-70, 1967.
2. Roberts, W.C. and Hammer, W.J.: Cardiac pathology after valve replacement with a tilting disc prosthesis (Bjork-Shiley type). A study of 46 necropsy patients and 49 Bjork-Shiley prosthesis. Am. J. Cardiol. 37: 1024, 1976.
3. Gray, L.A., Jr., Fulton, R.L., Srivastava, T.N. and Glowers, N.C.: Surgical treatment of thrombosed Bjork-Shiley aortic valve prosthesis. J. Thorac. Cardiovasc. Surg. 71: 429, 1976.
4. Sullivan, J.M., Harken, D.E. and Gorlin, R.: Pharmacologic control of thromboembolic complications of cardiac-valve replacement. N. Engl. J. Med. 284: 1391, 1971.

5. Harker, L.A. and Slichter, S.J.: Studies of platelet and fibrinogen kinetics in patients with prosthetic heart valves. N. Engl. J. Med. 283: 1302, 1970.
6. Weily, H.S. and Genton, E.: Altered platelet function in patients with prosthetic mitral valves. Effects of sulfinpyrazone therapy. Circulation 42:967, 1970.
7. Weily, H.S., Steele, P.P., Davies, H., Pappas, G. and Genton, E.: Platelet survival in patients with substitute heart valves. N. Engl. J. Med. 290: 534, 1974.
8. Steele, P., Weily, H.S., Davies, H., Pappas, G. and Genton, E.: Platelet survival time following aortic valve replacement. Circulation 51: 358, 1975.
9. Aster, R.H.: Effect of anticoagulant and ABO incompatibility on recovery of transfused human platelets. Blood 26: 732, 1965.
10. Baggenstoss, A.H. and Titus, J.L.: Rheumatic and collagen disorders of the heart. In Gould, S.E. (ed.): Pathology of the Heart and Blood Vessels, 3rd ed. Springfield, Il.: Charles C Thomas, 1968.
11. Steele, P.P., Rainwater, J.O. and Genton, E.: Favorable effects of sulfinpyrazone on thromboembolism in patients with rheumatic heart disease. Clin. Res. 27: 205A, 1979.
12. Steele, P., Carroll, J., Overfield, D. and Genton, E.: Effect of sulfinpyrazone on platelet survival time in patients with transient cerebral ischemic attacks. Stroke 8: 396, 1977.
13. Steele, P., Rainwater, J. and Vogel, R.: Platelet suppressant therapy in patients with prosthetic cardiac valves: Relationship of clinical effectiveness to alteration of platelet survival time. Circulation, in press.

Discussion

Dr. Folts: Did you happen to measure the hematocrit or red cell fragility periodically in these patients? As you know, the red cells are damaged as the poppet seats and release their ADP. This is supposed to add to the pannus formation which then leads to embolic complications. Thus the hematocrit would be of significance and fragility even more so.

Dr. Steele: Prosthetic valves hemolyze red blood cells. The biggest offender is the Beall valve, and if anything, platelet survival time is less abnormal with the Beall valve in patients without an embolism than it is in other mitral prosthetic valves that don't have as much of a hemolytic component. Therefore I don't think there's any relationship. There wasn't any relationship between platelet survival time and the degree of hemolysis. Virtually everybody, except patients with Beall valves, has normal hematocrits; that valve unfortunately carries with it a tremendous problem of blood hemolysis, but a high rate of embolization as might have been expected didn't result.

Dr. Fontanilles: In the cases in which you administered sulfinpyrazone concomitantly with oral anticoagulant (in your case, I think it was always warfarin), when the patient was well adjusted to warfarin and you started giving sulfinpyrazone, did you have any problems of interaction, considering that sulfinpyrazone is very highly protein-bound?

Dr. Steele: Yes, real problems. We customarily suggest decreasing the weekly dose of warfarin by half on initiation of sulfinpyrazone and then restoring prothrombin time, as desired. This will invariably entail a substantially lower dose of warfarin. During the blinded trial, the patients, as well as their physicians, understood this and consequently everybody had their warfarin dose decreased. Thus we were made ignorant of what the ultimate level of warfarin necessary to establish prothrombin time was. That procedure was not associated with any risk of embolization; in other words, in placebo patients, that was not the time when they embolized. That would take place within 2 to 4 weeks. Of course, with placebo patients the dose of warfarin almost invariably went back to its previous level.

Dr. Sherry: Dr. Steele, I assume that you have measured the effect of aspirin on platelet survival under these conditions. Have you done any clinical studies of the effect of aspirin alone in preventing thromboembolic complications associated with either prosthetic heart valves or rheumatic valvular disease?

Dr. Steele: Aspirin has probably been shown to decrease thromboembolism effectively in patients with aortic prosthetic valves. I believe the dosage was four tablets a day. In our experience, that dosage in either prosthetic valve patients or patients with coronary disease is associated with a modest alteration of platelet survival, considerably less striking an effect on platelet survival than that of sulfinpyrazone. However, when aspirin is combined with dipyridamole, the effects appear to be equivalent. To the extent to which embolization in these patients with either rheumatic heart disease or prosthetic cardiac valves depends on alteration of platelet survival time, I would predict that sulfinpyrazone would be more effective than aspirin.

Dr. Sherry: It is my understanding that Dr. Harker has published observations in which there is no effect of aspirin on platelet survival, yet you imply that you did see a modest improvement. If there is no effect of asprin alone and yet there is a reduction in the number of thromboembolic complications with aspirin alone, then the relationship of platelet survival to the prevention of thromboembolic complications is less clear.

Dr. McDonald: Dr. Steele, I am concerned about the process which involved selecting from the patients in whom platelet survival was measured, a group in which it was at the lowest level, that is, 0.2 days below your defined range of normal, prescribing a treatment, measuring platelet survival again, and finding that it has been lengthened. Where there is a range of possible values, if you happen to select the short measurement at the beginning, are you not at risk of finding prolonged survival no matter what you do when you measure it again? Could your results show a statistically significant decrease in one group after 48 months, because you started with short survival? Is there a quite significant chance that when you repeat the survival measurements, you will obtain a lower result? What is your reproducibility of platelet survival in a given subject from time to time?

Dr. Steele: Without an intervention, 0.2 days.

Dr. McDonald: How did you select 0.3 days as being the significant change?

Dr. Steele: I meant to say that I considered a change of 0.2 days to be an effect of sulfinpyrazone on the test. If it was a change of 0.1 day or no change at all, then it was considered not to be an effect of sulfinpyrazone on platelet survival time.

Dr. Robson: In the previous communication, we learned that aspirin teased out a sex difference in terms of TIAs. I am curious to know if you could detect any difference between sexes in the response to sulfinpyrazone? Did it perhaps favor the male or did it not?

Dr. Steele: No, I didn't see it. Rheumatic heart disease is more prevalent in women, but the patients that were involved in this study were much more frequently men. The emboli occurred about equally in both groups. Of the 11 patients with prosthetic valves who subsequently embolized, 9 were men and 2 women; of the 19 patients with rheumatic heart disease who embolized, 4 were women and 15 men. I think those proportions are quite comparable to the frequency of men and women in the population in the study. I have not seen any differential effect of sex on response of platelet survival time.

Dr. Oliver: Is there any possibility that the improvement with the sulfinpyrazone group could be due to some independent factor on myocardial status? Is there any evidence of a reduced incidence of atrial fibrillation in the sulfinpyrazone group. Was there a reduced incidence of failure or in new valve replacement? Are you quite satisfied that the improvement is entirely on the assumed basis of an effect on platelet survival? Could there be another factor?

Dr. Steele: I do not think that any other aspect of the natural history of rheumatic heart disease was changed, either favorably or unfavorably. The occurrence of new atrial fibrillation and of mitral valve replacements was equally divided among the three treatment groups. The conversion of paroxysmal atrial fibrillation to fixed atrial fibrillation was fairly constant. Patients were, by and large, not very ill; there were a lot of class I and class II, and a substantial portion of class 0, cases. This was because I wanted to avoid mitral valve replacement during the four years of the study. The fact that 33 patients had had to have mitral valve replacement reflected a general error in patient selection on our part (since we felt that had to be discontinued at that point), but they were about equally divided among the three groups.

Dr. McDonald: Were the platelet survival measurements made by persons who were blinded with respect to drug treatment?

Dr. Steele: Yes, we were all blinded.

Dr. Sherry: It's intriguing that sulfinpyrazone would have a more striking effect than aspirin in improving a shortened platelet survival, when we're dealing with platelets apparently aggregating and causing thrombi to form on prosthetic valves, where there is no real vascular surface. Has anybody studied whether any of the metabolites of sulfinpyrazone are able to prevent thrombin-induced platelet aggregation?

Dr. Wallis: Sulfinpyrazone itself has no effect *in vitro* or *ex vivo* on thrombin-induced aggregation. *In vitro* the sulfone and the parahydroxy metabolite have no effect on thrombin-induced aggregation. We have not yet tested the thioether, but *ex vivo* when thioether is in high concentration in guinea pig blood, there is no effect on thrombin-induced aggregation. In general, one could conclude that none of the metabolites has an effect on thrombin-induced aggregation.

The Anturane Reinfarction Trial

Erwin H. Margulies, Ph.D.

The objective of the Anturane Reinfarction Trial was to compare the effects of sulfinpyrazone (Anturane) versus placebo on cardiac mortality in patients who had experienced a recent acute myocardial infarct. The double-blind randomized trial was conducted at 26 clinical centers throughout the United States and Canada from September 1975 to August 1978. All scientific and operational policies were set by an external Policy Committee chaired by Dr. Sol Sherry. The Operations Committee, which was comprised of members of the CIBA-GEIGY Corporation, was responsible for the day-to-day conduct of the trial.

Methods

Patient Eligibility

Male and female patients, 45 to 70 years of age, were eligible for entry into the trial at 25 to 35 days following a qualifying acute myocardial infarction. Diagnoses were established on the basis of positive compatible electrocardiographic (ECG) findings, the presence of typical symptoms of chest pain, and two of three serum enzyme levels (serum glutamic oxaloacetic transaminase, lactic dehydrogenase, and creatinine phosphokinase) elevated to greater than twice the upper normal levels within 72 h of the onset of symptoms. Patients were excluded from entering the trial if they had a history of coronary surgery or cardiomegaly at the time of randomization, if they required regular administration of dipyridamole, clofibrate, or aspirin, or if they required concomitant anticoagu-

Erwin H. Margulies, Ph.D., Medical Department, Pharmaceuticals Division, CIBA-GEIGY Corporation, Summit, N.J.

lant therapy beyond the time of entry into the trial. Patients with untreated hypertension were also excluded.

Observation Period

Patients were to be observed for a minimum of 1 year and a maximum of 2 years following the acute myocardial infarction. When initial results of the trial were published in February 1978 [1], the average observation period was 8.4 months per patient. Upon conclusion of the trial, the average follow-up period was approximately 16 months.

Study Population Size

When the initial data were published, 1,620 patients had entered into the Anturane Reinfarction Trial. Of these, 101 patients were excluded from the analysis because they were found not to meet entry criteria or had less than 7 days' initial exposure to trial therapy. An additional 44 newly entered patients were excluded from analysis because only baseline data were available for them. Thus, 1,475 patients were eligible for analysis — 742 in the placebo group and 733 in the sulfinpyrazone group. Of those eligible patients, 214 had withdrawn from the trial, 113 for medical and 101 for nonmedical reasons. Both types of withdrawals were fairly equally distributed between the two therapy groups. Medical reasons for withdrawal were intercurrent medical problems, the use of unacceptable concomitant medication, or adverse drug reactions. Only 2% of the patients in both the sulfinpyrazone and placebo groups were withdrawn from the trial for adverse reactions.

Patient Characteristics

Of the trial patients 86.4% were male and 13.6% were females. A study of approximately 100 baseline characteristics indicated that the two treatment groups were comparable. Of all trial patients 45.8% were 45 to 55 years of age and 54.2% were 56 to 70 years of age; age distribution between treatment groups was almost identical. The mean age of patients in the sulfinpyrazone group was 56.8 years, and in the placebo group it was 56.6 years. For the most salient baseline characteristics of past medical history concerning prior myocardial infarction, angina pectoris, hypertension, pulmonary embolism, thrombophlebitis, stroke, claudication, diabetes, and smoking habits prior to infarction, there were no statistically significant differences between treatment groups [1].

Cardiac Mortality Categories

Prior to the conduct of the trial, three categories of cardiac mortality were defined: sudden cardiac death, myocardial infarction, and "other" cardiac deaths. Sudden cardiac deaths either occurred within 60 min of the onset of symptoms or were unobserved deaths. Myocardial infarction deaths were categorized as such on the basis of postmortem or clinical findings. "Other" cardiac deaths were those resulting from congestive heart failure, documented arrhythmia, or cardiogenic shock.

Results and Discussion

Initial Results

When the initial results were published, all deaths had been cardiac in nature, with the exception of one which resulted from cerebrovascular causes. Of the total deaths, 61% were categorized as sudden death, 30% as myocardial infarction, and 7.3% as "other." (The percentage of sudden deaths is in agreement with the postinfarction mortality data available in the literature [2].) The annualized mortality according to treatment group and cause of death is given in Table 1. For all cardiac deaths, mortality was reduced 48.5% in the sulfinpyrazone group, with the greatest reduction, 57.2%, occurring in sudden cardiac deaths.

Table 1. Reduction in Mortality in Sulfinpyrazone Treatment Group According to Cause of Death: Initial Results

Cause of Death	Annualized Rate (%)		Reduction (%)
	Placebo	Sulfinpyrazone	
All Causes	9.5	5.1	46.4
Cardiac	9.5	4.9	48.5
Sudden Death	6.3	2.7	57.2
Myocardial Infarction	2.6	1.8	30.8
"Other"	0.7	0.4	

Continuation of the Trial

Prior to publication, all trial investigators were informed of the nature of the results. They were requested to explain them to the trial patients and attempt to obtain a written reinformed consent to continue in the trial in a double-blind fashion until the requirements of the protocol were met, namely, a minimum of 1 year's observation for all trial patients. The Policy Committee felt this to be an ethically sound approach since the data had been collected over the early months following myocardial infarction. It was during this time that the efficacy of sulfinpyrazone in the reduction of cardiac death had been established. However, at the time of publication, no trial patients would be within this early high-risk period since patient accession into the trial was halted approximately 7 months prior to the reporting of the results. Therefore, it was felt that no patient was being asked to place himself at any undue risk. Only seven patients of all those actively in the trial at that time refused to continue in the double-blind trial.

Issues Raised by the Initial Publication

Multiple Data Analyses. Following publication of the initial results, several issues were raised. One concerned multiple data analyses prior to publication. In accordance with preestablished policies, upon enrollment of approximately 1,200 patients the Operations Committee and a statistical consultant assessed all collected data. Upon finding significant differences in cardiac mortality between the therapy groups, they recommended review of the data base by the Policy Committee. After detailed review of the data, when approximately 1,500 eligible patients had entered the trial and significant differences in cardiac mortality were still apparent, the Policy Committee terminated patient enrollment as of July 31, 1977.

Ineligible Patients and Unanalyzable Events. Another area of concern was the limitation of the statistical analysis to eligible patients and analyzable events. This meant that ineligible patients and unanalyzable events were excluded from the primary analysis. The exclusion of patients from statistical analysis in any trial is a practice that is not generally agreed upon; however, since these exclusions were on the basis of definitions set prior to the initiation of the trial, this approach was considered an acceptable methodology. It was felt that by excluding patients that were ineligible according to the trial protocol, as well as those events that were considered unanalyzable, the sensitivity of the trial would be increased, thus maximizing the chances for revealing true effects.

Cardiac Rhythm Abnormalities. The initial publication reported more cardiac rhythm abnormalities at trial entry in the placebo group (15%) than in the sulfinpyrazone group (11%). These abnormalities were defined by computerized ECG determinations taken at 1 month postinfarction, and not by use of cardiac rhythm strips or Holter monitoring. A routine, resting, 12-lead ECG is not an entirely reliable basis for establishing the presence of cardiac rhythm abnormalities. In any case, this possible imbalance in the presence of rhythm abnormalities at baseline could have in no way affected the trial results. The death rate for patients in the sulfinpyrazone group who had no baseline rhythm abnormalities was 4.0%, whereas for those with rhythm abnormalities it was 2.9%. For placebo-treated patients, the annualized death rate was 7.4% for those without rhythm abnormalities and 6.6% for those with rhythm abnormalities. Eight patients with rhythm abnormalities at baseline died, six in the placebo group and two in the sulfinpyrazone group. A similar distribution was found in patients without rhythm abnormalities. Thus, within the confines of this trial, the presence of rhythm abnormalities defined at baseline did not seem to be a substantial risk factor in terms of subsequent mortality.

Final Results

At the conclusion of the Anturane Reinfarction Trial, there had been 62 deaths in the placebo group and 44 deaths in the sulfinpyrazone group, reflecting a 29% reduction in total mortality. All of these deaths, with the exception of one, were cardiac in nature. As with the initial results, the greatest reduction (43%) in death rate occurred in the sudden cardiac death category (Table 2), and there was an overall decrease of 32% in cardiac death rate.

Mortality Patterns

In interpreting these results, a number of relevant factors should be considered. Following myocardial infarction, mor-

Table 2. Reduction in Mortality in Sulfinpyrazone Treatment Group
According to Cause of Death: Final Results

Cause of Death	Total	Number of Deaths		Reduction (%)
		Placebo	Sulfinpyrazone	
All Causes	106	62	44	29.0
Cardiac				
Sudden Death	59	37	22	40.5
Myocardial Infarction	35	18	17	
"Other"	11	7	4	

tality patterns can be described as having two distinct phases [3]. From the first through the sixth month, there is a "high-risk" mortality period during which annualized cardiac mortality is about 10% to 12%. Following this high-risk period, there is a dramatic reduction in the annualized cardiac mortality by approximately one half. From about the eighth month postinfarction through the next 4 to 5 years, the annualized mortality ranges between 3% and 5%. It is extremely important to analyze the results of the Anturane Reinfarction Trial in light of these distinctly different mortality phases.

These considerations must also be taken into account when comparing the trial with other postinfarction mortality studies. The approaches used in several trials differ in that, unlike the Anturane Reinfarction Trial which studied patients with a common starting point (entering the high-risk period), other trials have enrolled patients at times varying from 2 to 60 months following the acute event. This approach provides a diverse collection of patients under observation during different phases following an acute myocardial infarction and exposed to different risks of mortality.

Results According to Risk Periods

Based on the above, the results of the Anturane Reinfarction Trial were examined in a temporal fashion, considering mortality data within 6-month time frames (Tables 3 and 4). In so doing, it becomes clear that the benefit of sulfinpyrazone in the prevention of cardiac deaths, particularly sudden cardiac deaths, is established during the high-risk phase (1 through 7 months following the acute myocardial infarction). Thereafter,

Table 3. Total Deaths

| Time of | Number of Deaths | | |
Measurement	Placebo	Sulfinpyrazone	Difference
6 mo	36	16	—20
Initial Report*	44	25	—19
12 mo	44	31	—13
18 mo	59	41	—18
24 mo	62	44	—18

*Average observation period = 8.4 mo.

the benefit established during the initial period is maintained during the lower mortality period from 8 to 24 months, but never improved upon.

This is not to conclude that sulfinpyrazone is without benefit during the lower mortality phases. In view of the fewer patients in the later periods of observation and the substantially lower mortality after the seventh month postmyocardial infarction, the number of patients was simply insufficient to determine whether continuous therapy would be beneficial in preventing subsequent cardiac deaths. It is clear, however, that the benefit accrued during the high-risk period was not lost in the subsequent mortality phases.

It therefore seems that the effect of sulfinpyrazone in this trial was to eliminate certain risk factors during the high-mortality phase, thus establishing a lower mortality of approximately half that for the placebo group — a rate which was maintained relatively constant throughout the 24-month observation period.

Table 4. Sudden Deaths

| Time of | Number of Deaths | | |
Measurement	Placebo	Sulfinpyrazone	Difference
6 mo	25	6	—19
Initial Report*	29	13	—16
12 mo	29	16	—13
18 mo	36	20	—16
24 mo	37	22	—15

*Average observation period = 8.4 mo.

Statistical Significance of Data
by Risk Periods

Because of these temporal considerations, two sets of statistical analyses best represent the trial data. The first (Data Set 1) consists of data for patients with an average observation period of 8.4 months, representing in essence the early high-risk mortality period. For those data, there is a statistically significant difference between results for the sulfinpyrazone and placebo groups, which yields an adjusted Cox "p" value of 0.025 for all trial deaths and 0.015 for sudden cardiac deaths. Data Set 2, which represents the total trial data, incorporating both the early high-risk and later low-risk mortality periods, shows a difference between groups with a "p" value of 0.076 (Cox adjusted technique) for all trial deaths and 0.041 for sudden cardiac deaths.

Although the focus of statistical analysis for this trial was on eligible patients experiencing analyzable events, it has also been expanded to include both ineligible patients and unanalyzable events. When this was done, the effects of sulfinpyrazone in the prevention of sudden cardiac death at trial end were not diminished. For all events among eligible patients, the Cox adjusted analysis results in a "p" value of 0.035. When all events among all patients (including ineligible patients) were analyzed, a statistically significant benefit for sulfinpyrazone in the prevention of sudden death was evident (p=0.032).

Conclusions

On the basis of the data accumulated from this trial and the subsequent statistical analyses, the following conclusions have been drawn:

1. Sulfinpyrazone (200 mg, four times daily) given 25 to 35 days following an acute myocardial infarction, reduced the cardiac death rate by approximately 50% during the subsequent 6 months. Thereafter, the initial benefit was maintained, but not improved upon.

2. The primary effect of sulfinpyrazone was to prevent sudden death during the period of very high risk which extends through the seventh month postmyocardial infarction. This amounted to a 74% reduction during the first 6 months of therapy, but without additional observed benefit thereafter.

3. The administration of sulfinpyrazone to survivors of an acute myocardial infarction converts the period during which there is a very high risk of sudden death among such patients to the lower risk state observed during the end of the first year and thereafter.

References

1. The Anturane Reinfarction Trial Research Group: Sulfinpyrazone in the prevention of cardiac death after myocardial infarction. New Engl. J. Med. 298: 289-295, 1978.
2. Weinblatt, E., Shapiro, S., Frank, C., et al.: Prognosis of men after myocardial infarction: Mortality and first recurrence in relation to selected parameters. Am. J. Public Health 58: 1329-1347, 1968.
3. Bigger, J.T., Heller, C.A., Wenger, T.L., et al.: Risk stratification after acute myocardial infarction. Am. J. Cardiol. 42: 202-210, 1978.

Discussion

Dr. Sackett: In terms of my definitions of explanatory and intervention trials, the fashion in which the trial was set up and analyzed, would, in my view, be an appropriate example of an explanatory analysis in which the 7-day exclusion was certainly valid. My questions relate primarily to the extrapolation of the results into intervention, and for that reason I am interested in some of your subanalyses with respect to groups that we found to be unresponsive to the medications used in the TIA trial. More specifically, could you give some information about your point estimates for risk reduction among women, hypertensives, and diabetics in your trial.

Dr. Margulies: These data have not been released to the investigators yet and consequently it's inappropriate to release them here. In terms of male versus female patients, an extremely low number of female patients were in the trial, and I'm not sure that any comparisons would be valid. It's something that we have analyzed and will make commentary about at the appropriate time.

Dr. Oliver: For your Data Set 2 — all patients and all events (and that presumably includes the group in the 7-day rule at either end of the study) — was there a significant difference in sudden death?

Dr. Margulies: Yes, $p=0.032$.

Dr. Oliver: When you include follow-up deaths, do you include follow-up deaths of those that were withdrawn?

Dr. Margulies: Yes.

Dr. Oliver: This exact type of information has come out from the beta blocker trials conducted in the United Kingdom and in Europe. They have shown that the beta blockers are effective in the approximately first 9 months because of the changing mortality which, of course, is very well documented, as you say. The analogy is striking. The practolol trial, which was bigger indeed than the Anturane trial and reasonably well conducted (at least according to some of the precepts put forth by Dr. Sackett), showed very similar results. It might be that this analogy needs to be considered in terms of the mechanism of action of Anturane.

There is another problem to consider, which is that according to the number of trials that are being done, you can get various misleading results. If the planned trial size is for 250 events and a 33% difference is expected between treatment and control groups and 20 trials are in progress, one of these will produce misleading results. On the other hand, if the trial design is for 25 events and again a 33% difference is expected between the treated and the control, then of 200 established trials (as you might have, for example, with short-term antiarrhythmic drugs), there could be as many as 150 misleading results. This is quite unarguable in terms of the statistics if the aim is to show a difference at the 5% level. Of course, the Anturane trial lies between these two, with approximately 100 events, and there has been only one trial, which makes assessment difficult. But one can do certain extrapolations from these figures, and it is possible that of ten trials with the same design as the Anturane trial, three could be misleading. It seems to me, then, that we should think of this trial in terms of a pilot study. What is really required are more trials.

Dr. Margulies: I think there is a definitive amount of work to be done by methodologists and clinicians alike. I totally agree with you that in terms of conventional clinical trials, one is certainly not enough and more need to be done. In terms of mortality trials, however, I am not altogether sure. I know from a personal point of view, I can never be involved in another trial utilizing sulfinpyrazone. For the clinician, there is another point of reference. It is an extremely involved question, and it might be somewhat unfair to simply put the issue to sleep by saying that one trial is not enough.

Dr. Sherry: It is very impressive that there is a reduction of 75% in the sudden death category for eligible patients with analyzable events within the first 6 months of entry into the Anturane Reinfarction Trial; have the data been analyzed in terms of all patients and all events for the first 6 months? We are dealing with two different mortality rates, that is, early and late, and in the interpretation one must evaluate these two independently. Does that first 6-month period, regardless of how you analyze the results, still show a very striking difference?

Dr. Margulies: It cannot be analyzed in terms of sudden death alone. The data for all patients and all events for 6 months can be analyzed, but I can't release the results at this time.

Dr. Folts: Many patients involved in a study, whether they're taking placebo or the test drug, over a period of months to years will alter their living habits. Did you follow a social history as to life-style, change in eating habits, exercise programs, or a change in smoking habits in the two groups?

Dr. Margulies: We did follow diet patterns for patients in the trial, and we saw nothing of substantial interest there.

Dr. Folts: Did some enter exercise programs and some not? Did some stop smoking or some smoke less?

Dr. Margulies: No, we don't have that information.

Dr. Folts: It certainly would be a factor, wouldn't it?

Dr. Margulies: Absolutely, but any clinical trial can only do so much. In this one, it was decided that we couldn't include those factors. They are important questions, no doubt.

Dr. Domenet: This question of only one trial is a very important one. I am a little fearful, however, of the implications of doing 26 Anturane reinfarction studies. You did have, I think, 26 participating centers. Can you tell us whether the results from each of these centers all point the same way or in what way they diverge? The numbers wouldn't be sufficient to show statistically significant differences, but it would be interesting to know whether the trends are similar.

Dr. Margulies: The statisticians did look at the trials on an individual basis, in terms of compatibility of each center to the rest of the group. No single study center was incompatible in terms of the rest of the study centers. In terms of actual numbers of deaths per center, I think that is an inappropriate comparison to make, but it can be done.

Dr. Sherry: Could you comment on the review of the supposed difference in rhythm abnormalities at trial entry, when this was reanalyzed.

Dr. Margulies: We did, in fact, look on an individual basis at every patient identified as having a rhythm abnormality. We found that there were no significant ventricular dysrhythmias; the dysrhythmias were very minor indeed and had no association with mortality.

Dr. Clopath: Have you had a chance to examine histologically the hearts of those patients dying suddenly? If so, what did you find in the large and middle-sized coronary arteries and in the small branches? Could you find emboli there?

Dr. Margulies: We don't have histological information. We do have pathological data, postmortem findings, on a subsample of patients that is really not large enough for drawing any inferences. Obtaining postmortem data in a clinical trial is notoriously difficult and proved to be so again in this study.

Clinical Studies:
Chairman's Summary

Sol Sherry, M.D.

This particular session of the symposium has focused on certain clinical studies in which the antithrombotic properties of sulfinpyrazone were under evaluation.

In observations reported earlier we have learned that sulfinpyrazone has a potent effect in inhibiting platelet aggregation and release induced by collagen, as well as following certain antigen-antibody reactions. Perhaps even more importantly, sulfinpyrazone has a protective effect on the endothelial cell, thus providing complementary effects on the platelet-vessel wall interaction. Such duality of actions may be pertinent to the prevention by sulfinpyrazone of vascular injury and thrombus formation.

Dr. Walsh, in the first paper, reviewed the interface between the interaction of the platelet and the coagulation mechanism, which is also pertinent to the pathogenesis of thrombosis. His studies are trail-blazing in this area. It is intriguing that while neither sulfinpyrazone nor aspirin appears to have a well-defined effect on platelet coagulant activities, the combination of aspirin and sulfinpyrazone may prove to have an effect.

In the second paper Dr. Sackett reviewed some of the philosophical prinicples in trial design, i.e., whether a trial is to be designed as an explanatory or intervention trial. This was followed by an analysis of the Canadian Cooperative Neurological Study. In this trial aspirin in combination with sulfinpyrazone significantly reduced the incidence of stroke or death among males, particularly in the presence of certain risk factors

Sol Sherry, M.D., Professor and Chairman, Department of Medicine, Temple University School of Medicine, Philadelphia, Pa.

but not others. Sulfinpyrazone alone did not appear to have an effect under the particular conditions of the study.

Dr. Steele reviewed his observations on the sulfinpyrazone treatment of patients with prosthetic cardiac valves. It has been shown that anticoagulants are not very effective in reducing the significant incidence of thromboembolic complications following mitral valve replacement.

Studies have shown a shortened platelet survival time in patients with mitral valve replacement and this shortening is greater in those who suffer from thromboembolic complications. Similar but less extensive changes were noted in patients with aortic valve replacement. Sulfinpyrazone treatment improves platelet survival in a large percentage of patients with prosthetic valves, but not all. Those in whom there was improvement in platelet survival with sulfinpyrazone treatment appeared to be protected from subsequent thromboembolism; those in whom platelet survival was not affected by sulfinpyrazone continued to have thromboembolic complications.

Patients with rheumatic heart disease who also had a shortened platelet survival had a high risk of thromboembolic complications. The use of sulfinpyrazone in a large group of patients with rheumatic heart disease and shortened survival demonstrated a significant improvement in platelet survival and an associated reduction in thromboembolic complications.

The results indicate that sulfinpyrazone is an effective antithrombotic agent in many patients with prosthetic heart valves or rheumatic valvular disease who have thromboembolic complications.

Finally, the results of the Anturane Reinfarction Trial at its conclusion were described by Dr. Margulies. These observations support the earlier reported conclusion that Anturane reduces significantly the mortality from sudden death and that this reduction is primarily or perhaps exclusively limited to the first 6 months after trial entry, i.e., within the first 7 months following the index infarction. These data appear to fit in well with the differing mortality rates during the early months after a myocardial infarction and at the end of the first year and thereafter.

Symposium Summary

Summary Comments

Sol Sherry, M.D.

The objective of this symposium has been to update knowledge on the pharmacological actions of sulfinpyrazone (Anturane) which might explain why this drug proved so effective in reducing sudden death in the recently concluded Anturane Reinfarction Trial. In this respect the symposium has provided much new knowledge about the actions of sulfinpyrazone, several of which could relate to its effectiveness in the Anturane Reinfarction Trial. However, it is apparent that despite our advancing knowledge of the multiple actions of this drug *in vivo*, the exact mechanism(s) underlying the reduction in sudden death remains unclear at this time.

The Anturane Reinfarction Trial was undertaken with the expectation that sulfinpyrazone would inhibit platelet thromboemboli from occurring at sites of vascular injury or stenosis in the coronary tree, thereby perhaps eliminating an important mechanism for sudden death, i.e., platelet microemboli triggering ventricular fibrillation. In addition, this agent was likely to reduce death from an acute transmural myocardial infarction by preventing platelets from initiating an acute coronary thrombosis at the site of an acutely fissured or ruptured atheromatous plaque. Supporting these expectations was the known molecular action of sulfinpyrazone, namely, that this agent blocks the collagen-activated prostaglandin pathway in platelets by competitively inhibiting the cyclooxygenase which converts arachidonic acid to the cyclic endoperoxides. (This pathway leads to the synthesis and release of such powerful platelet aggregators and vasoconstrictors as thromboxane A_2.) This action is similar in net effect to that of aspirin, although the latter's molecular

Sol Sherry, M.D., Professor and Chairman, Department of Medicine, Temple University School of Medicine, Philadelphia, Pa.

mechanism is different, i.e., aspirin irreversibly inactivates the cyclooxygenase by acetylating it into an inactive enzyme.

As far as sulfinpyrazone is concerned, we have learned at this symposium that its effect *in vivo* may be enhanced and prolonged by a conversion of a portion of the sulfinpyrazone during passage through the liver into other active intermediates, e.g., the thioether analog, which is ten times more potent than the native drug.

Considering that only sudden death was reduced significantly in the Anturane Reinfarction Trial, and that the triggering event leading to ventricular fibrillation (the presumed cause of the majority of sudden deaths) is unknown, the question can be raised as to whether the effect of sulfinpyrazone in this trial might be independent of any effect on platelets. For example, it might be more directly related to a previously undescribed action of sulfinpyrazone on electrophysiological phenomena which control the appearance of ventricular arrhythmias and particularly fibrillation.

Thus, four other possibilities were raised during the discussion: hypouricemia, as induced by this uricosuric agent, may raise the threshold for ventricular reentry arrhythmias (the drug has not been shown to have an effect on isolated Purkinje fibers, thus changes in automaticity can be eliminated as the mechanism of action); an effect of sulfinpyrazone in reducing infarct size and thereby decreasing the risk of subsequent death; a direct effect of sulfinpyrazone on reentry arrhythmias; and a suppressive action by sulfinpyrazone on the synthesis or release of prostaglandins, other than those derived from the platelet, which could trigger abnormal electrophysiological phenomena.

The papers presented by Povalski, Moschos, and Kelliher and the comments of Oliver have addressed this question from the viewpoint of studies in various animal models. It is clear that sulfinpyrazone does indeed have an "antiarrhythmic" action. This action is not dependent on hypouricemia, since it can be demonstrated after a single IV injection of sulfinpyrazone. Moreover it cannot be attributed to any reduction in infarct size, as infarct size bore no association with the sulfinpyrazone effect, and in any case, it has never been established that larger infarcts carry a greater risk for sudden fatal arrhythmias than smaller ones.

Thus we are left with the other possibilities as an explanation for the antiarrhythmic action of sulfinpyrazone, i.e., the ability of this drug to inhibit ischemia-induced conduction delays, to raise the threshold for premature ventricular beats, to reduce the incidence of ventricular tachycardias, and to diminish the likelihood of ventricular fibrillation.

Since these effects can be demonstrated immediately following acute occlusion of a coronary artery, it has been suggested that inhibition of platelet prostaglandins by sulfinpyrazone could hardly account for its action, and that the antiarrhythmic effect must be mediated through another mechanism. However, Kelliher has suggested that released prostaglandins may still prove to be the primary mechanism for serious arrhythmias arising in association with acute ischemia of the myocardium. He cites earlier studies showing that certain prostaglandins can stimulate β-receptors and lead to the release of norepinephrine, and that β-receptor blocking agents inhibit the action of these prostaglandins. Thus, platelet prostaglandins other than thromboxane A_2 might be released in response to ischemia in the absence of platelet aggregation and sufficiently stimulate the β-receptor to induce a reentry arrhythmia. Alternatively, as suggested in the discussion, the source of such prostaglandins may be the endothelial cell or the ischemic tissue itself. Certainly, sulfinpyrazone's action as a prostaglandin synthesis inhibitor is not restricted to the platelet, for such biologically active substances are fairly ubiquitous in their source of origin. (The observations on platelets, however, are the most often advanced since these cell fragments can be readily isolated and studied.) In support of the hypothesis that sulfinpyrazone's action as an antiarrhythmic is mediated through its inhibitory effect on prostaglandin synthesis (whatever the source) are the observations that plasma catecholamine levels after ischemia are reduced in sulfinpyrazone-treated animals as compared to controls.

In addition to the studies presented here, it should be noted that Epstein of the National Heart, Lung, and Blood Institute has found that sulfinpyrazone and aspirin produced a significant increase (50%) in collateral flow to the epicardium of an acutely ischemic myocardium (personal communication). His studies indicated that while these drugs do not reduce the amount of myocardium that ultimately becomes necrotic, there is a reduction in the incidence of malignant arrhythmias during acute experimental infarction. Since this observation has been made with both sulfinpyrazone and aspirin, which share a common action in prostaglandin synthesis, it further supports the concept that the incidence of malignant arrhythmias following acute ischemia to the myocardium may be prostaglandin-induced and may well tie in the known molecular mechanism of action of sulfinpyrazone with its recently established antiarrhythmic effect.

The hypothesis that prostaglandins mediate the malignant arrhythmias that may arise in association with an acutely ischemic myocardium and that sulfinpyrazone's antiarrhythmic effect is mediated by a reduction in the prostaglandin concentration should be capable of testing. If acute ischemia causes the release of prostaglandins, increased levels should be detected in the coronary sinus blood, and the highest levels should be detected in those animals who suffer a malignant arrhythmia. Furthermore, the pattern of the prostaglandins in the coronary sinus blood might well indicate whether the source is the platelet. The answer to the latter question (the platelet as a source) could be greatly facilitated by simultaneous measurement of specific platelet proteins, e.g., PF4 (this can be detected in microquantities by highly specific radioimmunoassays). The latter question also can be approached by determining whether the sulfinpyrazone effect is still present in animals previously rendered thrombocytopenic.

The animal models used to establish the antiarrhythmic effect of sulfinpyrazone, while helping to explain how this drug works *in vivo*, may have little relevance to the causative mechanism leading to sudden death in the patients in the Anturane Reinfarction Trial. Perhaps more relevant is the model described and studied by Folts. Here there is no sudden total occlusion of the coronary artery with extensive myocardial necrosis but only a partial stenosis without significant tissue damage. This model is more analagous to the usual findings in patients who die suddenly, i.e., the presence of one or more partially stenosed coronary vessels. In his studies, Folts has shown that partial stenosis leads to cyclical flow patterns which can be directly related to the formation and disintegration of platelet aggregation and plugs.

As expected, in his studies sulfinpyrazone limits the aggregation of the platelets and of more extensive plugs, eliminates in great part the cyclical changes in flow, and prevents the severe ischemic episodes which are capable of triggering a malignant arrhythmia.

At present I would interpret the experimental observations as offering the following explanation for the action of sulfinpyrazone in reducing sudden death. This drug works in two ways: it eliminates platelet thromboembolism as a causative mechanism in sudden death (admittedly, this mechanism may be operative in only a percentage of the cases of sudden death) and equally, if not more importantly, it raises the threshold for reentry arrhythmias during ischemic episodes, regardless of cause. While the mechanism for the latter action is still unclear, it may be related to its effect on prostaglandin-mediated catecholamine release.

In Margulies' summary of the findings at the end of the Anturane Reinfarction Trial, it was pointed out that the major, if not total, effect of sulfinpyrazone was observed during the first 6 months after trial entry (25 to 35 days following the index infarction). It was also noted that the mortality rate during the first half year after an infarct is much higher (double or more) than that during the latter half of the year or during subsequent years. At present it is not clear whether sulfinpyrazone eliminates only those factors that enhance the risk of dying suddenly in the first 6 to 7 months or if its effect continues but is masked by the low mortality (3% to 5%) which begins in the latter part of the first year. Resolving this question may prove to be difficult.

Of considerable interest, however, is that the break in the mortality curve to a lower and steady state, which occurs about 6 to 7 months after a myocardial infarction, is not restricted to this disorder alone. Rather, it is seen among patients who have had the recent onset of a serious ischemic episode (Prinzmetal's angina, ventricular tachycardia, successful resuscitation after cardiac arrest, etc.). Each of these groups of patients is at high risk of sudden death during the first half year. Since sulfinpyrazone was so effective in preventing sudden death after an acute myocardial infarction, the question can be asked as to whether it would have a similar effectiveness during the period of high risk following other serious ischemic episodes.

The lack of effect of sulfinpyrazone in the Canadian Neurological Study should not be construed as in conflict with the results achieved in the Anturane Reinfarction Trial. Stroke and sudden death are due to entirely different mechanisms: the former is probably a thrombotic event, whereas the latter is most often due to a malignant ventricular arrhythmia. The disparate results would seem to indicate that sulfinpyrazone is not as effective in preventing an acute arterial thrombosis as one had hoped it might be. Whether a combination of an anticoagulant with sulfinpyrazone would have the desired effect remains to be investigated. It should also be noted that the Canadian Neurological Study did not investigate the high-risk period, i.e., the first year after the onset of a transient ischemic attack.

Finally, there are other pharmacological actions of sulfinpyrazone, as brought out in this symposium, which may prove to be of considerable importance in medical therapy. This drug's well-recognized action on prostaglandin synthesis is shared by aspirin and several other drugs (e.g., indomethacin), but it also has other actions not shared by these agents. Its uricosuric action appears to be similar to that of probenecid, but it is still poorly understood since the mechanism of uric acid (or urate) reabsorption, which sulfinpyrazone blocks, has not been investigated to any extent. It is suspected that this reabsorption involves an active transport mechanism involving a carrier protein. Since the reaction of a carrier protein with its substrate has similarities to the formation of an enzyme-substrate complex, sulfinpyrazone may well serve as a competitive inhibitor for the reaction of uric acid (or urate) with the carrier protein.

We also learned in this symposium that sulfinpyrazone can readily be distinguished from other inhibitors of prostaglandin synthesis by its ability to prevent the sublethal Forssman reaction. Since the thrombocytopenia in this case is complement-dependent, and since complement activation usually involves cell injury, it appears that sulfinpyrazone in some obscure way has the ability to protect against cell damage. A somewhat analogous effect was described by Cooper in his studies on the action of sulfinpyrazone in preventing a complement-mediated pulmonary dysfunction in sheep. Here the infusion of complement-activated plasma produced pulmonary hypertension (presumably from granulocyte aggregates and the effects of their extruded lysosomes) and an associated granulocytopenia which was eliminated in those animals pretreated with sulfinpyrazone.

The fascinating studies reported by Harker also deal with a protective effect of sulfinpyrazone on cell injury. However, in these studies, complement activation played no role, since the direct cytotoxic effects of homocysteine and hyperlipidemia on endothelial cells in tissue culture could be largely prevented by sulfinpyrazone.

Whatever the mechanism for this protective effect on cell injury, it may well be playing a role in a number of the other interesting studies reported in this symposium: the shortened duration of white thrombus formation by sulfinpyrazone after a supposed ADP-induced thrombus by laser beam injury in the bat wing and hamster cheek pouch; the prolongation of survival of cardiac transplants in rats treated with azathioprine supplemented with sulfinpyrazone; and the restoration toward normal of the shortened platelet survival observed in patients with rheumatic valvular disease or prosthetic valve implants.

These studies may have important therapeutic implications. Will sulfinpyrazone be useful in the prevention of arteriosclerosis, will it be useful in the management of patients in whom immune mechanisms involving complement activation and tissue injury are responsible for significant pathological sequelae, will it have a role to play in preventing organ graft rejection? The elaboration of the mechanism(s) whereby sulfinpyrazone is capable of preventing cell injury may well determine the ultimate role of this drug in clinical therapeutics.

Subject Index

Acetyl group, platelet, 71
Adenine nucleotides, 252
Adenosine diphosphate (ADP). *See* Platelet
aggregation, ADP-induced.
Adenylate cyclase, platelet, 39
Ag-B loci, 230
Aggregation. *See* Platelet aggregation.
Anesthesia depth, cardiac experiments, 251
Angina
Prinzmetal's, 69-70, 331
stable vs. unstable, 146-47
Animal species
baboon, 87-88, 119, 133, 142
bat, 101ff
cat, 74, 193ff
dog(s)
allograft rejection in, 132
complement levels in, 247
coronary occlusion in, 153ff
coronary stenosis in, 212ff
myocardial ischemia in, 212ff, 249-50
sulfinpyrazone metabolism in, 142
thromboxane A_2 receptor, lack of, in,
35
guinea pig, 3ff, 20-25, 29-32, 76, 142
hamster, 101ff
man, 25-29, 32, 34-35, 257ff, 275ff,
295ff, 311ff
mice, 13
monkey(s)
atherosclerosis in, 88-89, 98
cynomolgus, 122
platelet plugs in, 226
rhesus, 142
pigs, 113ff, 121, 221, 226, 293-94
rabbit(s), 43ff, 59-60, 63, 76
graft survival in, 245
sex difference in aspirin response in,
286, 293
sulfinpyrazone metabolism in, 128, 131,
134, 142
sulfinpyrazone metabolite platelet-
binding in, 35
uric acid, serum, in, 97

rat, 122-23, 125-26, 133, 142, 230ff
sheep, 55ff, 76, 189
swine, miniature, 122, 124-25, 127-29,
131, 133-34, 142
Antiarrhythmic action
aspirin, 166-68, 172
sulfinpyrazone, 147, 167, 193, 202,
249-53, 327ff
Antibody
anti-factor-XI, 258
anti-human-endothelial-cell, 85
Forssman, 3ff
humoral, in renal allograft patients, 240
levels, circulating
in cardiac transplant, rats, 223, 243
in rats, 232
Anticoagulant therapy, 270-71
warfarin, with prosthetic aortic valves,
295
Antigen-antibody
complexes, 240
reaction, 3, 16, 239, 241-42
Antithrombin III, 258
Antithymocyte globulin, 229
Anturane Reinfarction Trial (ART), 147,
193, 290-91, 331ff
cardiac rhythm abnormalities in, 315, 322
ineligible patients in, 314
mortality by risk period in, 318-19
unanalyzable events in, 314, 317
Aorta
vs. iliac artery, rabbit, 141
rat, 51, 54, 122-23
Aortic endothelial cells. *See* Endothelial
cells.
Aortic valve replacement. *See* Prosthetic cardiac valve.
Arachidonate, sodium. *See* Arachidonic
acid.
Arachidonic acid, 19ff, 40ff, 195, 202
in different species, 74
in different tissues, 74
Arrhythmia(s)
automatic, Purkinje tissue, 151, 328

335